Diversity Issues in the Diagnosis, Treatment, and Research of Mood Disorders

Edited by
Sana Loue and Martha Sajatovic

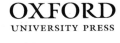

OXFORD
UNIVERSITY PRESS

2008

OXFORD
UNIVERSITY PRESS

Oxford University Press, Inc., publishes works that further
Oxford University's objective of excellence
in research, scholarship, and education.

Oxford   New York
Auckland   Cape Town   Dar es Salaam   Hong Kong   Karachi
Kuala Lumpur   Madrid   Melbourne   Mexico City   Nairobi
New Delhi   Shanghai   Taipei   Toronto

With offices in
Argentina   Austria   Brazil   Chile   Czech Republic   France   Greece
Guatemala   Hungary   Italy   Japan   Poland   Portugal   Singapore
South Korea   Switzerland   Thailand   Turkey   Ukraine   Vietnam

Published by Oxford University Press, Inc.
198 Madison Avenue, New York, New York 10016

www.oup.com

Oxford is a registered trademark of Oxford University Press

Library of Congress Cataloging-in-Publication Data
Diversity issues in the diagnosis, treatment, and research of mood disorders /
edited by Sana Loue and Martha Sajatovic.
    p. ; cm.
Includes bibliographical references and index.
ISBN: 978-0-19-530818-1
1. Affective disorders—Cross-cultural studies.   2. Minorities—Mental health.
[DNLM: 1. Mood Disorders—therapy.   2. Biomedical Research.
3. Cross-Cultural Comparison.   4. Mood Disorders—diagnosis. WM 171 D618 2007]
I. Loue, Sana.   II. Sajatovic, Martha.
RC537.D54 2007
616.85'27—dc22   2007011341

9 8 7 6 5 4 3 2 1

Printed in the United States of America
on acid-free paper

Contents

Contributors

IQBAL AHMED, MD, John A. Burns School of Medicine, University of Hawaii, Honolulu, HI

SHERYL E. ALLEN, MD, MS, Medical College of Wisconsin, Milwaukee, WI

DECLAN T. BARRY, PhD, Yale University School of Medicine, New Haven, CT

MARK BEITEL, PhD, Yale University School of Medicine, New Haven, CT

ELIZABETH CARPENTER–SONG, MA, ABD Case Western Reserve University, Cleveland, OH

ESPERANZA DIAZ, MD, Robert Wood Johnson Medical School, University of Medicine and Dentistry of New Jersey, Piscataway, NJ

GERI DONENBERG, PhD, Institute for Juvenile Research, University of Illinois at Chicago, Chicago, IL

JAVIER ESCOBAR, MD, Robert Wood Johnson Medical School, University of Medicine and Dentistry of New Jersey, Piscataway, NJ

MATTHEW A. FULLER, PharmD, Louis Stokes Cleveland Department of Veterans Affairs Medical Center, Case Western Reserve University, School of Medicine, Cleveland, OH

LORIN GARDINER, MD, University of Washington School of Medicine, Seattle, WA

PETER GUARNACCIA, PhD, Institute for Health, Health Care Policy, and Aging Research,

Rutgers University, New Brunswick, NJ

RAYMOND HARRIS, PhD, University of Washington School of Medicine, Seattle WA

CRISTINA I. HUEBNER, MA, Caring Health Center, Springfield, MA

CAREY JACKSON, MD, MPH, MA, University of Washington School of Medicine, Seattle, WA

AMY M. KILBOURNE, PhD, MPH, VA Ann Arbor Serious Mental Illness Treatment Research and Evaluation Center, Ann Arbor MI

ELIZABETH J. KRAMER, SC.M., New York University School of Medicine, New York, NY

JEFFREY L. LONGHOFER, PhD, LISW, Mandel School of Applied Social Sciences, Case Western Reserve University, Cleveland, OH

SANA LOUE, JD, PhD, MPH, School of Medicine, Case Western Reserve University, Cleveland, OH

HUMBERTO MARIN, MD, Robert Wood Johnson Medical School, University of Medicine and Dentistry of New Jersey, Piscataway, NJ

MATT MENDENHALL, MSW, LISW, PH.D. Candidate, Mandel School of Applied Social Sciences, Case Western Reserve University, Cleveland, OH

MEGAN NORDQUEST SCHWALLIE, MA, The University of Chicago, School of Social Service Administration, Chicago, IL

IGDA MARTINEZ PINCAY, PsyM, Institute for Health, Health Care Policy and Aging Research, Rutgers University, New Brunswick, NJ

CYNTHIA I. RESENDEZ, MD, Weill Medical College of Cornell University, New York, NY

MARTHA SAJATOVIC, MD, University Hospitals Case Medical Center, Case Western Reserve University, School of Medicine, Cleveland, OH

AMY E. WEST, PhD, University of Illinois at Chicago, Chicago, IL

JOSEPH J. WESTERMEYER, MD, PhD, MD, PhD, Minneapolis VA Medical Center, and University of Minnesota, Minneapolis, MN

EARNESTINE WILLIS, MD, MPH, Medical College of Wisconsin, Milwaukee, WI

DOUG ZATZICK, MD, MPH, University of Washington School of Medicine, Seattle, WA

Diversity Issues in the Diagnosis, Treatment, and Research of Mood Disorders

1

Using Care With Culture

ELIZABETH CARPENTER–SONG, MEGAN NORDQUEST
SCHWALLIE, & JEFFREY L. LONGHOFER

If what we make of a book such as *The Spirit Catches You* is a set of
stereotypes about what "they" think, or a bunch of rules about how to deal
with "them," like so many specialized tools to be stashed in a briefcase
and trotted out each time one of "them" shows up, then we will certainly
fail to keep alive the empathetic curiosity that allows one to be thought-
fully alert to difference.
—Taylor (2003, p. 179)

Increasingly, mental health practice demands acknowledgment of the role of
culture in the mediation of the interpretation and experience of mental disorder. In fact, the "main message" of the Surgeon General's recent (U.S. Department of Health and Human Services, 2001) report on culture, race, and
ethnicity was that "culture counts." A long tradition of research in medical
anthropology and cross-cultural psychiatry has demonstrated the multiplicity of
ways in which culture is both a site of production and a mediator of symptoms
in mental disorders.

In contrast to a view of mental disorders that posits them as more or less
uniform universal disease processes, it is imperative to take seriously the role of
culture in shaping mental disorders. From the start, it should be noted that we
take culture to be an emergent phenomenon. We view culture, "in its broadest
dimensions, as shared symbols and meanings that people create in the process
of social interaction. . . . It thereby orients people in their ways of feeling,
thinking, and being in the world" (Jenkins & Barrett, 2004, p. 5). Following
Kleinman (1988a) and Jenkins (1998, p. 357; Jenkins & Barrett, 2004, pp. 6–7),
we argue that culture must be understood to influence nearly every aspect of
mental illness, including

- how illnesses are identified, defined, and made meaningful
- how illnesses vary with respect to timing and onset
- symptomatology
- the course and outcome of illnesses
- how individuals and collectivities respond to and experience mental illness
- utilization of and response to treatment.

Awareness of the cultural mediation of psychopathology is particularly important in considerations of mood disorders. Mood disorders, such as depression and bipolar disorder, pose unique challenges to clinicians and patients alike. For a diagnosis to be rendered, a distinction must be made between normal feelings of sadness and happiness and their extreme, pathological counterparts. Teasing this out is no easy task. As Arthur Kleinman (1988a) has observed, "Depression, after all, can be a disease, a symptom, or a normal feeling" (p. 16). Kleinman's statement calls attention to the multiple referents that emotion words possess. Some of the difficulty in diagnosing mood disorders seems to stem from this indexical overlap that results in a slippage between the everyday language of *emotion* and the clinical language of *mood*. Lutz (1990) argues for a dialectical relationship between everyday and scientific ideas about emotion. Appreciation of such a dialectic holds unique clinical relevance for mood disorders given the blurring of everyday and clinical understandings occurring within the context of their identification and diagnosis.

Beyond linguistic difficulties, identification of mood disorders is further complicated by the fluid and fleeting nature of everyday emotional life. On any given day, one might experience joy upon hearing a child's first word, frustration while stuck in a traffic jam, and sadness upon receiving the news that an elderly parent has taken a fall. Our emotional experience and expression are mediated by personal temperament, social roles and interactions, as well as broader cultural expectations and meanings. We recognize variation in temperament when we categorize others as "melancholic," someone who "looks on the bright side," or someone who is a "hot head," a "downer," or "happy-go-lucky." Similarly, certain social roles and contexts allow or inhibit expression of emotion. Take the employee who has just been reprimanded by her boss. Although she may feel angry and overwhelmed, it is unlikely that she will raise her voice, cry, or slam a door in her boss's presence. Less obvious are the ways in which cultural expectations and meanings may affect the experience and expression of moods and emotions. For instance, in contrast to the dominant American sentiments to "get over it" and "move on" in relation to the death of a loved one, orthodox Judaism calls for more protracted mourning rituals for immediate family.

The clinical burden of distinguishing between normal and pathological moods and emotions is thus inherently substantial. When one factors in differences in ethnic and cultural background and/or language barriers, this already heavy load is made even more daunting. Attempts to redress such barriers are manifest in the most recent attempts to incorporate "culture" in clinical practice. These efforts have centered on demands for culturally appropriate care and cultural competence in clinical encounters.

In this chapter we first provide an overview of recent calls for "culturally competent" clinical practice. Then we turn to the anthropological record to provide evidence for the necessity of situating symptoms in cultural context. Having acknowledged the value of the provision of culturally appropriate care, we elaborate on specific weaknesses of current models of cultural competence.

We conclude with recommendations for how to listen for culture within clinical encounters.

"CULTURE" IN HEALTH CARE: CALLS FOR CULTURAL COMPETENCE

Cultural competence has been defined as:

> a set of congruent behaviors, knowledge, attitudes, and policies that come together in a system, organization, or among professionals that enables effective work in cross-cultural situations. "Culture" refers to integrated patterns of human behavior that include the language, thoughts, actions, customs, beliefs, and institutions of racial, ethnic, social, or religious groups. "Competence" implies having the capacity to function effectively as an individual or an organization within the context of the cultural beliefs, practices, and needs presented by patients and their communities. (Cross et al., as quoted in Lee & Farrell, 2006, p. 9)

In their overview of key trends, Betancourt and colleagues (2005) identify the goal of cultural competence as "creat[ing] a health care system and workforce that are capable of delivering the highest quality care to every patient regardless of race, ethnicity, culture, or language proficiency" (p. 499). Brach and Fraserirector (2000) argue that "the idea of cultural competency is an explicit statement that one-size-fits-all health care cannot meet the needs of an increasingly diverse American population" (p. 183). They also identify multiple levels at which cultural competency can be defined and operate, arguing that cultural competency must go beyond cultural awareness or sensitivity to include specific skills and techniques. Second, they note that cultural competency can refer to an ongoing commitment to institute appropriate practices and policies for diverse populations (Brach & Fraserirector, 2000).

Cultural competence agendas have arisen in the context of increasing diversity within the United States (Betancourt et al., 2005; Brach & Fraserirector, 2000). Clinicians are thus likely to treat patients who may have limited English language proficiency, different care-seeking patterns and expectations for care, and culturally specific orientations that may influence adherence (Berger, 1998; Betancourt et al., 2005, pp. 499–500). In addition, patient–provider communication has also been linked to patient satisfaction, adherence, and health outcomes (Betancourt et al., 2005, p. 500; Stewart, 1999). Moreover, service utilization and treatment adherence may be promoted by culturally appropriate services (Snowden & Hu, 1997; Takeuchi, Sue, & Yeh, 1995; U.S. Department of Health and Human Services, 1999, p. 182).

Much of the contemporary discussion of the importance of considering culture in clinical practice also stems from increasing awareness of dramatic health disparities among ethnic minority populations in the United States. Focusing on the role and impact of patient race and ethnicity, Cooper and Roter (2003) cite studies that have found that physicians deliver less information, less supportive talk, and less proficient clinical performance to black and

Hispanic patients and patients of lower socioeconomic status than to more advantaged patients. Recent reports (Smedley, Stith, & Nelson, 2003; U.S. Department of Health and Human Services, 2001) call attention to striking disparities and the disproportionate burden of mental illness borne by racial and ethnic minorities. More specific to mental health services, the Surgeon General's report on culture, race, and ethnicity identifies four primary disparities:

1. Minorities have less access to and availability of mental health services.
2. Minorities are less likely to receive needed mental health services.
3. Minorities in treatment often receive a poorer quality of mental health care.
4. Minorities are underrepresented in mental health research (U.S. Department of Health and Human Services, 2001).

The report concludes that "[m]ore is known about disparities than the reasons behind them" (U.S. Department of Health and Human Services, 2001, p. 3).

Disparities specific to the appropriate diagnosis and treatment of mood disorders are particularly troublesome. For example, the Surgeon General's report on culture, race, and ethnicity (U.S. Department of Health and Human Services, 2001) notes that African Americans tend to be diagnosed more often with schizophrenia than with affective disorders in comparison with white Americans. Clinician bias is cited as a possible contributing factor to this differential. This finding is noteworthy given that the stigma attached to serious mental disorders such as schizophrenia can be socially debilitating as a result of the associations with dangerousness, violence, incompetence, and bizarre behavior (Hinshaw & Cicchetti, 2000). For Latino populations, the report (United States Department of Health and Human Services, 2001) recounts similar findings: Hispanics have been found less likely to receive a diagnosis of depression or a prescription for antidepressant medication in comparison with white Americans. Such discrepancies in the diagnosis and treatment of mood disorders point to significant problems in the application of current diagnostic guidelines and treatment protocols.

Understanding disparities is best accomplished by considering the multiplicity of factors that contribute to the production of inequality. Sources of disparities are likely to be complex, existing at the level of individual patients and providers, and of health care systems, as well as historical influences on the contemporary context of health seeking and caregiving (Smedley et al., 2003). Alegria and colleagues (2002) have shed some light on possible explanations for disparities in utilization of specialty mental health services among minority populations. In their analysis of data derived from the 1990–1992 National Comorbidity Survey (NCS), they found a lower level of access to specialty mental health care among poor Latinos compared with poor non-Latino whites. They identified five factors that could explain such differences: language fluency, cultural differences such as self-reliance, access to Medicaid specialty services in Latino neighborhoods, differences in recognition of mental health problems, and lower quality of mental health care among Latinos. Furthermore, they found that nonpoor African Americans were less likely than their white counterparts to use specialty mental health services. Alegria and colleagues (2002) suggest that African Americans may have fewer financial resources at their disposal, that there exists greater mistrust and experiences of racism among African American patients, and that regional variations in access to care may also exist.

LOST IN TRANSLATION

Calls for culturally appropriate care in forms of cultural competency models acknowledge the potential for cultural misunderstandings to affect clinician–patient interactions. Such misunderstandings may result in incomplete assessments, diagnostic errors, treatment inadequacies, and unsuccessful treatment alliances (Kirmayer, Groleau, Guzder, Blake, & Jarvis, 2003). The anthropological record is replete with examples of the dangers of miscommunication in clinical practice.

Interethnic and cross-cultural variations in the meaning assigned to particular states underscore the difficulty in attributing validity to supposedly universal psychiatric categories. Kleinman (1988a) identifies the common cross-cultural experiences and elaborations of trance and possession states as posing a particular challenge to the validity of "medicalization." Discussing Filipino experience, Tompar-Tiu and Sustento–Seneriches (1995) note that healers' trance and possession states are not considered pathological in the context of Philippine culture.

Likewise, Obeyesekere (1985) argues that the generalized hopelessness that Brown and Harris (1978) take to be the basis of depressive disorder is positively valued in Sri Lanka as the foundational insight about the nature of the everyday world. The Western depressive would likely be the good Buddhist. The unique and locally constituted experiences of and reactions to illness cross-culturally are also exemplified in Gaines and Farmer's (1986) discussion of dysphoric affect in Catholic Mediterranean culture. Similar to the argument put forth by Obeyesekere (1985), Gaines and Farmer (1986) provide a case study of a woman living in a housing project outside central Paris to demonstrate that consideration of cultural meanings may complicate an otherwise clear-cut diagnosis of clinical depression. Gaines and Farmer (1986) provide a cultural and historical context for the woman's typical mode of emotional and interactional operation, showing how, within the Catholic Mediterranean tradition, rhetoric of complaint and suffering is an ennobling social practice in which individuals become "visible saints," social cynosures within the community. Thus, the authors advise caution in using Western diagnostic checklists without checking for cultural context that may produce a confounding effect.

Further highlighting the necessity of situating behaviors in cultural context, the danger of misdiagnosis is made clear by cross-cultural evidence regarding bereavement patterns. Among some Southeast Asian clients, the ability to see or talk to deceased relatives may be reflective of a cultural orientation to the supernatural rather than a delusion (Uba, 1994). Similarly, Kleinman (1988a) has found that hearing the voice of a dead spouse may be a normal experience of bereavement for some Native Americans as opposed to a hallucination.

Jenkins and Valiente's (1994) consideration of *el calor*, a sensation of intense heat in the body, among Salvadoran women refugees also points to the danger of reducing collective experiences of trauma to signifiers of individual psychopathology. Clinical misunderstandings of *el calor* may have potentially serious consequences for patients. To that end, Jenkins and Valiente (1994) report an incident during which a patient was overcome by intense heat while waiting for the resident to come into the hospital examination room. The patient removed her blouse and soaked it in cold water to relieve the sensation of intense bodily heat. Not aware of *el calor*, when the resident entered the room, he read the situation as a psychotic episode, transferring her immediately to the local state psychiatric hospital, where she remained without her family's knowledge and without an interpreter for several days.

The biomedical diagnosis and treatment of *el calor* creates significant clinical confusion. For example, several Salvadoran women reported what they view as common misdiagnoses, including menopause or high blood pressure (Jenkins & Valiente, 1994). Similarly, psychiatric renderings of the experience of *el calor* included depression, panic attacks, generalized anxiety, and posttraumatic stress disorders (Jenkins & Valiente, 1994). Yet, like the bereavement experiences discussed earlier, it should be noted that *el calor* may, in some circumstances, be understood as a nonpathological, culturally normative experience (Jenkins & Valiente, 1994). The statement of one Salvadoran women, "*No pienso que es enfermedad*" ("I don't think it's sickness") (Jenkins & Valiente, 1994, p. 175) reflects the problematic constellation of collective experiences of violence, emotional responses, and mental disorders.

WHERE THEY FALL SHORT

A recent editorial in *Anthropology News* points out the anthropological underpinnings of the cultural competence movement (Green, 2006). Tying cultural competency to racism, anthropologist James Green references the evolution of the term *cultural competence* from *ethnic competence* in the various editions of his own book *Cultural Awareness in the Human Services* (Green, 1982, 1999). Green (2006) notes that although the concept was rooted in optimism, cultural competence failed because, for many social and health service workers, "culture" was "little more than a trait list" (p. 3). Green (2006) expresses his dismay that cultural competency training has diminished into a requirement to be fulfilled for continued financial support. He now finds *competence* itself a dangerous term because it diminishes the complexity and uncertainty that would inherently be part of culturally sensitive care, and instead suggests *cultural responsibility* and *cultural humbleness* as more appropriate and telling terms (Green, 2006, p. 3).

Despite the well-intentioned foundations of cultural competency, the way in which "culture" is understood and deployed in such models falls short on

several counts. First, "culture" is often presented as static. Anthropologist Ja-
nelle Taylor (2003) trenchantly critiques the "canonical text for cultural competence efforts," *The Spirit Catches You and You Fall Down* by Anne Fadiman
(1997), on the basis that the book presents culture as a "reified, essential, static
thing" (Taylor, 2003, p. 160). Similarly, anthropologist Susan Shaw (2005) has
argued that "essentializing" narratives of culture add to the "commodification
and reification of culture" (p. 292). Taylor (2003) proceeds to note that static
understandings of culture are inconsistent with the current state of culture
theory within anthropology. Accordingly, culture is reduced to a property of (certain) individuals. As such, cultural competency discourses do not view culture
as an emergent process and product of human interaction. This treatment of
culture is guilty of what Jenkins and Barrett (2004) describe as an attempt to
"reduce [culture] to something it is not, a quantifiable 'cultural factor' or a
'cultural variable'" (p. 4). Consequently, cultural competency discourses leave
little room for cultural change (Taylor, 2003).

In addition to limiting possibilities for change, cultural variation is, by extension, eclipsed by static definitions of culture. Such a statement may seem
paradoxical insofar as cultural competence efforts are predicated on notions of
cultural difference. Efforts to provide culturally competent care, particularly
those characterized by attempts to achieve "ethnic resemblance" between patient and provider, depend on "racialized" notions of culture and assertions of
fundamental differences among ethnic groups (Rattansi, 1992; Shaw, 2005). In
their article "Is Cultural Competency a Backdoor to Racism?," S. Agnes Lee
and Michelle Farrell (2006) demonstrate how the implementation of cultural
competency models and curricula is often the proposed solution for numerous
racial and ethnic disparities in U.S. health care. The authors argue that the
inability of such models and programming "to capture the diverse and fluid
nature of culture and self-identity" only reifies existing racial categories rather
than deconstructing barriers to health care (Lee & Farrell, 2006, p. 9). By not
acknowledging the flexible, emergent quality of culture, such efforts fail to address diversity adequately *within* cultural groups (Santiago–Irizarry, 1996; Shaw,
2005). As Santiago–Irizarry's (1996) ethnography of a Latino mental health
clinic illustrates, one-size-fits-all mobilizations of "culture" are likely to lack
relevance for clients as well as practitioners.

Beyond lacking relevance for those involved, uncritical use of "culture" in
clinical practice may unwittingly render the patient's culture as that which is
problematic. In this vein, Santiago–Irizarry (1996) identifies a tension in efforts
to institutionalize culturally sensitive psychiatric practice. On the one hand,
such efforts may be understood as attempts to redress medical hegemony. Yet
on the other hand, she avers that such efforts may "medicalize" dimensions of
ethnically specific behaviors as psychological symptoms. Moreover, she critiques the construction of Hispanics as an "at-risk" population. The main thrust
of her argument rests on her identification of the double-edge sword of "vulnerability," such that this characterization "marks the genesis of the paradoxical
notion of culture as both source of dysfunction and therapeutic panacea"
(Santiago–Irizarry, 1996, p. 6). Similarly, Lambert and Sevak (1996) caution

against the slippage that may exist in medical contexts between recognition of cultural difference and perceived deviance from a middle-class Anglo norm. Furthermore, they note the danger of reducing complex health beliefs and practices to presumed fundamental cultural differences.

Oversimplifications of "culture" also manifest in the conflation of culture with race or ethnicity. (We recognize the complexity of the concepts race and ethnicity. For thorough coverage of the meanings of each of these terms, please refer to the American Anthropological Association's Race Project website [http://raceproject.aaanet.org]. The project website provides a comprehensive bibliography addressing the subject.) Redressing this error, in part, Alegria and colleagues (2002) caution against limiting efforts to understand sources of disparities in mental health care utilization to the effects of race or ethnicity alone. Instead, they advocate a more complex view that integrates minority status alongside considerations of socioeconomic status and geographic region. Moreover, Ortner (1998) has cautioned that even if there is a recognition of a "fusion" between race, ethnicity, and class, class remains "hidden" in the United States. Indeed, the contributions of class, gender, age, and geography may well be more salient than "race" or "ethnicity" to an individual's identity, and his or her experience and interpretation of distress.

By emphasizing cultural difference, cultural competency efforts may also obscure important similarities. Notably, similarities *across* patient populations may reveal important structural features of clinical encounters. In seeking to improve clinical practice, researchers would do well to remain aware of the ways in which imbalances of power may be endemic to interactions between patients and providers (Fisher & Groce, 1990; Mishler, 1984; West, 1984a, b; West & Frankel, 1991). Lambert and Sevak (1996) have suggested the limited explanatory utility of linking differentials in health care experiences to "culture," instead calling attention to the rift between biomedicine and lay understandings of health and illness. Likewise, Betancourt and colleagues (2005) note that barriers in clinical communication are not confined to minority groups, but may just be "more pronounced in these cases" (p. 500).

Finally, from the perspective of medical anthropology, cultural competency discourses often fail to recognize Western medicine itself as a cultural system. This necessitates broadening of conceptions of the importance of interpreters or culture brokers in the clinical encounter to be mindful of the language and culture of medicine itself. Breakdowns and slippages in communication in the clinical encounter can tell us much about assumptions embedded within contemporary medical practice. Discussing the training and socialization of physicians, Good and colleagues (2003) note that the "medical gaze" quickly becomes the dominant knowledge frame in medical school, with efficiency highly valued. In this respect, medical students and attending physicians are "most caring of patients who are willing to become part of the medical story they wish to tell and the therapeutic activities they hope to pursue" (Good et al., 2003, p. 595). More broadly, Gaines (1992) has pointed out that Western biomedicine (of which U.S. psychiatry is a part) is itself a cultural construction to be considered within historical context. Gaines (1992) traces the distinct but historically situated cultural meanings present in the nomenclature system of the *Diagnostic and Statistical Manual of Mental Disorders* (DSM), showing it to be a product of a professional ethnopsychiatry rather than a culture-free science. In this respect, he argues against a view of U.S. psychiatric disease categories as natural and universal.

OUR RECOMMENDATIONS

For decades, medical anthropologists have offered critiques of contemporary medicine (Hahn & Gaines, 1995; Mishler, 1984; Singer & Baer, 1995). The current climate of *cultural competence* creates a new venue in which to apply our expertise as students of culture. Our reservations regarding cultural competence, however, must move beyond the level of critique to recommendation, to be clinically relevant. Furthermore, while subjecting clinical practice to cultural critique, anthropologists ought to be mindful of the relative luxuries of their positions as researchers, observers, and interviewers, who need not identify problems, offer therapeutic advice, or treat patients.

We acknowledge the practical realities of contemporary mental health practice. In addition to the challenges inherent in diagnosis and effective treatment, clinicians now must contend with the additional burdens of substantial time and economic constraints. For example, Kleinman (1988a) has pointed out that a diagnosis must be made for both patient and clinician to receive reimbursement in the current insurance/health management organization (HMO)/managed care climate. In addition, patients are increasingly facile at invoking (and sometimes demanding) psychiatric diagnoses. The advent of direct-to-consumer advertisement of psychopharmaceuticals has facilitated such uncritical and casual use of psychiatric labels in popular culture. Patients increasingly come to the clinical encounter with a prepackaged self-diagnosis and treatment plan informed by commercials and print media, entertainment, and the Internet.

We also recognize the potential for a detailed, nuanced patient story to be daunting within the constraints of contemporary mental health practice. The challenge, therefore, is to engage with complexity without the dual problems of either oversimplification or the stagnation of effective treatment interventions. Models of cultural competence posit culture as something to *know* rather than something to *be ready for*. We argue that culturally appropriate care need *not* require an encyclopedic knowledge of the world's cultures and their specific ethnomedical and ethnopsychiatric systems of knowledge.

In *The Birth of the Clinic*, Foucault (1973) notes that the rise of modern medicine can be traced to a fundamental shift in the orientation of the clinician to the patient. At the heart of the practice of the premodern physician was the question: How do you feel? Foucault maintains that this question, grounded in the totality of the experience of the ill individual, becomes transformed at the inception of modern medicine to the question of: Where does it hurt? Anthropologist Tanya Luhrmann (2000) makes a similar observation specific to the contemporary practice of psychiatry. Specifically, the training process encourages psychiatrists to "think of psychiatric illness as an organic disease, a 'thing' underlying and generating the symptoms" (p. 25).

In contrast to a "culture-free" process of indexing constellations of behaviors first as symptoms and second as disease, we argue that diagnosis must be understood as a process embedded in the complex interplay of biology and culture. In this vein, we look to Kleinman's (1988a) understanding of psychiatric diagnosis as an interpretation of an individual's experience. Accordingly, the diagnostic process is reciprocally produced by clinician and patient. Although we argue that this is the case for all clinical encounters, the observation holds particular salience in clinical practice involving care of patients from other cultures or underrepresented populations.

We recommend that clinical encounters be viewed as two-way learning encounters. We advocate *openness* on the part of the clinician as well as a *willingness* to seek clarification when patients present unusual or unfamiliar complaints. This requires a shifting role for clinicians as *both* trained professionals and lifelong "students." To this end, we recommend the incorporation of dimensions of anthropological technique into clinical practice.

In a final chapter of the groundbreaking *The Illness Narratives*, Arthur Kleinman (1988b) provides a "practical clinical methodology" for humane health care of the chronically ill. Kleinman's model not only allows for uncertainty and complexity within the clinical encounter, but embraces such aspects as a part of the "existential experience of illness as much as that of healing" (Kleinman, 1988b, p. 228). He suggests three anthropological techniques—a miniethnography, a brief life history, and the elicitation and negotiation of an explanatory model—to facilitate a clinical encounter.

Within the miniethnography, the clinician seeks to understand the illness from the patient's and family's points of view. Here the clinician uses empathy, observational skills, interpretation and analytic skills, and self-reflection first to reconstruct the patient's (and family's) illness narrative and social context, and then to note important and/or reoccurring patterns and relationships in a patient's life. Along with the miniethnography, the life history then provides the patient the chance to narrate his or her life as broadly as he or she wishes. It creates the space for the clinician to be an active listener, a biographer, who finds each detail the patient wishes to provide to be valuable to the clinical encounter. The process of recording the patient's life history along with the miniethnography may further help the practitioner to identify important patterns (Kleinman, 1988b).

Kleinman (1998b) then suggests the elicitation of the patient's explanatory model through a series of open-ended questions concerning the explanation for and causation of the illness. However, he cautions that the explanatory model is not a "direct rendering" of the patient's words (Kleinman, 1988b, p. 240). It must instead be understood as the practitioner's interpretation of the patient's illness story. An explanatory model is informed by both patient and family nonverbal communication as well as by the miniethnography and life history. After the elicitation of the patient's explanatory model, the practitioner must present his or her own biomedical model. This process involves skill on the part of the clinician, because he or she must translate the biomedical model into lay terms understandable to the patient. Kleinman (1988b) states this means understanding that miscommunication is not simply a "lack of effective knowledge," but rather the possession of different kinds (p. 242). The last step of the process is then the negotiation stage, during which the clinician and patient must confer and collaborate as colleagues on decisions regarding treatment of the illness.

This entire process is valuable because it allows the clinician to be self-reflective and evaluative of the various constructions that provide the foundations for his or her own explanation of illness. As a whole, Kleinman (1988b) finds that using these three anthropological techniques provides for a kind of medical psychotherapy in which the clinician's active involvement and interest in the patient's life provide for a therapeutic "remoralization" of both patient and practitioner (p. 246).

In a similar vein, other scholars have highlighted the value of anthropological theory and ethnographic inquiry to the provision of culturally appropriate mental health care. Seely (2004) suggests an adaptation of the ethnographic method for use in intercultural psychotherapy. She uses three case studies to illustrate how clinically adapted ethnographic inquiry focused on contextualizing clients' distress in their native culture can be helpful in determining cultural resistances to treatment, legitimizing concepts unique to the client's culture, and diffusing some of the power and "positionality" inherent to the therapist–client relationship. The success of both Kleinman and Seely's methodologies in the treatment of diverse populations rests upon clinicians' commitment to be open to illness conceptions and normative practices different from their own, and a willingness to learn from their patient.

CONCLUDING REMARKS

In this chapter we have argued for an appreciation of the complex ways in which culture may mediate the expression and experience of mental disorders and treatment. Although we applaud efforts to bring culture into clinical practice, the manner in which "cultural competence" has taken shape falls short in light of anthropological understandings of culture. In addition to considering problems wrought by cultural misunderstandings between client and provider, we have highlighted the importance of the language and culture of medicine in the production of clinical miscommunication. In this respect, we point to the complexity of clinical "barriers" to recommend that clinical encounters be viewed as two-way learning encounters characterized by *openness* on the part of the clinician as well as a *willingness* to seek clarification when patients present unusual or unfamiliar complaints. What we hope, therefore, that what readers of this volume take away is an increased awareness of the diversity of ethnomedical and ethnopsychiatric systems of knowledge. The specific examples provided in this volume ought not to be viewed as conditions or syndromes to be memorized, but rather as vivid illustrations of the myriad ways in which "culture counts."

REFERENCES

Alegria, M., Canino, G., Rios, R., Vera, M., Calderon, J., Rusch, D., et al. (2002). Inequalities in use of specialty mental health services among Latinos, African Americans, and non-Latino whites. *Psychiatric Services, 53*(12), 1547–1555.

Berger, J. T. (1998). Culture and ethnicity in clinical care. *Archives of Internal Medicine, 158,* 2085–2090.

Betancourt, J. R., Green, A. R., Carrillo, J. E., & Park, E. R. (2005). Cultural competence and health care disparities: Key perspectives and trends. *Health Affairs, 24*(2), 499–505.

Brach, C., & Fraserirector, I. (2000). Can cultural competency reduce racial and ethnic health disparities? A review and conceptual model. *Medical Care Research and Review, 57,* 181–217.

Brown, G. W., & Harris, T. (1978). *Social origins of depression: A study of psychiatric disorder in women.* London, UK: Tavistock Publications.

Cooper, L. A., & Roter, D. L. (2003). Patient–provider communication: The effect of race and ethnicity on process and outcomes of healthcare. In B. D. Smedley, A. Y. Stith, & A. R. Nelson (Eds.), *Unequal treatment: Confronting racial and ethnic disparities in health care* (pp. 552–593). Washington, DC: National Academies Press.

Fadiman, A. (1997). *The spirit catches you and you fall down: A Hmong child, her American doctors, and the collision of two cultures.* New York: Farrar, Straus, and Giroux.

Fisher, S., and Groce, S. (1990). Accounting practices in medical interviews. *Language in Society, 19*(2), 225–250.

Foucault, M. (1973). *The birth of the clinic: An archaeology of medical perception.* New York: Pantheon Books.

Gaines, A. D. (1992). From *DSM-I* to *III-R*; voices of self, mastery and the other: A cultural constructivist reading of U.S. psychiatric classification. *Social Science and Medicine, 35*(1), 3–24.

Gaines, A. D., & Farmer, P. E. (1986). Visible saints: Social cynosures and dysphoria in the Mediterranean tradition. *Culture, Medicine and Psychiatry, 10*(4), 295–330.

Good, M. D., James, C., Good, B., & Becker, A. (2003). The culture of medicine and racial, ethnic, and class disparities in healthcare In B. D. Smedley, A. Y. Stith, & A. R. Nelson (Eds.), *Unequal treatment: Confronting racial and ethnic disparities in health care* (pp. 594–625). Washington, DC: The National Academies Press.

Green, J. W. (1982) *Cultural awareness in the human services.* Englewood Cliffs, NJ: Prentice-Hall.

Green, J. W. (1999). *Cultural awareness in the human services: A multi-ethnic approach* (3rd ed.). Boston, MA: Allyn & Bacon.

Green, J. W. (2006). On cultural competence. *Anthropology News, 47*(5), 3.

Hahn, R. A., & Gaines, A. D. (Eds.). (1995). *Physicians of Western medicine: Anthropological approaches to theory and practice.* Dordrecht: Kluwer Academic Publishers.

Hinshaw, S., & Cicchetti, D. (2000). Stigma and mental disorder: Conceptions of illness, public attitudes, personal disclosure, and social policy. *Development and Psychopathology, 12,* 555–598.

Jenkins, J. H. (1998). Diagnostic criteria for schizophrenia and related psychotic disorders: Integration and suppression of cultural evidence in *DSM-IV*. *Transcultural Psychiatry*, 35(3), 357–376.

Jenkins, J. H., & Barrett, R. J. (2004). Introduction. In J. H. Jenkins & R. J. Barrett (Eds.), *Schizophrenia, culture, and subjectivity: The edge of experience* (vol. 11, pp. 1–25). New York: Cambridge University Press.

Jenkins, J. H., & Valiente, M. (1994). Bodily transactions of the passions: *El calor* among Salvadoran women refugees. In T. J. Csordas (Ed.), *Embodiment and experience: The existential ground of culture and self* (pp. 163–182). New York: Cambridge University Press.

Kirmayer, L. J., Groleau, D., Guzder, J., Blake, C., & Jarvis, E. (2003). Cultural consultation: A model of mental health service for multicultural societies. *Canadian Journal of Psychiatry*, 48(3), 145–153.

Kleinman, A. (1988a). *Rethinking psychiatry*. New York: Free Press.

Kleinman, A. (1988b). *The illness narratives: Suffering, healing, and the human condition*. New York: Basic Books.

Lambert, H., & Sevak, L. (1996). Is "cultural difference" a useful concept? Perceptions of health and the sources of ill health among Londoners of South Asian origin. In D. Kelleher & S. Hiller (Eds.), *Researching cultural differences in health* (pp. 124–159). London, UK: Routledge.

Lee, S. A., & Farrell, M. (2006). Is cultural competency a backdoor to racism? *Anthropology News*, 47(3), 9–10.

Luhrmann, T. M. (2000). *Of two minds: The growing disorder in American psychiatry*. New York: Alfred A. Knopf.

Lutz, C. (1990). Engendered emotion: Gender, power, and the rhetoric of emotional control in American discourse. In C. Lutz & L. Abu-Lughod (Eds.), *Language and the politics of emotion* (pp. 69–91). New York: Cambridge University Press.

Mishler, E. (1984). *The discourse of medicine: The dialectics of medical interviews*. Norwood, NJ: Ablex.

Obeyesekere, G. (1985). Depression, Buddhism, and the work of culture in Sri Lanka. In A. Kleinman & B. Good (Eds.), *Culture and depression: Studies in anthropology and cross-cultural psychiatry of affect and disorder* (pp. 134–152). Los Angeles, CA: University of California Press.

Ortner, S. B. (1998). Identities: The hidden life of class. *Journal of Anthropological Research*, 54(1), 1–17.

Rattansi, A. (1992). Changing the subject? Racism, culture, and education. In J. Donald & A. Rattansi (Eds.), *"Race," culture, and difference* (pp.11–48). London, UK: Sage.

Santiago–Irizarry, V. (1996). Culture as cure. *Cultural Anthropology*, 11(1), 3–24.

Seely, K. (2004). Short-term intercultural psychotherapy: Ethnographic inquiry. *Social Work*, 49(1), 121–130.

Shaw, S. J. (2005). The politics of recognition in culturally appropriate care. *Medical Anthropology Quarterly*, 19(3), 290–309.

Singer, M., & Baer, H. (1995). *Critical medical anthropology*. Amityville, NY: Baywood Publishing.

Smedley, B. E., Stith, A. Y., & Nelson, A. R. (Eds.). (2003). *Unequal treatment: Confronting ethnic and racial disparities in health care*. Washington, DC: National Academies Press.

Snowden, L. R., & Hu, T. W. (1997). Ethnic differences in mental health services among the severely mentally ill. *Journal of Community Psychology*, 25, 235–247.

Stewart, M. (1999). Evidence on patient–doctor communication. *Cancer Prevention and Control, 3,* 25–30.

Takeuchi, D. T., Sue, S., & Yeh, M. (1995). Return rates and outcomes from ethnicity-specific mental health programs in Los Angeles. *American Journal of Public Health, 85,* 638–643.

Taylor, J. S. (2003). The story catches you and you fall down: Tragedy, ethnography, and "cultural competence." *Medical Anthropology Quarterly, 17*(2), 159–181.

Tompar–Tiu, A., & Sustento–Seneriches, J. (1995). *Depression and other mental health issues: The Filipino American experience.* San Francisco, CA: Josey-Bass.

Uba, L. (1994). *Asian Americans: Personality patterns, identity, and mental health.* New York: Guilford Press.

U.S. Department of Health and Human Services. (1999). *Mental health: A report of the Surgeon General.* Rockville, MD: U.S. Department of Health and Human Services.

U.S. Department of Health and Human Services. (2001). *Mental health: Culture, race, ethnicity—Supplement to mental health: Report of the Surgeon General.* Rockville, MD: U.S. Department of Health and Human Services.

West, C. (1984a). *Routine complications: Troubles with talk between doctors and patients.* Bloomington, IN: Indiana University Press.

West, C. (1984b). When the doctor is a "lady": Power, status and gender in physician–patient encounters. *Symbolic Interaction, 7*(1), 87–105.

West, C., & Frankel, R. (1991). Miscommunication in medicine. In N. Coupland, H. Giles, & J. Wiemann, (Eds.), *Miscommunication and problematic talk* (pp.166–194). Newbury Park, CA: Sage Publications.

2

Issues in the Diagnosis and Assessment of Mood Disorders in Minorities

HUMBERTO MARIN & JAVIER I. ESCOBAR

The diagnosis and assessment of mental disorders in minority groups in the United States is gaining relevance as issues such as "health disparities" come to the forefront. In this process, the traditional ("colonial") view of minority is being gradually replaced by a new perspective that values cultural identities and advocates the implementation of culturally relevant interventions for groups outside mainstream American culture.

Key questions relevant to mental health issues such as mood disorders that arise in this debate include the following:

- Are the concepts/definitions of mood disorders as defined in Western societies universally applicable?
- To what degree are mood disorders influenced by biological and environmental factors?
- Even if biology (genotype) was the same in all regions, are there any differences in the presentation of these disorders by patients from different cultures (phenotypes)?
- Are these disorders perceived/recognized/explained differently by clinicians from different cultural backgrounds?

Although this review cannot provide a fully satisfactory answer to these queries, it is our intent to highlight major findings and controversies regarding official *DSM* categories of mood disorders when used across different groups and cultures. As precisely stated in a previous report, "received categories of psychiatric nosology are lenses through which clinicians see the world" (Kirmayer & Groleau, 2001) Thus, despite their shortcomings, Western definitions of mental disorders, exemplified in the *DSM* and the International Classification of Diseases

(ICD), remain our best tools for comparative studies, and this is the perspective we will use to frame our review and comments herein.

THE DEFINITION OF MINORITY

In North America, the concept of "minority" is relative and fluid, varying according to the field of analysis. In the area of mental health, it is often meant to designate individuals who are "socially disadvantaged." From an ethnic/cultural perspective, this definition generally applies to African Americans, Hispanics, Native Americans, and some Asian subgroups. However, in practice, it is virtually impossible to disentangle the contributions of specific ethnic/cultural factors from the large and rather amorphous set of social and economic factors that impact psychological functions and lead to emotional distress. Thus, when examining factors contributing to mood disorders in minorities, as well as their disadvantages related to proper prevention, detection, and treatment of these disorders, it is virtually impossible to separate the impact of culture from that of general socio-economic factors like poverty, isolation, and low educational level.

INTERNAL HETEROGENEITY OF ETHNIC GROUPS:
THE CASE WITH ASIANS

Some of the definitions of *minority* that are currently in use in North America are grossly impractical, oversimplified "umbrella" concepts. For example, under the label of Asian Americans we include at least two dozen heterogeneous groups, racially different, who speak multiple languages and practice radically different religions. This group includes Christians and Muslims from the Near East, who are already quite different among themselves, as well as Far Eastern peoples like Japanese or Koreans. In turn, some of these nationalities, such as Indian or Chinese, also include several subgroups, each with sufficient racial or cultural distinctiveness to warrant separation into different echelons.

Later we show that in the case of Hispanics, dramatic differences are seen across subgroups and generations regarding their mental health status. A similar process is occurring with Asians. A recent study comparing Chinese, Filipino, and white youths found that ethnicity predicted depression whereas generational differences predicted coexisting somatic symptoms and substance use disorders, highlighting the importance of focusing studies on specific subgroups and generations of Asian American youth (Willgerodt & Thompson, 2006).

Although studies in this area have included many minorities, some important groups are missing. One particular group in North America that has been largely ignored in studies on mental disorders and their treatment is that of Arab Americans (Ericsson & Al-Timimi, 2001). Such an omission is regrettable, although not surprising in view of current world events.

HISPANICS: A MOST HETEROGENEOUS GROUP

In the United States, minority groups are not monoliths, and Hispanics are a good example of this. A term of convenience, *Hispanic* serves as an umbrella to individuals whose origin extends to more than 20 countries and who are enormously diverse in terms of social, economic, and educational factors. There are common tenets such as language, close-knit family systems, and the "mores and motivations" from the Catholic Church that still justify a common ethnocultural identification for this group. However, Hispanics are very heterogeneous in areas that may impact the incidence, presentation, course, and treatment of mood disorders. These include birthplace, level of acculturation, genetic elements, race, health care access/utilization, and language (Marin, Escobar, & Vega, 2006).

The Latino "Paradox"

A surprising observation, given the many disadvantages affecting immigrants of Hispanic heritage, is that being born in the United States and having a higher level of identification and affinity with U.S. mainstream culture (high acculturation) is a consistently documented risk factor for mood and other psychiatric and physical disorders in U.S. Hispanics (Vega, Kolody, Aguilar–Gaxiola, Alderete, Catalano, & Caraveo–Anduaga, 1998). This also seems to hold true for other ethnic groups. For example, a recent estimate using data from the 1998–2003 National Health Interview Surveys (NHIS) shows that U.S.-born black and Hispanic adults are more likely to experience serious psychological distress than their immigrant counterparts (Dev & Lucas, 2006).

Curiously, for some minority groups such as Asians, the tendency may be the opposite. A study with immigrants from Korea, Japan, and China (Yeh, 2003) showed that those immigrants who identified more closely with U.S. culture reported fewer mental health symptoms than those immigrants who continue to have a strong identification with their countries of origin. Language differences seem to be the critical factor for this observation (Yeh, 2003). Also, a community survey of immigrants from India found that immigrants who reported greater social and cultural U.S. ties and fewer traditional ones, independent of other social and demographic variables, had better mental health scores than their less acculturated peers (Mehta, 1998). Moreover, under conditions of high parent–child conflict, less acculturated Asian youths seem to be at higher risk for suicidal behaviors than their more acculturated counterparts (Lau, Zane, & Myers, 2002). Thus, it has been stated that "differences in the impact of length of stay in the United States on immigrant health suggest that the role of acculturation in understanding immigrant health is complex and may differ for various race/ethnicity groups" (Dev, & Lucas, 2006).

ETHNICITY AND ASSIMILATION INTO THE DOMINANT SOCIETY

The degree of assimilation and social stability over time is likely to differ across various North American and European minority groups. For example, individuals belonging to minorities with distinctive physical features (skin color) will likely assimilate more slowly, particularly if language is at stake (e.g., the case currently with African immigrants to Spain).

African Americans

African Americans have been identified as a separate group for centuries, and yet they have assimilated well into the "melting pot." However, they continue to face problems such as discrimination. There seems to be a gender effect because at least one study showed that elderly African American males suffer more than females from the stressful effects of racism (Utsey, Payne, Jackson, & Jones, 2002).

U.S. Hispanics

The more recent diaspora of people of Hispanic origin has led to problems in rapid assimilation that appear to be mainly related to language. Some subgroups, particularly the better educated, "light-skinned" ones, seem likely to assimilate faster, as is the case with the Cuban American population of southern Florida. This may be because their main external difference—language—tends to disappear in a very few generations. Difficulty communicating with health providers is a big hurdle to health care, and this is reported by about one third of Latinos in the United States. However, this issue affects primarily foreign-born Latinos, of which 42% report this difficulty, compared with only 8% of the U.S. born (Pew Hispanic Center/Kaiser Family Foundation, 2002). Less assimilated immigrant Hispanic elders report a higher depression rate than their more acculturated counterparts (Gonzalez, Haan & Hinton, 2001). Besides this, some disadvantaged Hispanic subpopulations seem to be at higher risk for mental illness (e.g., the elderly, illegal aliens, and segregated or impoverished sectors) (Black, Markides, & Miller, 1998; Bromberger, Harlow, Avis, Kravitz, & Cordal, 2004; Dunlop, Song, Lyons, Manheim, & Chang, 2003; Saluja, Iachan, Scheidt, Overpeck, Sun, & Giedd, 2004).

Asian Americans

In some Asian groups, like Southeast Asians and Koreans, the risk for psychological distress seems to increase with age (Iwamasa & Hilliard, 1999). Despite their great educational success and the fact that they are now overrepresented in the professional classes, many Asians in the United States continued to be perceived as "permanent outsiders" or "perpetual foreigners," as has been the case with African Americans in many areas of the country (Mio, 2004). These are examples of *persistent discrimination*, despite successful assimilation and linguistic proficiency.

DIFFERENCES IN MOOD DISORDERS IN HISPANIC AND ASIAN SUBGROUPS

Significant differences have been found among Hispanic subgroups regarding the frequency of mood disorders. In the Hispanic Health and Nutrition Examination Survey (H-HANES) that took place in 1982–1984, Puerto Ricans showed a significantly higher frequency of depression than Mexicans and Cuban Americans (Moscicki, Rae, Regier, & Locke, 1987). This is a curious finding if we consider that Puerto Ricans have considerably higher access to mental health care than the other two subgroups, and significantly less stress related to immigration status than Mexicans. It is a complex issue, and one wonders whether Puerto Ricans' racial admixture may lead them to experience more racism and rejection. Significant intragroup differences regarding use of mental health services also have been reported within Hispanic and Asian American minorities. Puerto Ricans and Cubans use significantly more services than Mexicans and other Hispanic subgroups (Weinick, Jacobs, Cacari Stone, Ortega, & Burstin, 2004). A study on use of mental health services by Asian Americans found that, compared with whites, East Asians and Filipinos used significantly more services whereas Southeast and other Asians used roughly the same or less. The authors conclude that aggregating Asian subpopulations into a single group in services research is no longer appropriate (Barreto & Segal, 2005).

Suicide

Overall, in the United States, minorities show indexes of suicide that are significantly less than those of the general population. However, certain subgroups seem particularly vulnerable, showing relatively high rates of mood disorders and mood disorder-related behaviors such as suicide ideation and attempts. According to the Youth Risk Behavior Survey of the Centers for Disease Control and Prevention (CDC), in 1999, Latino youth were significantly more likely to have attempted suicide, made a suicide plan, or seriously considered suicide than young African and European Americans (Canino & Roberts, 2001) Asian women seem to have the highest suicide rate according to ethnicity (Chen, Chen, & Wang, 2002).

Psychological Distress

The causes and severity of psychological distress seem to differ among minority groups and even among their subgroups and generations. For Hispanics as a whole, the stressful effect of acculturation probably weighs significantly less than the effect of assimilating risky behaviors, and the result is a net loss in mental health with acculturation. The opposite seems to be true for Asians, with the benefits of acculturation outweighing the loss of protective culturally determined behaviors. For African Americans, the main source of psychological distress is not as much acculturation as it is perceived rejection (racism) and socioeconomic factors.

The Incidence of Mood Disorders across Countries and Cultures

A recent review of studies of the frequency of mood disorders with strict criteria for relevance found a 36-fold (0.61% to 22%) variation in the prevalence of major depression and a 15-fold (0.1% to 1.5%) variation in the prevalence of bipolar I disorder in different locations (Warach, Goldner, Somers, & Hsu, 2004). A cross-national study with 38,000 community subjects in 10 countries (United States, Canada, Puerto Rico, France, West Germany, Italy, Lebanon, Taiwan, Korea, and New Zealand) reported significant variations in the frequency of major depression. Major depression lifetime rate extremes were 1.5% in Taiwan and 19.0% in Beirut. However, significant differences also appeared between countries of not-so-distant culture and development, like the United States (5.2%) and France (16.4%). The lifetime rate for bipolar disorder ranged from 0.3% in Taiwan to 1.5% in New Zealand, with only seven sites considered (Weissman, Bland, Canino, Faravelli, Greenwald, Hwu, et al., 1996). A major methodological problem in some of these studies is the inability to control for the effect of other critical variables (such as the ongoing wars and conflicts in the Middle East) on rates of distress and mood symptoms. The presence at a given time of too many of these extraneous factors significantly decreases the usefulness of these multinational studies. For example, a recently published study on of the prevalence and predictors of depression in primary care in six countries, which included a Russian site (St Petersburg), showed that 75% of subjects there could not afford treatment when needed (Simon, Fleck, Lucas, Bushnell, & LIDO Group, 2004). One has to assume that this reality would affect the willingness of individuals to report symptoms and look for care. Thus, unless we have study samples large enough in each location to examine the relative importance of multiple variables, the results will probably continue to be confusing and unreliable.

Large Population Surveys in the United States: Findings and Shortcomings in Relation to Ethnicity

In the United States, studies have repeatedly found that the frequency of depression in Latinos and African Americans is similar to, or lower than, the frequency in non-Hispanic whites, despite higher risk factors for many disorders present in those minority populations. It is possible that methodological issues (use of instruments originally developed for middle-class European American populations), as well as cultural and ethnic issues (including language) and practical issues (the evasive character of undocumented Hispanics and the poorer Hispanics and blacks) may contribute to these atypical findings. However, in the case of U.S. Hispanics, one would expect that the high percentage of foreign-born Hispanics with their lower frequency of depression and other disorders may tilt the results for the whole group. A study using the database from the third National Health and Nutrition Examination Survey found that the prevalence of major depression was higher in whites than African Americans and Hispanic Americans; the opposite pattern was found for dysthymic disorder (Riolo,

Nguyen, Greden, & King, 2005). The NCS replication showed lower overall-rates for Hispanics compared with non-Hispanic whites in the areas of anxiety, mood, impulse control, and substance use disorders, as well as for any disorder (Kessler, Berglund, Demler, Jin, Merikangas, & Walters, 2005). Recently, a large survey, the National Epidemiologic Survey on Alcoholism and Related Conditions (NESARC), found a 12-month rate of Major Depressive Disorder of 5.53% for whites, 4.27% for Hispanics, and 4.52% for African Americans (Hasin, Goodwin, Stinson, & Grant, 2005). However, in the 1998–2003 NHIS mentioned earlier, among U.S.-born adults, Hispanics were more likely to experience serious psychological distress (4.4%) than either black adults (3.3%) or white adults (2.7%) (Dev & Lucas, 2003). In general, there exists a consensus that mental disorders tend to be undercounted in minority groups, including African Americans.

The extremely low rates of depression found among the Chinese, both in China and in the United States, deserve special discussion. For example, a community survey of Chinese-origin respondents in Los Angeles found a *DSM-III* lifetime major depression rate of just 6.9% (Takeuchi, Chung, Lin, et al., 1998). In the international study reported earlier (Weissman, Bland, Canino, Faravelli, Greenwald, Hwu et al., 1996), the prevalence of depression in Taiwan was only 1.5%. Among the possible factors contributing to this low reporting of depression among the Chinese, stigma, a tendency to report distress through somatic outlets, and culturally relevant concepts such as neurasthenia have been offered as potential explanations, together with issues of detection and identification, stoicism, and family and group support (Parker, Gladstone, & Kuan, 2001).

A caveat is needed here. Even if is true that Hispanics, and probably other minorities, have a lower risk for mood disorders, after they develop a disorder it tends to be more persistent (Breslau, Kendler, Su, Gaxiola–Aguilar, & Kessler, 2005; Golding & Lipton, 1990). This sounds logical, particularly when taking into account their less favorable environment, reduced access to services, and lower quality of such services. Thus, if mood disorders are present, there is a lower chance for their opportune detection and treatment.

Two issues relevant to the cross-cultural study of mood disorders are the particular *meaning* of mental or mood disorder and the *language of distress* operating in each cultural group.

Explanatory Models of Disease

Patients seek care with a repertoire of attitudes and complaints in efforts to convey what they view as a problem and its probable causes. Often, patients and physicians differ in their perspectives on these issues, particularly with regard to the attribution on what or who is responsible for the problem. Cultural differences in this regard have been repeatedly demonstrated and, in the case of ethnic minorities, these differences are also influenced by the degree of identification with the mainstream, dominant culture (level of acculturation). Even within a single ethnic group, diverging, even contradictory explanations of mental disorder may be elicited, as shown in a recent study on conceptual models of depression comparing South Asian immigrants with European Americans (Karasz, 2005). These explanatory models for mood disorders have an impact on treatment outcomes, including medication adherence (Bollini, Tibaldi, Testa, & Munizza, 2004).

"Language of Distress"

The concept of language of distress was born from studies on somatic presentations and has permeated the discussion about differences in somatic symptoms associated with mood disorders across cultures. Although there are many reports documenting higher levels of somatic presentations in the case of non-Western and Latino populations, what seems to differ is the type of presentation ("functional syndromes" such as fibromyalgia, chronic fatigue, or irritable bowel vs. conversion or dissociative symptoms), the phenomena being quite ubiquitous (Kirmayer, 2001). Regardless of the true incidence of these presentations, in the United States, the expectation from clinicians working with minority groups with mood disorders is that they will present or emphasize somatic symptoms (see below). We discuss this in more detail later.

THE DIAGNOSIS AND DETECTION OF MOOD DISORDERS IN MINORITY GROUPS

Diagnostic Bias

Several studies in the United States suggest that Hispanics and African Americans are more likely to receive a diagnosis of psychotic disorder and less likely to receive one of mood disorder than whites. In the 1980s, a review of the medical records of 76 bipolar patients showed that Hispanic (Puerto Rican) and African American patients were more likely than whites to be misdiagnosed as schizophrenic, particularly if they were young and experienced auditory hallucinations (Mukherjee, Shukla, Woodle, Rosen, & Olarte, 1983). This finding regarding African Americans became so common that a 1982 report of a study was titled "Another Study of Manic-Depression among Poor Blacks" (Freed, 1982). Unfortunately, this trend continues to be quite prevalent (Strakowski, Keck, & Arnold, 2003). A Texas study monitoring 936 inpatients with at least four hospitalizations found that 44% of Hispanics initially diagnosed as schizophrenic underwent a diagnosis change—a rate double that of whites and African Americans (Chen, Swann, & Burt, 1996). A study of an inpatient national sample of elderly veterans found that African Americans and Hispanics were more likely than whites to have a diagnosis of psychotic disorder (Kales, Blow, Bingham, Copeland, & Mellow, 2000).

In the United States, minority patients (of African, Asian, and Hispanic provenance) with mood disorders are more likely to use denial as a coping mechanism, and present with somatic complaints rather than psychological ones. This tendency for Hispanics and other minorities to somatize distress has been repeatedly documented in the literature, although such is also confounded with social class.

An American study, using a personality inventory in claims for workers' compensation, found that Hispanics were more likely to somatize than whites (DuAlba & Scott, 1993). In a study in California, depressed Latino and African American women scored significantly higher than whites on somatization indexes (Myers, Lesser, Rodriguez, Mira, Hwang, Camp, et al., 2002). For Asian Indians, a qualitative study reports that religious beliefs and stigmatization of mental illness predispose to somatization, denial of psychological symptoms, and delayed seeking of professional help (Conrad & Pacquiao, 2005).

Reliability/Validity of Assessment Tools in Minority Populations

Research-oriented screening questionnaires, diagnostic interviews, and instruments measuring symptom severity or change for mood disorders are intimately linked to the diagnostic criteria used to classify these disorders. A frequent critique of general work in this area is that the more precise and stringent these definitions are (a worthy goal of good research), the more "real" patients they will leave out (a fact that seriously limits clinical applications of the research). This problem is expected to be magnified when restrictive classifications are applied to cultural/ethnic groups outside the mainstream. For this reason, the very limited usefulness of these instruments to establish cross-cultural differences or commonalities must always be borne in mind.

The use of clinical instruments poses an additional thorny question: Do these instruments distort the diagnosis or severity of a mental condition in individuals belonging to different cultures? Although we do not have clear examples of this with regard to mood disorders, a widely used instrument to measure cognition—the Mini Mental State Examination—has been repeatedly shown to yield erroneous, inflated rates of dementia in groups such as Hispanics (Escobar, Burnam, Karno, Forsythe, Landsverk, & Holding, 1986; Espino, Lichtenstein, Palmer, & Hazuda, 2001). Thus, particular caution must be exercised in the transfer of clinical instruments across cultures.

Barriers to the Identification and Treatment of Mood Disorders in Minority Patients

Minorities have had historically less access to health care and mental health care than the general U.S. population. Health coverage is an important factor here, but there are other influences such as stigma, nonmedical conceptualization of illness, poor health literacy, mistrust of or ignorance about the medical establishment, and practical issues like geographic isolation, lack of transportation, job schedule, and family responsibilities (Table 2.1). There are significant variations across and within groups for access and insurance coverage, and Hispanics (particularly those who are foreign born) are disadvantaged in this regard (Dev & Lucas, 2006; Escalante, Barrett, del Rincon, Cornell, Phillips, & Katz, 2002; Marin, Escobar, & Vega, 2006; Matthews & Hughes, 2001).

Table 2.1 Common Barriers to the Identification and
Treatment of Mood Disorders in Minority Patients

Objective Barriers
- Health insurance (lack of health insurance,
  access to services but reduced access to medication/therapy,
  health insurance with no parity for mental disorders, etc.)
- Linguistic barriers
- Socioeconomic barriers (inability to pay the copayment,
  inability to get leave from work or childcare to go to the health
  facility, etc.)
- Geographic barriers (geographic isolation, lack of transportation,
  health care facilities in unfamiliar or intimidating environments)

Subjective Barriers
- Mistrust about the medical establishment
  (e.g., African Americans)
- Nonmedical conceptualization of illness
  and poor health literacy
- Ignorance about the navigation
  of health care services
- Illegal stay in the country or intimidation
  of lawful residents
- Stigma
- Fatalism and stoicism

How to Address Barriers to the Identification
and Treatment of Mood Disorders in Minority Patients

Effective solutions to these health care barriers seem easy to outline, but hard
to implement. Possible solutions include expanding health insurance coverage,
funding charity care, and enhancing access to effective treatments such as
medications. Access can be improved by establishing links with the community
and, ideally, locating services in communities adding features such as extended
hours of operation and adapting the services to the customs of local minorities
(e.g., accepting walk-ins or scheduling appointments in person in addition to the
telephone). Linguistic barriers deserve special consideration because they continue to exert an effect even after most other barriers have been overcome. Linguistic barriers are significant for many Hispanics and Asians, and also for some
Caribbean and African immigrants. Almost one half of U.S. Hispanics use Spanish as their primary language. Low English proficiency significantly decreases the
use of health and mental health services in Hispanic children and adults (Marin,
Escobar, & Vega, 2006). A study among Chinese Americans found that language-
based discrimination influenced the patterns of mental health use, shifting it
toward informal services and seeking help from friends (Spencer & Chen, 2004).

Practical solutions offered to deal with a language barrier include using bi-
lingual/bicultural professional staff members, using interpreters, providing language skill training for existing staff, and using internal language banks, phone-
based interpreter services, or written translations. It must be pointed out that the
last three options should be used only as backup or emergency stop-gap measures.

Primary Care

An important final consideration in this chapter is the fact that minority patients are more likely to receive treatment for mental disorders in primary care and less likely to receive treatment from specialists. Thus, proper identification of minority patients with mood disorders in primary care is critical, because minority patients (including children, adults, and older adults) seem to be at higher risk for nondetection of their mood disorders in primary care settings (Borowsky, Rubenstein, Meredith, Camp, Jackson–Triche, & Wells, 2000; Chung, Teresi, Guarnaccia, Meyers, Holmes, Bobrowitz, et al., 2003; Heneghan, Johnson Silver, Bauman, & Stein, 2000; Schmaling & Hernandez, 2005).

Full integration of mental health into primary care, a highly desirable goal, seems out of the question in our current health care system. However, a number of effective chronic care models for depression have been successfully implemented in primary care, and new models of collaboration between mental health and primary care clinicians are being tested at several sites, including some in depressed minorities with comorbid medical conditions like cancer (Unutzer, Katon, Callahan, Williams, Hunkeler, Harpole, et al., 2002; Dwight–Johnson, Ell, & Lee, 2005).

CONCLUSIONS AND RECOMMENDATIONS

Minority groups are heterogeneous. Therefore, in the assessment of minority patients with mood disorder, clinicians should use cultural-specific information, but should not let it obscure the individual patient. For each patient, it is important to get information on nationality and subgroup, immigration status and years in the United States, language, acculturation, personal beliefs on illness and treatment, and current socioeconomic characteristics, because all these factors may affect the presentation of mood disorders.

Linguistic barriers should never be minimized. The ideal solution to them is to use culturally and linguistically proficient mental health care providers. However, this is hardly generalizable. As a second best option, a professional translator in situ should be used whenever indicated. Use of family members or relatives as translators is best avoided because of confidentiality issues and distortion/censorship of the information. It has been repeatedly demonstrated that, for complex reasons, including excessive confidence in their language proficiency, health care providers fail to use translators, and this bears heavily on quality of care.

Remember that minority patients are more likely to receive mental health treatment in primary care, to have their mood disorders unrecognized, to present with somatic complaints for mood disorders, and to report psychotic symptoms in the absence of a thought disorder. Be alert to any symptom suggestive of mood disorder, but do not jump to the diagnosis of a psychotic disorder.

If you are in a primary care psychiatry setting, minimize referrals. Minority patients are significantly more likely than average to be "lost in transit."

Patients from disadvantaged minorities have less access to care and, after they are in care, they have fewer visits. The time window to treat them is shorter than average. Thus, be careful but not timid when making a diagnosis and establishing treatment for minority patients with mood disorders. Also remember that minority patients can benefit more than average from enhanced interventions such as family education, supplemental case management, collaborative care, or quality improvement interventions, as opposed to treatment as usual.

REFERENCES

Barreto, R. M., & Segal, S. P. (2005). Use of mental health services by Asian Americans. *Psychiatric Services, 56*(6), 746–748.

Black, S. A., Markides, K. S., & Miller, T. Q. (1998). Correlates of depressive symptomatology among older community-dwelling Mexican Americans: The Hispanic EPESE. *Journal of Gerontology Series B–Psychological Sciences & Social Sciences, 53*(4), S198–S208.

Bollini, P., Tibaldi, G., Testa, C., & Munizza, C. (2004). Understanding treatment adherence in affective disorders: A qualitative study. *Journal of Psychiatric & Mental Health Nursing, 11*, 668–674.

Borowsky, S. J., Rubenstein, L. V., Meredith, L. S., Camp, P., Jackson–Triche, M., & Wells, K. B. (2000). Who is at risk of nondetection of mental health problems in primary care? *Journal of General Internal Medicine, 15*(6), 381–388.

Breslau, J., Kendler, K. S., Su, M., Gaxiola–Aguilar, S., & Kessler, R. C. (2005). Lifetime risk and persistence of psychiatric disorders across ethnic groups in the United States. *Psychological Medicine, 35*, 317–327.

Bromberger, J. T., Harlow, S., Avis, N., Kravitz, H. M., & Cordal, A. (2004). Racial/ethnic differences in the prevalence of depressive symptoms among middle-aged women: The Study of Women's Health across the Nation (SWAN). *American Journal of Public Health, 94*(8), 1378–1385.

Canino, G., & Roberts, R. E. (2001). Suicidal behavior among Latino youth. *Suicide and Life-Threatening Behavior, 31*(Suppl.), 122–131.

Chen, J.- P., Chen, H., & Wang, C. B. (2002). Depressive disorders in Asian American adults. *Western Journal of Medicine, 176*, 239–244.

Chen, Y. R., Swann, A. C., & Burt, D. B. (1996). Stability of diagnosis in schizophrenia. *American Journal of Psychiatry, 153*, 682–686.

Chung, H., Teresi, J., Guarnaccia, P., Meyers, B.S., Holmes, D., Bobrowitz, T., et al. (2003). Depressive symptoms and psychiatric distress in low income Asian and Latino primary care patients: Prevalence and recognition. *Community Mental Health Journal, 39*(1), 33–46.

Conrad, M. M., & Pacquiao, D. F. (2005). Manifestation, attribution, and coping with depression among Asian Indians from the perspectives of health care practitioners. *Journal of Transcultural Nursing, 16*(1), 32–40.

Dev, A. N., & Lucas, J. W. (2006). Physical and mental health characteristics of U.S.- and foreign-born adults: United States, 1998–2003. *Advance Data from Vital and Health Statistics, CDC, Mar 1*, (369), 1–19.

DuAlba, L., & Scott, R. (1993). Somatization and malingering for workers' compensation applicants: A cross-cultural MMPI study. *Journal of Clinical Psychology, 49*(6), 913–917.

Dunlop, D. D., Song, J., Lyons, J. S., Manheim, L. M., & Chang, R. W. (2003). Racial/ethnic differences in rates of depression among preretirement adults. *American Journal of Public Health*, 93(11), 1945–1952.

Dwight-Johnson M., Ell K., & Lee P.-J. (2005). Can collaborative care address the needs of low-income Latinas with comorbid depression and cancer? Results from a randomized pilot study. *Psychosomatics*, 46,224–232.

Ericsson, C. D., & Al-Timimi, N. R. (2001). Providing mental health services to Arab Americans: Recommendations and considerations. *Cultural Diversity and Ethnic Minority Psychology*, 7(4), 308–327.

Escalante, A., Barrett, J., del Rincon, I., Cornell, J. E., Phillips, C. B., & Katz, J. N. (2002). Disparity in total hip replacement affecting Hispanic Medicare beneficiaries. *Medical Care*, 40(6), 447–450.

Escobar, J. I., Burnam, A., Karno, M., Forsythe, A., Landsverk, J., & Holding, J. M. (1986). Use of the Mini-Mental State Examination (MMSE) in a community population of mixed ethnicity: cultural and linguistic artifacts. *Journal of Nervous & Mental Disease*, 174, 607–614.

Espino, D. V., Lichtenstein, M. J., Palmer, R. F., & Hazuda, H. P. (2001). Ethnic differences in Mini-Mental State Examination (MMSE) scores: Where you live makes a difference. *Journal of the American Geriatrics Society*, 49, 538–548.

Freed, E. (1982). Another study of manic-depression among poor blacks. *American Journal of Psychiatry*, 139(1), 141–142.

Golding, J. M., & Lipton, R. I. (1990). Depressed mood and major depressive disorder in two ethnic groups. *Journal of Psychiatric Research*, 24(1), 65–82.

Gonzalez, H. M., Haan, M. N., & Hinton, L. (2001). Acculturation and the prevalence of depression in older Mexican-Americans: Baseline results of the Sacramento area Latino study on aging. *Journal of the American Geriatrics Society*, 49(7), 948–953.

Hasin, D. S., Goodwin, R. D., Stinson, F. S., & Grant, B. F. (2005). Epidemiology of major depressive disorder: Results from the National Epidemiologic Survey on Alcoholism and Related Conditions. *Archives of General Psychiatry*, 62, 1097–1106.

Heneghan, A. M., Johnson Silver, E., Bauman, L. J., & Stein, R. E. (2000). Do paediatricians recognize mothers with depressive symptoms? *Paediatrics*, 106(6), 1367–1373.

Iwamasa, G. Y., & Hilliard, K. M. (1999). Depression and anxiety among Asian American elders: A review of the literature. *Clinical Psychology Review*, 19(3), 343–357.

Kales, H. C., Blow, F. C., Bingham, C. R., Copeland, L. A., & Mellow, A. M. (2000). Race and inpatient psychiatric diagnoses among elderly veterans. *Psychiatric Services*, 51(6), 795–800.

Karasz, A. (2005). Cultural differences in conceptual models of depression. *Social Sciences & Medicine*, 60, 1625–1635.

Kessler, R. C., Berglund, P., Demler, O., Jin, R., Merikangas, K. R., & Walters, E. E. (2005). Lifetime prevalence and age-of-onset distributions of *DSM-IV* disorders in the National Comorbidity Survey replication. *Archives of General Psychiatry*, 62, 593–602.

Kirmayer, L. J. (2001). Cultural variations in the clinical presentations of depression and anxiety: implications for diagnosis and treatment. *Journal of Clinical Psychiatry*, 62(Suppl. 13), 22–28.

Kirmayer, L. J., & Groleau, D. (2001). Affective disorders in cultural context. *Psychiatric Clinics of North America*, 24(3), 465–478.

Lau, A. S., Zane, N., & Myers, H. F. (2002). Correlates of suicidal behavior among Asian American outpatient youths. *Cultural Diversity and Ethnic Minority Psychology*, 8(3), 199–213.

Marin, H., Escobar, J. I., & Vega, W. A. (2006). Mental illness in Hispanics: A review of the literature. *Focus, IV*(1), 23–37.

Matthews, A. K., & Hughes, T. L. (2001). Mental health service use by African American women: Exploration of subpopulation differences. *Cultural Diversity and Ethnic Minority Psychology, 7*(1), 75–87.

Mehta, S. (1998). Relationship between acculturation and mental health for Asian Indian immigrants in the United States. *Genetic, Social & General Psychology Monographs, 124*(1):61–78.

Mio, J. S. (2004). Asians on the edge: The reciprocity of allied behavior. *Cultural Diversity and Ethnic Minority Psychology, 10*(1), 90–94.

Moscicki, E. K., Rae, D. S., Regier, D. A., & Locke, B. Z. (1987). The Hispanic Health and Nutrition Survey: Depression among Mexican Americans, Cuban Americans, and Puerto Ricans. In M. Garcia & J. Arana (Eds.), *Research agenda for Hispanics* (pp. 145–159). Chicago, IL: University of Illinois Press.

Mukherjee, S., Shukla, S., Woodle, J., Rosen, A. M., & Olarte, S. (1983). Misdiagnosis of schizophrenia in bipolar patients: A multiethnic comparison. *American Journal of Psychiatry, 140*(12), 1571–1574.

Myers, H. F., Lesser, I., Rodriguez, N., Mira, C.B., Hwang, W.C., Camp, C., et al. (2002). Ethnic differences in clinical presentation of depression in adult women. *Cultural Diversity and Ethnic Minority Psychology, 8*(2), 138–156.

Parker, G., Gladstone, G., & Kuan, T. C. (2001). Depression in the planet's largest ethnic group: The Chinese. *American Journal of Psychiatry, 158,* 857–864.

Pew Hispanic Center/Kaiser Family Foundation. (2002). *2002 National survey of Latinos: Summary of findings.* Menlo Park, CA: Henry J Kaiser Foundation.

Riolo, S. A., Nguyen, T. A., Greden, J. F., & King, C. A. (2005). Prevalence of depression by race/ethnicity: Findings from the National Health and Nutrition Examination Survey III. *American Journal of Public Health, 95*(6), 998–1000.

Saluja, G., Iachan, R., Scheidt, P. C., Overpeck, M. D., Sun, W., & Giedd, J. N. (2004). Prevalence of and risk factors for depressive symptoms among young adolescents. *Archives of Pediatric and Adolescent Medicine, 158,* 760–765.

Schmaling, K. B., & Hernandez, D. V. (2005). Detection of depression among low-income Mexican Americans in primary care. *Journal of Health Care for the Poor and Underserved, 16*(4), 780–790.

Simon, G. E., Fleck, M., Lucas, R., Bushnell, D. M., & LIDO Group. (2004). Prevalence and predictors of depression treatment in an international primary care study. *American Journal of Psychiatry, 161,* 1626–1634.

Spencer, M. S., & Chen, J. (2004). Effect of discrimination on mental health service utilization among Chinese Americans. *American Journal of Public Health, 94*(5), 809–814.

Strakowski, S. M., Keck, P. E., & Arnold, L. M. (2003). Ethnicity and diagnosis in patients with affective disorders. *Journal of Clinical Psychiatry, 64,* 747–754.

Takeuchi, D. T., Chung, R. C.-Y., Lin, K. M., et al. (1998). Lifetime and twelve-month prevalence rates of major depressive episodes and dysthymia among Chinese Americans in Los Angeles. *American Journal of Psychiatry, 155,* 1407–1414.

Unutzer, J., Katon, W., Callahan, C. M., Williams, J.W., Hunkeler, E., Harpole, L., et al. (2002). Collaborative care management of late-life depression in the primary care setting. *Journal of the American Medical Association, 288*(22), 2836–2845.

Utsey, S. O., Payne, Y. A., Jackson, E. S., & Jones, A. M. (2002). Race-related stress, quality of life indicators, and life satisfaction among elderly African Americans. *Cultural Diversity and Ethnic Minority Psychology, 8*(3), 224–233.

Vega, W. A., Kolody, B., Aguilar–Gaxiola, S., Alderete, E., Catalano, R., & Caraveo–Anduaga, J. (1998). Lifetime prevalence of *DSM-III-R* psychiatric disorders among urban and rural Mexican Americans in California. *Archives of General Psychiatry*, 55, 771–778.

Warach, P., Goldner, E. M., Somers, J. M., & Hsu, L. (2004). Prevalence and incidence studies of mood disorders: A systematic review of the literature. *Canadian Journal of Psychiatry*, 49(2), 124–138.

Weinick, R. M., Jacobs, E. A., Cacari Stone, L., Ortega, A. N., & Burstin, H. (2004). Hispanic healthcare disparities: Challenging the myth of a monolithic Hispanic population. *Medical Care*, 42, 313–320.

Weissman, M. M., Bland, R. C., Canino, G. J., Faravelli, C., Greenwald, S., Hwu, H.G., et al. (1996). Cross-national epidemiology of major depression and bipolar disorder. *Journal of the American Medical Association*, 276(4), 293–299.

Willgerodt, M. A., & Thompson, E. A. (2006). Ethnic and generational influences on emotional distress and risks behaviors among Chinese and Filipino American adolescents. *Research in Nursing & Health*, 29, 311–324.

Yeh, C. J. (2003). Age, acculturation, cultural adjustment, and mental health symptoms of Chinese, Korean, and Japanese youths. *Cultural Diversity and Ethnic Minority Psychology*, 9(1), 34–48.

3

Culture-Specific Diagnoses and Their Relationship to Mood Disorders

PETER GUARNACCIA & IGDA MARTINEZ PINCAY

It may well be that the dichotomy between "us" and "them" in regard to discussions of culture-bound syndromes has been too quickly drawn; between, that is, the non-Western peoples, the "underdeveloped" peoples, the "primitives" (who have the "exotic" and the "culture-bound" syndromes) and the western world, the "developed world," the "civilized" world.
—Hughes (1985, p. 11)

This chapter examines the relationship between culture-specific diagnoses and mood disorders. How researchers and clinicians refer to cultural syndromes related to mood disorders is a contentious issue. We open our chapter with a brief discussion of the history and controversies (as the quote from Hughes [1985] that opens this chapter indicates) surrounding these labels. We then discuss the relationship between a well-documented range of cultural categories of distress and mood disorders. A key point that we want to make early and often is that there is no one-to-one relationship between these cultural categories and psychiatric disorders as codified in either the American (*DSM-IV* [American Psychiatric Association, 1994]) or international (ICD-10 [World Health Organization, 1992]) diagnostic systems.

The relationship between cultural categories and psychiatric diagnoses needs much more careful investigation. We offer a program of such research based on our previous work (Guarnaccia & Rogler, 1999). Another key issue is that only a few of the many cultural forms of expressing distress have received sustained research attention integrating cultural and psychiatric research methods. We focus our review on those syndromes, particularly *ataques de nervios*, neurasthenia, and *susto*, which have received the most intensive research and have been shown to be associated in some ways with depression and anxiety. We end the chapter with some suggestions for responding to culture-specific diagnoses in clinical settings and for the incorporation of these syndromes into future versions of the diagnostic manuals.

THE MEANING OF CULTURE-SPECIFIC DIAGNOSES

Cross-cultural mental health researchers have introduced a number of terms to refer to and describe culture-specific forms of expressing and diagnosing emotional distress. The problem of multiple labels itself is indicative of the problems associated with the identification of the phenomenon. The label of *culture-bound syndrome* emerged as an alternative to earlier characterizations of cultural expressions of distress in pejorative language. More recent writing has critically examined the appropriateness of the culture-bound syndrome label.

The term *culture-bound syndrome* was introduced by Yap (1969) almost 40 years ago to describe "forms of psychopathology produced by certain systems of implicit values, social structure and obviously shared beliefs indigenous to certain areas" (Yap, 1969, cited in Levine & Gaw, 1995:524). Several authors (Hughes, 1985; Levine & Gaw, 1995; Prince & Tcheng–Laroche, 1987; Simons, 1985) have reviewed the different names, often pejorative, that were used prior to Yap's usage: *exotic psychoses, ethnic psychoses, psychogenic psychoses,* and *hysterical psychoses.* The general preference for Yap's usage is the result of his efforts to avoid biases inherent in the earlier labels, which carried assumptions about the "irrational" behavioral and thought patterns of "exotic" people from non-Western cultures. The use of *culture-bound syndromes* was intended to be less judgmental and more descriptive.

Recent critiques have pointed out that the culture-bound syndrome label, which practically always refers to forms of distress among persons in societies other than the United States or Europe, is not devoid of troublesome assumptions. Trouble stems from the assumption that if the syndromes that are culture bound belong to "them," those that are "culture-free" belong to "us" (Bartholomew, 2000; Hahn, 1995). The dichotomy, of course, is patently false. Culture suffuses all forms of psychological distress, the familiar as well as the unfamiliar (Mezzich, Kleinman, Fabrega, & Parron, 1999b; Rogler, 1997).

The relegation of the culture-bound syndromes to the next-to-last appendix of the *DSM-IV* (American Psychiatric Association, 1994) reinforces the notion that the glossary is in some sense a "museum of exotica" (Mezzich et al., 1999b); there, the syndromes are isolated from other parts of the manual (Lewis–Fernandez & Kleinman, 1995). Many of the descriptions of specific syndromes in the glossary do suggest links between the culture-bound syndrome and *DSM* disorders. The *DSM-IV* defines culture-bound syndrome as follows:

> The term culture-bound syndrome denotes recurrent, locality-specific patterns of aberrant behavior and troubling experience that may or may not be linked to a particular *DSM-IV* diagnostic category. Many of these patterns are indigenously considered to be illnesses, or at least afflictions and most have local names.... culture-bound syndromes are generally limited to specific societies or culture areas and are localized, folk, diagnostic categories that frame coherent meanings for certain repetitive, patterned and troubling sets of experiences and observations. (American Psychiatric Association, 1994, p. 844)

The term *syndrome* fits the experiences designated by culture-bound syndromes. Their listing in the *DSM-IV* glossary makes it clear that each represents a constellation of symptoms and experiences within a cultural group or cultural area. The syndromes have coherence within their respective cultural settings, where they are explained according to local understandings of illness.

The notion of a syndrome being bound by culture is more problematic. The attribution of "boundedness" emerged early in the history of the term in studies that focused on a particular cultural group in a particular community and found a behavior pattern that appeared unique. The behavior pattern had a specific popular label, but the pattern itself did not readily fit the experience of Western observers, whether they were missionaries, anthropologists, or clinicians (Bartholomew, 2000). The observers often believed that the communities in question had somehow been socially isolated and, therefore, saw patterns of distress as unique and locality bound. Considering the massive cultural diffusions that have occurred throughout human history, the concept of boundedness has rarely been tenable.

It would be more accurate to say that many of these syndromes have developed or spread within broad cultural areas and that they are labeled and elaborated in accord with cultural ideas and norms. Although syndromes may originate in particular cultural areas, they have spread widely with migrations and have been incorporated into indigenous concepts of illness, thus qualifying the concept of boundedness. In the contemporary global market of intensified cultural exchanges, exportable syndromes become detached from geographic areas. Their boundedness inheres not in specific locales, but among ethnic groups and in the sociocultural patterns of which they form a part, whether in their countries of origin or in new homes.

The term *folk illness* sometimes is used by anthropologists as an alternative designation that does not carry the conceptual baggage of the term *culture-bound syndrome*. Folk illnesses are meaningful because "their symptomatology expresses a patterned relationship to the society's salient cultural values" (Hughes, Simons, & Wintrob, 1997, p. 998). One drawback to this label is that the descriptor *folk* connotes illness among the common people, or that sector of the population that is "untutored or unrefined" (Morris, 1981). Its usage repeats the early ethnocentrism of labels by referring to potentially devalued social statuses.

Idiom of distress (Nichter, 1981) has gained some popularity in anthropology. The use of the term *idiom* links the study of these categories to linguistic concerns that are central in anthropology. The term *idiom* also does not presuppose pathology. Similarly, the use of *distress* indicates that although the experience may be upsetting to the person and his or her social network, and may reflect suffering on the part of the ill person, the condition may not be viewed as a disorder within the social network and community.

Related concerns are reflected in another term, *popular illness*, which connotes a category of distress recognized in the community but not in professional nosology (Good & Good, 1982; Guarnaccia, 1993). This label recognizes some parallelisms between popular illnesses within the lay sector of the health care system and the biomedical nosology of the professional sector (Kleinman, 1980). *Popular* derives from the Latin words *popularis* (of the people) and *populus* (people). The term's emphasis is the personal experience and understanding of distress from the perspective of the sufferer, which parallels the professional understanding of the problem as disease (Hahn, 1995; Kleinman, 1980). Although the term *popular illness* has the advantage of this important parallelism, it has not entered professional discourse on this topic.

The editors of this book provided the term *culture-specific diagnoses* to highlight the parallel between these syndromes and psychiatric diagnoses. This term emphasizes the importance of studying these syndromes within their cultural context. There continues to be no clear consensus on what label to use. Usage cannot be centrally mandated. Because culture-bound syndrome was adopted for the title of the *DSM-IV* glossary, this term maintains a certain privileged status, although it is a contested privilege. It is contested both because of difficulties inherent in discussions of these experiences and in relating such phenomena to psychiatric diagnostic categories. Throughout this chapter, we will use several of these terms, depending on the context of the discussion.

A REVIEW OF KEY CULTURE-SPECIFIC DIAGNOSES AND THEIR RELATIONSHIP TO MOOD DISORDERS

DSM and ICD categories do not easily subsume most culture-specific diagnoses, although studies of the relationship between culture-specific diagnoses and psychiatric diagnoses show that there are sometimes close associations between the two. There would not be a question of the relationship between culture-specific diagnoses and psychiatric diagnoses had previous attempts to subsume the cultural syndromes into standard psychiatric nomenclature been successful. The conditional statement in the *DSM-IV* that these syndromes "may or may not" be linked to a psychiatric diagnosis, makes clear that the relationship between the cultural syndromes and psychiatric disorders is complex and still needs considerable research. Our position is that *DSM* and ICD categories do not easily subsume most culture-specific diagnoses, although such syndromes are sometimes closely associated with psychiatric diagnoses in what may be termed a *comorbid* relationship.

In this section we review some of the major culture-specific diagnoses for which we have ample research information that addresses the issues of their relationship to mood disorders. All these syndromes are referenced in "Glossary of Culture-Bound Syndromes" in the *DSM-IV* (American Psychiatric Association, 1994, pp. 844–849). We begin each discussion of the cultural syndrome with its definition from the *DSM-IV*. We then briefly review the research literature on the syndrome, identifying its relationship to mood disorders. We include *ataques de nervios* (attacks of nerves), neurasthenia, and *susto* (fright). In addition, we discuss an innovative and important study by Manson and colleagues (1985) that examined the relationship between several Hopi forms of illness and the diagnoses of depression.

Ataque de Nervios (Attack of Nerves)

The *DSM-IV* glossary of culture-bound syndromes includes the following definition of *ataque de nervios* based on the research programs of Guarnaccia

(Guarnaccia, Canino, Rubio-Stipec, & Bravo 1993; Guarnaccia, Rivera, Franco, & Neighbors, 1996; Guarnaccia, Lewis–Fernandez, & Rivera Marano, 2003) and Lewis–Fernandez and colleagues (Lewis–Fernandez, 1994, 1996; Lewis–Fernandez, Guarnaccia, Martinez, Salman, Schmidt, & Liebowitz, 2002), and written by these two researchers.

> An idiom of distress principally reported among Latinos from the Caribbean, but recognized among many Latin American and Latin Mediterranean groups. Commonly reported symptoms include uncontrollable shouting, attacks of crying, trembling, heat in the chest rising into the head, and verbal or physical aggression. Dissociative experiences, seizurelike or fainting episodes, and suicidal gestures are prominent in some attacks but absent in others. A general feature of an *ataque de nervios* is a sense of being out of control. *Ataques de nervios* frequently occur as a direct result of a stressful event relating to the family (e.g., news of a death of a close relative, a separation or divorce from a spouse, conflicts with a spouse or children, or witnessing an accident involving a family member). People may experience amnesia for what occurred during the *ataque de nervios*, but they otherwise return rapidly to their usual level of functioning. Although descriptions of some *ataques de nervios* most closely fit the *DSM-IV* description of panic attacks, the association of most *ataques* with a precipitating event and the frequent absence of the hallmark symptom of acute fear or apprehension distinguish them from panic disorder. *Ataques de nervios* span the range from normal expressions of distress not associated with having a mental disorder to symptom presentations associated with the diagnoses of anxiety, mood, dissociative, or somatoform disorders. (American Psychiatric Association, 1994, p. 845)

The research programs of Guarnaccia, Lewis–Fernandez, and colleagues (Guarnaccia et al., 1996, 2003; Lewis–Fernandez, 1998) have documented the cultural coherence and meanings of *ataques de nervios* as a cultural syndrome among Puerto Ricans and other Caribbean Latinos. Our work has identified loss of control of emotions, behaviors, and a social world out of control as the core experiences of *ataques de nervios*. This loss of control is a result of major dislocations in the family and other close social networks. We have also identified older women from lower socioeconomic status as being particularly likely to express their emotional distress through this idiom (Guarnaccia et al., 1993). Our work suggests a popular nosology based on various categories of *nervios*, several of which require more systematic research, as we have done for *ataques de nervios* (Guarnaccia et al., 2003).

At the same time, our work has clearly shown that people who experience *ataques de nervios* are more vulnerable to developing a psychiatric disorder, particular along the anxiety–depression spectrum (Guarnaccia et al., 1993; Lewis–Fernandez et al., 2002; Liebowitz, Salman, Jusino, Garfinkel, Street, Cardenas, Silvestre, Fyer, Carrasco, Davies, Guarnaccia, & Klein, 1994; Salman, Liebowitz, Guarnaccia, Jusino, Garfinkel, Street, et al., 1998). Although much speculation by psychiatrists focused on *ataques* being a culturally shaped version of a panic attack, Lewis–Fernandez and colleagues (2002) systematically demonstrated that most *ataques* did not meet the criteria for panic attacks and that they were associated with a range of disorders.

The association of *ataques de nervios* with mood disorders was clearly established in the initial adult epidemiology study in Puerto Rico that examined *ataques* in relation to *DSM* disorders (Guarnaccia et al., 1993). In that study of 912 subjects selected to represent the island of Puerto Rico, 20% of those who reported an *ataque* also met criteria for major depressive disorder (using research interview criteria) compared with 2% of those who did not report an *ataque* (odds ratio (OR), 9.84). Similarly, 28% of those who reported an *ataque* met criteria for dysthymic disorder compared with 9% of those who did not report an *ataque* (OR, 3.63). Overall, 30% of those who reported an *ataque de nervios* met research criteria for any of the mood disorders assessed in the study, compared with 6% of those who did not report an *ataque* (OR, 6.18). Of those who met research criteria for any of the anxiety disorders, 40% were in the *ataque* group compared with 14% in the no *ataque* group (OR, 4.02). This epidemiological study revealed that there was a strong association with meeting research criteria for both mood and anxiety disorders among those who reported an *ataque de nervios*.

A subsequent study among Puerto Ricans and Dominicans in the Washington Heights neighborhood of Manhattan at the Hispanic Treatment Program of the New York State Psychiatric Institute provided clearer delineation of the relationship of different *ataque* features to psychiatric disorders (Salman et al., 1998). This study included 156 clinical subjects, of whom 109 reported an *ataque de nervios*. Of this group, 33 met criteria for an affective disorder (primarily major depressive episode; $n = 26$) and 69 met criteria for an anxiety disorder (most frequently, panic disorder; $n = 45$). The identification of *ataque* subtypes in this study aided in establishing its relationship to particular psychiatric disorders. Among those participants in the study whose *ataques de nervios* were characterized by intense fearfulness and feelings of asphyxia and chest tightness, diagnoses of panic disorder were more common. Those whose *ataques* were more dominated by the emotion of anger and aggressive behavior, such as breaking things, were more likely to meet criteria for co-occurring mood disorders. These studies provide an empirical basis for uncovering specific linkages between *ataques de nervios* and psychiatric disorders within the structure of comorbid relationships.

More recent work has examined the comorbidity of *ataques de nervios* with psychiatric disorder in Puerto Rican children (Guarnaccia, Martinez, Ramirez, & Canino, 2005). This research built on a large epidemiological study in Puerto Rico (Canino, Shrout, Rubio–Stipec, Bird, Bravo, Ramirez, et al., 2004) that examined representative samples of children in the community and in the mental health service system. The prevalence of *ataque de nervios* was 9% ($n = 1897$) in the community sample and 26% ($n = 767$) in the clinical sample. As in the adult study, children in Puerto Rico who reported an *ataque de nervios* were more likely to meet research diagnostic criteria for both mood and anxiety disorders. Children in the community who reported an *ataque de nervios* were almost eight times more likely to meet criteria for any mood disorder and five times more likely to meet criteria for any anxiety disorder than children who did not report an *ataque*. Similarly, in the clinical sample, children who reported an *ataque* were six times more likely to meet criteria for any mood disorder and 3.5 times more likely to meet criteria for any anxiety disorder.

The combined findings of these studies support a strong relationship between *ataques de nervios* and both mood and anxiety disorders. These studies also suggest that different characteristics of *ataque* profiles are associated with the different psychiatric diagnoses. The overall research program on *ataques de nervios* provides a model for assessing the relationship between culture-specific diagnoses and psychiatric disorders (Guarnaccia & Rogler, 1999). The findings of strong relationships with both mood and anxiety disorders also lends support for the need for a mixed anxiety–depression diagnosis for multicultural populations.

Neurasthenia

The definition of neurasthenia in China (*shenjing shuairuo* in Chinese) depends heavily on the work of Kleinman (1977, 1982, 1986) on the relationship among neurasthenia, depression, and somatization.

> In China, a condition characterized by physical and mental fatigue, dizziness, headaches, other pains, concentration difficulties, sleep disturbance, and memory loss. Other symptoms include gastrointestinal problems, sexual dysfunction, irritability, excitability, and various signs suggesting disturbance of the autonomic nervous system. In many cases, the symptoms would meet the criteria for a *DSM-IV* mood or anxiety disorder. This diagnosis is included in the *Chinese Classification of Mental Disorders, Second Edition* (CCMD-2). (American Psychiatric Association, 1994, p. 848)

The ICD-10 includes neurasthenia as one of the disorders in the main section of the manual, as opposed to in a glossary of culture-bound syndromes. It is incorporated in the section on neurotic, stress-related, and somatoform disorders under the category "other neurotic disorders (F48)" (http://www.who.int/classifications/apps/icd/icdonline/gf40.htm). Given the long association of neurasthenia with depression, it is somewhat surprising to see it categorized in the ICD-10 with primarily anxiety and somatoform disorders. The ICD-10 contains the following description of neurasthenia (F48.0):

> Considerable cultural variations occur in the presentation of this disorder, and two main types occur, with substantial overlap. In one type, the main feature is a complaint of increased fatigue after mental effort, often associated with some decrease in occupational performance or coping efficiency in daily tasks. The mental fatiguability is typically described as an unpleasant intrusion of distracting associations or recollections, difficulty in concentrating, and generally inefficient thinking. In the other type, the emphasis is on feelings of bodily or physical weakness and exhaustion after only minimal effort, accompanied by a feeling of muscular aches and pains and inability to relax. In both types a variety of other unpleasant physical feelings are common, such as dizziness, tension headaches, and feelings of general instability. Worry about decreasing mental and bodily well-being, irritability, anhedonia, and varying minor degrees of both depression and anxiety are all common. Sleep is often disturbed in its initial and middle phases but

hypersomnia may also be prominent. (http://www.who.int/classifications/apps/icd/
icd10online/gf40.htm, accessed 6/4/2007)

Several studies in China have found a strong comorbidity between neurasthenia and mood disorders, as well as somatization. Kleinman (1986) in his studies
in both mainland China and Taiwan found considerable overlap between the
diagnosis of neurasthenia and depressive disorders. In his study of 100 Chinese
patients diagnosed with neurasthenia, 93 also had a depression diagnosis, with 87
meeting criteria for major depressive disorder. Sixty-nine of the patients were also
diagnosed with an anxiety disorder and 25 with a somatoform disorder. In Taiwan,
22 of 51 patients with neurasthenia also met criteria for a major depressive disorder, which was the most common psychiatric diagnosis in this group of patients.

More recently, Chang and colleagues (2005) report on the relation between
shenjing shuairuo and DSM-IV disorders in a Chinese primary care clinic. The
study included 139 patients, most of rural Chinese origin, who presented with
unexplained somatic complaints. These patients were assessed using the Structured Clinical Interview for Diagnosis (SCID), the Brief Symptom Inventory
(BSI), and the Short Form 36 (SF-36) to assess functional impairment. Of the 49
patients who were diagnosed using the cultural definition of shenjing shuairuo, 26
met criteria for the ICD-10 diagnosis of neurasthenia, with a focus on symptoms of
fatigue or weakness. Of those who met criteria for a DSM-IV diagnosis, all were in
the somatoform disorders spectrum. Twenty-two did not meet criteria for a DSM-
IV diagnosis. This study indicates an evolution of the use of shenjing shuairuo,
neurasthenia, and depression in China so that these categories have become more
differentiated. The study also found that those diagnosed with a primary mood
disorder experienced more impairment than those with shenjing shuairuo. Chang
and colleagues (2005) argue for seeing shenjing shuairuo as a somatocognitive–
affective syndrome that remains culturally salient among laypersons in China and
is not easily captured by either mood or somatoform disorders.

An epidemiological study of neurasthenia by Zheng and colleagues (1997) of
Chinese Americans found similar distinctions between neurasthenia and DSM
disorders. Using ICD-10 criteria for neurasthenia, they identified 112 (6.4%)
subjects with neurasthenia out of a sample of 1747 Chinese Americans residing in Los Angeles. More than half ($n = 63$, 56%) did not meet criteria for a DSM-
III-R diagnosis. Compared with those with depression and anxiety diagnoses, they
reported fewer psychological symptoms on the Symptom Checklist -90-Revised
(SCL-90-R), but similar levels of somatization symptoms. Their conclusion is that
neurasthenia is a distinct clinical condition with only partial comorbidity with
DSM diagnoses.

Neurasthenia, like ataque de nervios discussed earlier, is a complex syndrome
with only partial overlap with DSM psychiatric disorders. Although Kleinman's
(1982, 1986) earlier research identified a strong link between neurasthenia and
depression in China, more recent research in China and among Chinese Americans has identified changing understandings of the syndrome and differing relationships between neurasthenia and psychiatric disorders. Given that many

people who report or meet criteria for neurasthenia do not meet criteria for any *DSM* disorder, neurasthenia is better understood as a distinct category for organizing the experience of distress among people of Chinese origin. If they do also meet criteria for a *DSM* disorder, it is as likely to be a somatoform disorder rather than a mood disorder. These findings further complicate the relationship between culture-specific diagnoses and mood disorders. They also raise questions about the clarity of the boundaries among mood, anxiety, and somatoform disorders.

Susto—Fright or Soul Loss

The following description of *susto* depends heavily on the ethnography of Rubel and colleagues (1984), as well as a study by Taub (1992). More recent work by Weller, Baer, and colleagues (2002, 2005) provides new insights into the relationship of *susto* to mental disorders.

> A folk illness prevalent among some Latinos in the United States and among people in Mexico, Central America, and South America. *Susto* is also referred to as *espanto, pasmo, tripa ida, perdida del alma,* or *chibih. Susto* is an illness attributed to a frightening event that causes the soul to leave the body and results in unhappiness and sickness. Individuals with *susto* also experience significant strains in key social roles. Symptoms may appear any time from days to years after the fright is experienced. It is believed that in extreme cases, *susto* may result in death. Typical symptoms include appetite disturbances, inadequate or excessive sleep, troubled sleep or dreams, feeling sadness, lack of motivation to do anything, and feelings of low self-worth or dirtiness. Somatic symptoms accompanying *susto* include muscle aches and pains, headache, stomachache, and diarrhea. Ritual healings are focused on calling the soul back to the body and cleansing the person to restore bodily and spiritual balance. Different experiences of *susto* may be related to major depressive disorder, posttraumatic stress disorder, and somatoform disorders. Similar etiological beliefs and symptom configurations are found in many parts of the world. (American Psychiatric Association, 1994, pp. 848–849)

Rubel and colleagues (1984) carried out a comprehensive study of *susto*, a Latin American folk illness associated with fright that has a long history of research. The researchers specifically rejected at the outset any hypotheses about the correlation between *susto* and biomedical categories, choosing to focus on understanding the local context and meaning of the illness before attempting to identify relationships with biomedically defined disorders (Rubel et al., 1984, p. 7). Based on their own previous work on *susto*, they hypothesized that the major cause of *susto* would be social stressors, particularly those resulting from an inability to carry out social roles. The authors used multiple methods to study those identified as suffering *susto*, including detailed ethnographic interviews with sufferers about their experience with and understanding of the illness, medical histories and examinations, psychiatric assessment using a symptom scale called the 22-Item Screening Score for Measuring Psychiatric Impairment, and a measure of social stress.

Their major findings were that people suffering *susto* experienced more feelings of inadequacy in social role performance, that they suffered more diseases and had higher rates of fatality from those diseases, and that they were no different from control subjects on the measure of psychiatric impairment. *Susto* was not associated, however, with any specific disease; *susto* sufferers appeared to be susceptible to a range of disorders and experienced a range of symptoms. They concluded: "Now it is inadequate and inappropriate to conceive of *susto* as a form of unique social behavior on the one hand, or as a purely biomedical phenomena on the other" (Rubel et al., 1984, p. 122). Their study indicates the importance of studying folk illnesses on their own terms, and of investigating them from a range of perspectives using both in-depth interviews and clinical methods.

More recent work on *susto* (Taub, 1992) has delineated different dimensions of the *susto* experience and its relationship to different psychiatric disorders. Using anthropological and epidemiological methods to study *chibih* (the Zapotec term for *susto* in Oaxaca), Taub investigated the relationship between *susto* and Western-defined psychology. She recruited a sample of 40 women and carried out in-depth anthropological interviews and psychiatric assessments (Diagnostic Interview Schedule [DIS], Center for Epidemiological Studies–Depression Scale[CES-D]). Ten of the women had current *chibih* and 18 reported *chibih* in the past. Women with current or past *chibih* were much more likely to meet the DIS depression criteria (72% of those with lifetime *chibih* vs. 24% of those without) and were more likely to have CES-D scores in the range of likely casesness (CES-D score, >16 points).

Taub (1992) also identified three types of *chibih* that had different relationships with psychiatric diagnoses. An interpersonal *susto* characterized by feelings of loss, abandonment, and not being loved by family, with accompanying symptoms of sadness, poor self image, and suicidal ideation, seemed to be closely related to major depression. When the *susto* resulted from a traumatic event that played a major role in shaping symptoms and in emotional processing of the experience, the diagnosis of posttraumatic stress disorder (PTSD) was more appropriate. *Susto* that was characterized by several somatic symptoms that recurred and were chronic, and for which the person sought health care from several practitioners, resembled one of the somatoform disorders.

Weller and colleagues (2002) have conducted systematic studies of *susto* in different Latino communities in the United States, Mexico, and Guatemala as part of a larger study of folk and biomedical illnesses. Their first work involved a comprehensive description of *susto* based on studies with Mexican Americans in Texas, Mexicans in Guadalajara, Mexico, and *mestizos* in Guatemala. Although they note some regional variations in *susto*, some of the core experiences include that the illness is caused by a fright, but not necessarily soul loss, and that core symptoms include agitation, crying, nervousness, trembling, fear of unfamiliar places, and sleep disturbances. *Susto* was also seen as a serious illness that could cause diabetes and lead to death.

In a subsequent study, Weller and colleagues (2005) examined the relationships among *susto*, *nervios*, and depression symptoms in an urban clinic in Mexico. They surveyed 200 adults in a public primary care clinic. Sixty-nine percent reported having experienced *susto* and 65%, *nervios*. Using the Zung depression scale (ranging from 20–80 points, with a higher score meaning more depressed) to measure depression, they found that those who reported *susto* and *nervios* had higher rates of depressive symptoms than those who did not report these folk illnesses (42 points vs. 38 points, $p < .04$ for *susto*; 44 points vs. 34 points, $p < .0001$ for *nervios*). Those who reported both *susto* and *nervios* had higher depression scores. *Nervios* sufferers were more likely to be depressed than *susto* sufferers.

As with the previous syndromes we have discussed, *susto* has a complex relationship with psychiatric disorders as well as with medical conditions. *Susto* clearly indicates someone who is more vulnerable to distress and who has experienced more difficult life problems. Those with *susto* are more likely to suffer from psychological problems of varying types. Knowing the context of the fright and the social characteristics of the person may provide clues regarding whether the person is more likely to experience a mood, anxiety, or somatoform disorder.

Hopi Illnesses Related to Mood Disorders

Manson and colleagues (1985) developed the American Indian Depression Schedule (AIDS) specifically to assess concurrently Hopi illness categories and psychiatric diagnoses of depression, somatization, and alcohol-related behavior. The researchers first elicited Hopi illness categories that affected people's minds or spirits from a sample of 36 subjects selected to represent gender, age, and geographic diversity within the Hopi reservation. They then identified the affective, cognitive, and behavioral experiences associated with these syndromes using standard question frames designed to elicit key information systematically about these illnesses. Using this information and modified versions of the relevant sections of the Diagnostic Interview Schedule, they constructed the American Indian Depression Schedule that was then used in an epidemiological study of matched clinical ($n = 22$) and community samples ($n = 32$) of Hopis.

Manson and colleagues (1985) were able to examine the relationship among the Hopi illness categories and psychiatric disorders. One of the most important findings of this study was that although the key depression symptom of prolonged sadness correlated with one of the Hopi illnesses, other Hopi illnesses shared the somatic and psychosocial experiences of depression without this mood symptom criterion. Although there was overlap among the Hopi illnesses and several of the symptoms of depression, there was no one-to-one mapping between any of the Hopi illnesses and depression as a disorder. In addition, the prevalence of the Hopi illness categories indicated the importance of assessing these categories in addition to the most frequent mood disorders to gain a fuller understanding of the mental health of the Hopi. This study clearly demonstrated the importance of including culture-specific diagnoses in cross-cultural psychiatric research to improve the validity of such studies.

Summary

Without a more systematic and wide-ranging program of research on a broader range of culture-specific diagnoses, current approaches that only focus on classificatory exercises with culture-specific diagnoses do not, from our viewpoint, further our understanding of these syndromes. The strategy of trying to find the right classificatory scheme by basing it on similarity between one or two symptoms of the culture-specific diagnosis and of the psychiatric disorder is limited. It is particularly problematic when researchers privilege the *DSM* categories as the main organizing structure of relevance to culture-specific diagnoses. This approach is not likely to produce new insights into these syndromes on their own terms or in relation to psychiatric diagnosis. To resolve the cognitive dissonance created by the complex relationship between the culture-specific diagnoses and psychiatric disorders, cross-cultural mental health researchers need to carry out intensive research that illuminates these syndromes, rather than simply attempting to subsume them into psychiatric categories and obliterating them (Guarnaccia & Rogler, 1999; Hughes, 1985; Kleinman, 1978).

This section has provided some insights into the potential for understanding the relationship between culture-specific diagnoses and mood disorders, as well as other mental health problems. We examined research that focuses in depth on the relationship between a small number of cultural syndromes and mood disorders; however, there is still considerable work to do. The next section proposes a framework for research (Guarnaccia & Rogler, 1999) that would bring the study of culture-specific diagnoses into the mainstream of mental health research.

RESEARCH PROGRAM ON THE RELATIONSHIP BETWEEN CULTURE-SPECIFIC DIAGNOSES AND MOOD DISORDERS

> Whether or not there are "new" psychiatric illnesses to be found in folk cultures or nonmetropolitan populations is a question that first requires semantic resolution. Undoubtedly there are in certain cultures clinical manifestations quite unlike those described in standard psychiatric textbooks, which historically are based on the experiences of Western psychiatrists. In this sense, illnesses presenting so strangely may be regarded as "new." However, each of the same textbooks also espouses a system of disease classification that by its own logic is meant to be final and exhaustive. From this point of view, no more new illnesses are to be discovered, and any strange clinical condition can only be a variation of something already recognized and described. Two problems then arise: Firstly, how much do we know about the culture-bound syndromes for us to be able to fit them into standard classification; and secondly, whether such a standard and exhaustive classification in fact exists. (Yap, 1974, p. 86)

Yap (1969, 1974) challenged the field to learn more about the culture-bound syndromes so that their relationship to psychiatric disorders could be resolved, yet there is still far to go. This next section proposes a research program on culture-specific diagnoses that is faithful to the holistic nature of these syndromes, while at the same time applying the most current research approaches from a number of fields. This research effort comprises a series of key questions that need to be answered for understanding culture-specific diagnoses on their own terms and in relationship to psychiatric disorders. The questions are organized into the following four broad dimensions:

1. Nature of the phenomenon
2. Location in the social context
3. Relationship to psychiatric disorder
4. Social/psychiatric history of the syndrome

We provide a general approach to addressing each of these areas (these questions were originally proposed and discussed in Guarnaccia and Rogler [1999]). At the end of this review we propose a new fifth question on outcomes.

First Question: Nature of the Phenomenon

How do we characterize the syndrome within its cultural context? What are the defining features of the phenomenon? One way to begin studying a culture-specific diagnosis is to refer to the research literature in anthropology and psychiatry. The DSM-IV glossary of culture-bound syndromes has descriptions of 25 syndromes that cultural experts identified as particularly relevant to psychiatry. When a society's illness categories are not known by the researcher, a common elicitation technique is to do open-ended interviewing with key informants to identify the ways things can go wrong with people's minds, emotions, or spirits (this was the approach used by Manson and colleagues [1985]).

The salience of a culture-bound syndrome, the quickness and extent of its recognition within a cultural group, is more difficult to establish. Appearance in the literature provides some evidence of a category's salience, but this is not a foolproof standard. Clinical and epidemiological studies can provide a basis for documenting the salience of culture-bound syndromes. For example, the salience of *ataque de nervios* to Puerto Rican mental health was actively debated until a question on *ataques* was incorporated into an epidemiological study of adult mental health in Puerto Rico (Guarnaccia et al., 1993). In that community study in Puerto Rico, 145 of the 912 (16%) people interviewed reported having had at least one *ataque de nervios*. The large proportion of respondents who recognized the syndrome during the interview and who admitted to the experience in their lifetime attested to the salience of *ataques de nervios* to Puerto Ricans' mental health.

After the salience is documented, the subjective experiences associated with the syndrome—that is, the syndrome's phenomenology—needs examination. Investigations should focus on what it feels like to experience the syndrome: the physical sensations, emotions, and thoughts of the person while experiencing the syndrome. The questions in Kleinman's explanatory model (Kleinman, 1980, p. 106) can be very useful in developing prototypical descriptions of the syndrome, including information about the range in variation of that experience. They are intended to provide a starting point for assessment.

A fuller phenomenological portrait can be developed most effectively with representative samples of individuals who have experienced a culture-bound syndrome. Developing a complete picture of the syndromal experience is important, because a key feature in defining culture-specific diagnoses is eliciting the full symptom profile of the experience, not just a few predominant symptoms. A careful symptomatic description of the experience serves to distinguish it from other syndromes. Interviews about the phenomenology of the syndrome should allow for the systematic elicitation of symptoms using both open-ended questions and symptom checklists.

Second Question: Location in the Social Context

Who are the people who report this syndrome and what is their location in the social structure? What are the situational factors that provoke these syndromes? Fully characterizing the culture-specific diagnosis involves identifying the social characteristics and social position of people who suffer from the syndrome. Social structural factors determine who is most at risk for experiencing illness and disorder. Contextual factors influence when the syndrome is likely to occur and the social situations that provoke them. For example, *susto* is a syndrome that is defined by being provoked by a frightening experience. In many cases, the social context is central to diagnosing the syndrome.

Third Question: Relationship to Psychiatric Disorder

How is the cultural syndrome empirically related to psychiatric disorder? With the kinds of knowledge already identified in previous questions about a culture-specific diagnosis, researchers can then address the relationship between the syndrome and the psychiatric disorder. We call this *the comorbidity question* on the assumption that studying the syndrome's patterned relationship to psychiatric diagnoses is a more fruitful approach than attempting prematurely to subsume it into the official diagnostic categories. Systematic research, such as that described in the previous section, has identified strong correlations between culture-specific diagnoses and criteria for psychiatric disorder, but there is rarely a one-to-one relationship. Hughes and colleagues (1997) state this point eloquently:

> The phenomena of the culture-bound syndromes do not constitute discrete, bounded entities that can be directly translated into conventional Western categories. Rather, when examined at a primary level, they interpenetrate established diagnostic entities with symptoms that flood across numerous parts of the *DSM* nosological structure. (pp. 996–997)

Culture-specific diagnoses are often comorbid with a range of psychiatric disorders, as most psychiatric disorders are with each other (Kessler, McGonagle, Zhao, et al., 1994). Answers to the comorbidity question bring research on culture-specific diagnoses into the mainstream of psychiatric research.

Differences in the symptomatic, emotional, and contextual aspects of cultural syndromes, in turn, may signal different comorbid relationships, or lack of relationships, with psychiatric diagnoses. For mood disorders, one is clearly looking to see whether sadness is a key dimension of the cultural syndrome. However, as previously indicated in the review of syndromes, the cultural syndromes are more likely to share somatic symptoms with mood disorders than the primary symptom of sadness. At the same time, loss events, which have been shown to be key correlates of depression (Brown & Harris, 1978), are prominent experiences that provoke several of the syndromes that we reviewed. Thus, it is critical to understand how the syndrome fits within the life course of the person to identify fully the link with mood disorders.

Fourth Question: Social/Psychiatric History of the Syndrome

When the syndrome and psychiatric disorders are comorbid, what is the sequence of onset? How does the life history of the sufferer, particularly the experience of traumatic events, affect the sequence? The fourth question elaborates concerns raised in the third question, but emphasizes integrating the history of cultural syndromes with the history of psychiatric disorder. These experiences do not exist outside the life course of the person, and understanding them in that context provides additional insights into the relationship among the syndromes and disorders that cannot be understood in isolation. Knowing whether there has been a recent death of a loved one or a loss of a key social relationship, or whether the person is close by or in the country of origin (in the case of immigrants), is a key aspect of making an appropriate cultural and psychiatric diagnosis. To help interpret the current episode as normative distress or the sign of current or developing disorder, it would help to know whether there have been several episodes of the cultural syndrome or of other psychiatric problems in the person's life history.

The need for this type of integrative program has been recognized for 30 years, but has yet to be fully realized. As Kleinman (1978) pointed out in an early editorial,

> [n]ot only do cross-cultural psychiatry and psychology need to regularly assess and assimilate relevant anthropological approaches, but anthropology needs to do the same for developments in psychiatry and psychology. . . . the great gap in concepts, methods, style of doing research, orientation to practical therapeutic concerns, and findings that separates these three disciplines will not narrow significantly until each discipline becomes at least as interested in assembling an integrated picture of a complex, plural reality as it is in further isolating a much simpler account of a single dimension. (p. 208)

After this more phenomenological and epidemiological program has provided detailed understanding of the cultural syndrome, a key issue becomes how to intervene to aid the person in distress. Effective alleviation of suffering is both a key research and clinical concern. Important questions revolve around what treatments are offered. One question is, if the culture-specific diagnosis is effectively treated, does the person also experience relief of the mood disorder? Given the effectiveness of both psychotherapeutic and pharmacological treatments for mood disorders, if the mood disorder is resolved, does the culture-specific diagnosis resolve as well? Given the different conceptualizations of these types of disorders, with depression being seen as more psychobiological in psychiatry and cultural syndromes as more social–contextual in anthropology, one would not necessarily expect such neat resolution of the problem if only some dimensions are addressed. A research program focused on treatment and outcomes for culture-specific and psychiatric diagnoses would begin to address these questions, as well as relieve human suffering.

TOOLS FOR WORKING WITH CULTURE-SPECIFIC DIAGNOSES IN CLINICAL SETTINGS

Medical anthropology and cultural psychiatry have developed tools and per-spectives that are useful in assessing culture-specific diagnoses in clinical work and in negotiating between culture-specific diagnoses and psychiatric diagnoses. One such model includes the explanatory model questions developed by Klein-man (1980). Another more recent model is the *DSM-IV* Outline for Cultural Formulation, which was developed for and included in *DSM-IV* by the National Institute of Mental Health (NIMH) Culture and Diagnosis Work Group (Mez-zich et al., 1999b) and elaborated on by the Group for the Advancement of Psychiatry (GAP) Committee on Cultural Psychiatry (Group for the Advance-ment of Psychiatry, 2002). These frameworks are designed to help clinicians inquire about and better understand the cultural dimensions of their patients' presentations of their mental health problems.

The explanatory model questions were proposed by Kleinman (1980, p. 106) as a tool to aid clinicians in interviewing their patients about the cultural un-derstandings of their illnesses. This deceptively simple set of eight questions provides a framework for a brief clinical interview that can identify the presence and meaning of a culture-specific diagnosis. In particular, the first five questions are useful in this regard and include the following: What do you call your prob-lem? What do you think has caused your problem? Why do you think it started when it did? What does your sickness do to you? How severe is the sickness? These queries could easily fit into an intake or initial interview when a patient is first seen by a provider, and can help guide the clinician in determining the best assessment techniques and course of treatment for the patient.

For a particularly accessible and informative example of the use of these questions to elucidate a culture-specific diagnosis, we refer the reader to Anne Fadiman's *The Spirit Catches You and You Fall Down* (1997, p. 260–261). This book concerns a young Hmong girl with *quag da peg*, which are the Hmong words for the title of the book, and which is sometimes equivalent to the medical diagnosis of epilepsy. After detailing the miscommunications, misunderstand-ings, and conflicts between the family and their medical providers, Fadiman uses the explanatory model questions to highlight her understanding of spirit pos-session and soul loss for the Hmong family she has come to know. She realizes that had the doctors been able to ask these questions and understand the answers with the use of a skilled interpreter, they would have had a much better under-standing of the family's perspective on their daughter's illness. More research-oriented examples related to depression can be found in Kleinman's *Social Or-igins of Distress and Disease* (1986) and *The Illness Narratives* (1988).

A more specific set of questions concerning the relationship between culture-specific diagnoses and psychiatric diagnoses grew out of the work of the NIMH

Culture and Diagnosis Group (Mezzich et al., 1999b). This group provided wide-ranging cultural input to the development of *DSM-IV*. Two particular features of this input appear in Appendix I, "Outline for Cultural Formulation and Glossary of Culture-Bound Syndromes" (American Psychiatric Association, 1994, pp. 843–849). The "Outline for Cultural Formulation" was included in abbreviated form in the *DSM-IV* with no examples, and its juxtaposition to "Glossary of Culture-Bound Syndromes" led to the misleading impression that the formulation was only for those presenting with cultural syndromes (Lewis–Fernandez & Kleinman, 1995; Mezzich, Kirmayer, Kleinman, Fabrega, Parron, Good, et al., 1999a). For the purposes of this chapter, this linking is useful to clinicians, because our point is that clinicians need guidance on how to inquire about and understand culture-specific presentations of mental illness. However, we concur with those cited earlier that the cultural formulation is relevant to all clinical encounters.

The key area of the cultural formulation in this regard is the section on cultural explanations of the individual's illness (American Psychiatric Association, 1994, pp. 843–844). The major elements of inquiry include the predominant idioms of distress through which symptoms are communicated, the meaning and perceived severity of the individual's symptoms in relation to the norms of the cultural reference group, local illness categories used by the individual's family and community to identify the condition, the perceived causes or explanatory models that the individual and reference group use to explain the illness, and past and current experiences with popular and professional sources of care. Again, these areas can serve as a support for clinicians who seek to understand better their patients' perspectives on the symptoms, expressions, and difficulties they present.

There are several resources to which clinicians can turn for further guidance and examples using this formulation technique. The cultural formulation has been elaborated by the GAP Committee on Cultural Psychiatry in their publication *Cultural Assessment in Clinical Psychiatry* (Group for the Advancement of Psychiatry, 2002). Illustrative cases using the cultural formulation and discussing the implications of cultural understanding of mental health problems have been available in select issues of *Culture, Medicine and Psychiatry* starting in the mid 1990s (for example, see Lewis–Fernandez, 1996). Although there is no magic to these questions or to the process of eliciting answers to them from patients who have different cultural understandings of their illness from their provider, they provide a framework to aid the clinician in getting started.

After the information is elicited, the next key step is for the clinician to lead a negotiation process whereby the clinician and patient come to understand each others' perspectives on the mental health problem and come to agreement on how to proceed. Kleinman describes this approach in *The Illness Narratives* (1988, pp. 227–251). The process that Kleinman develops is first for the provider to elicit and understand the patient's explanatory model, and then to make clear the provider's explanatory model. The process then focuses on developing a treatment plan based on negotiation between the patient and provider models. This approach has been further elaborated in a variety of models developed for cultural competence training for physicians to aid them in this negotiation process (Like, 2005). The effects on quality of depression care from these approaches to assessing cultural understandings of culture-specific diagnoses and psychiatrist–patient negotiation are pressing areas for research.

TOWARD *DSM-V:* SOME MODEST PROPOSALS CONCERNING THE RELATIONSHIP OF CULTURE-SPECIFIC DIAGNOSES AND MOOD DISORDERS

We conclude this chapter with some suggestions for incorporating issues raised by our review of culture-specific diagnoses for inclusion in the mood disorders section of *DSM-V.* Our first recommendation is that the *DSM-V* should incorporate a mixed anxiety–depression diagnosis. This diagnosis already exists in ICD-10, code F41.2 (World Health Organization, 1999; see also http://www.who .int/classification/apps/icd/icd10online/gf40.htm): "This category should be used when symptoms of anxiety and depression are both present, but neither is clearly predominant, and neither type of symptom is present to the extent that justifies a diagnosis if considered separately." Further criteria include that the symptoms taken together should result in disability. The patient may first report physical symptoms, such as fatigue or pain, but (with further diagnostic assessment) depressed mood and anxiety are often present. This description fits with the presentation of cultural syndromes presented in the previous section of this chapter.

 DSM-IV includes a mixed anxiety–depression diagnosis in "Appendix B: Criteria Sets and Axes Provided for Further Study." The inclusion of this category grew out of the recommendations of the *DSM-IV* field trial (Zinbarg, Barlow, Liebowitz, Street, Broadhead, Katon, Roy–Byrne, Lepine, Teherani, Richards, Brantley, & Kraemer, 1994). The description of the disorder from the *DSM-IV* (American Psychiatric Association, 1994, p. 723) parallels the ICD-10 description, with some important differences. The *DSM-IV* description emphasizes the presence of depressed mood for at least a month, whereas the ICD-10 recognizes the presence of both depression and anxiety, and notes that the primary presentation may be somatic. The *DSM-IV* description is as follows:

> The essential feature [of mixed anxiety–depression disorder] is a persistent or recurrent dysphoric mood for at least one month. The dysphoric mood is accompanied by additional symptoms that also must persist for at least one month and include at least four of the following: concentration or memory difficulties, sleep disturbance, fatigue or low energy, irritability, worry, being easily moved to tears, hypervigilance, anticipating the worst, hopelessness or pessimism about the future, and low self-esteem or feelings of worthlessness. The symptoms must cause clinically significant distress or impairment in social, occupational, or other important areas of functioning. (American Psychiatric Association, 1994, p. 723)

The overview also notes that the disorder is particularly common in primary care settings, which is the basis of this description, and that the disorder is also common in outpatient community mental health settings (Barlow & Campbell,

2000; Kreuger, Markon, Chentsova–Dutton, Goldberg, & Ormel, 2003). Support for inclusion of this diagnosis comes from both the prevalence of mixed anxiety–depression symptoms associated with culture-specific diagnoses and the prevalence of these presentations in primary health and mental health care settings where most people seek mental health care, particularly multicultural patients. The requirement for the presence of one month of dysphoric mood as the essential symptom seems unwarranted given the mixed nature of the diagnosis and that many primary-care patients, particularly those who are recent immigrants, present distress through primarily somatic idioms recognized in the description of the disorder.

A second recommendation is to refine and expand the discussion of the outline for cultural formulation. The outline should be moved to the introductory section of the DSM-V, where it can be discussed in relation to the multiaxial system of diagnosis. This was always the intent of the NIMH Culture and Diagnosis Group—that the cultural formulation be seen as an adjunct to a complete multiaxial diagnosis. The discussion of the cultural formulation should be expanded using materials from the GAP publication on cultural assessment (Group for the Advancement of Psychiatry, 2002). A series of case examples of cultural formulations should be included as part of the supplementary materials developed to enhance the use of DSM-V. These could be drawn from the GAP publication, from the case series in *Culture, Medicine and Psychiatry*, and from other sources.

The glossary of culture-bound syndromes needs to be updated in two ways for DSM-V. Syndromes that are already present in the DSM-IV glossary need updating with more recent research, such as that presented in this chapter. In addition, more intensive research on a broader range of culture-specific diagnoses needs to be commissioned as part of the DSM-V field trials and other research endeavors. We have provided a framework for such a research effort. For example, *ataques de nervios* and neurasthenia were included in the recent NIMH-funded national Latino and Asian American mental health study (Alegria, Takeuchi, Canino, Duan, Shrout, Meng, et al., 2004a; Alegria, Vila, Woo, Canino, Takeuchi, Vera, et al., 2004b). Although it may still be appropriate to include these syndromes in an appendix to DSM-V, there should be a greater effort to link the syndromes to specific disorder chapters, such as those we have provided to mood disorders. As the research on other culture-specific diagnoses develops that allows for fuller characterization of those diagnoses as well as an assessment of their relationship to psychiatric diagnoses, this information should be incorporated into DSM-V and other official psychiatric diagnostic systems.

Given the growing cultural diversity of the United States in general, and the increasing attention to cultural competence in mental health care, one facet of improving care for multicultural populations is improving our understanding of the culture-specific diagnoses on their own, and in relationship to psychiatric diagnoses. Given the prevalence of depression and other mood disorders in clinical settings and community surveys, and the significant disability attributable to depressive disorders, better understanding of the relationship between culture-specific diagnoses and mood disorders is a research, clinical, and public health imperative.

REFERENCES

American Psychiatric Association. (1994). *Diagnostic and statistical manual of mental disorders* (4th ed.). Washington, DC: American Psychiatric Association.

Alegria, M., Takeuchi, D., Canino, G., Duan, N., Shrout, P., Meng, X. -L., et al. (2004a). Considering context, place and culture: The National Latino and Asian American Study. *International Journal of Methods in Psychiatric Research*, 13, 208–220.

Alegria, M., Vila, D., Woo, M., Canino, G., Takeuchi, D., Vera, M., et al. (2004b). Cultural relevance and equivalence in the NLAAS instrument: Integrating etic and emic in the cross-cultural measures for a psychiatric epidemiology and services study. *International Journal of Methods in Psychiatric Research*, 13, 270–288.

Barlow, D. H., & Campbell, L. A. (2000). Mixed anxiety–depression and its implications for models of mood and anxiety disorders. *Comprehensive Psychiatry, 41*(Suppl. 1), 55–60.

Bartholomew, R. E. (2000). *Exotic deviance: Medicalizing cultural idioms—From strangeness to illness.* Boulder, CO: University Press of Colorado.

Brown, G. W., & Harris, T. (1978). *Social origins of depression.* New York: Free Press.

Canino, G., Shrout, P. E., Rubio–Stipec, M., Bird, H. R., Bravo, M., Ramirez, R., et al. (2004). The *DSM-IV* rates of child and adolescent disorders in Puerto Rico: Prevalence, correlates, service use, and the effects of impairment. *Archives of General Psychiatry, 61,* 85–93.

Chang, D. F., Myers, H. F., Yeung, A., Zhang, Y., Zhao, J., & Yu, S. (2005). *Shenjing shuairuo* and the *DSM-IV*: Diagnosis, distress, and disability in a Chinese primary care setting. *Transcultural Psychiatry, 42,* 204–218.

Fadiman, A. (1997). *The spirit catches you and you fall down.* New York: Farrar, Strauss, Giroux.

Good, B., & Good, M. J. D. (1982). Toward a meaning-centered analysis of popular illness categories: "Fright illness" and "heart distress" in Iran. In A. J. Marsella & G. M. White (Eds.), *Cultural conceptions of mental health and therapy.* (141–166). Dordrecht, Holland: D. Reidel.

Group for the Advancement of Psychiatry. (2002). *Cultural assessment in clinical psychiatry.* Washington, DC: Group for the Advancement of Psychiatry.

Guarnaccia, P. J. (1993). Ataques de nervios in Puerto Rico: Culture bound syndrome or popular illness? *Medical Anthropology, 15,* 157–170.

Guarnaccia, P. J., Canino, G., Rubio–Stipec, M., & Bravo, M. (1993). The prevalence of ataques de nervios in the Puerto Rico Disaster Study: The role of culture in psychiatric epidemiology. *The Journal of Nervous and Mental Disease, 181,* 157–165.

Guarnaccia, P. J., Lewis–Fernandez, R., & Rivera Marano, M. (2003). Toward a Puerto Rican popular nosology: *Nervios* and *ataque de nervios. Culture, Medicine and Psychiatry, 27,* 339–366.

Guarnaccia, P. J., Martinez, I., Ramirez, R., & Canino, G. (2005). Are *ataques de nervios* in Puerto Rican children associated with psychiatric disorder? *Journal of the American Academy of Child and Adolescent Psychiatry, 44,* 1184–1192.

Guarnaccia, P. J., Rivera, M., Franco, F., & Neighbors, C. (1996). The experiences of ataques de nervios: Towards an anthropology of emotion in Puerto Rico. *Culture, Medicine and Psychiatry, 20,* 343–367.

Guarnaccia, P. J., & Rogler, L. H. (1999). Research on culture-bound syndromes: New directions. *American Journal of Psychiatry, 156,* 1322–1327.

Hahn, R. A. (1995). *Sickness and healing: An anthropological perspective*. New Haven, CT: Yale University Press.

Hughes, C. C. (1985). Culture-bound or construct-bound? The syndromes and *DSM-III*. In: R. C. Simons & C. C. Hughes (Eds.), *The culture-bound syndromes: Folk illnesses of psychiatric and anthropological interest* (pp. 3–24) Dordrecht, Holland: Reidel.

Hughes, C. C., Simons, R. C., & Wintrob, R. M. (1997). The "culture-bound syndromes" and *DSM-IV*. In T. Widiger, A. Frances, H. A. Pincus, M. B. First, R. Ross, & W. Davis (Eds.), *DSM-IV source book* (Vol. 3, pp. 991–1000). Washington, DC: American Psychiatric Press.

Kessler, R. C., McGonagle, K. A., Zhao, S., et al. (1994). Lifetime and 12-month prevalence of *DSM-III-R* psychiatric disorders in the United States: Results from the National Comorbidity Study. *Archives of General Psychiatry, 51*, 8–19.

Kleinman, A. M. (1977). Depression, somatization and the "new cross-cultural psychiatry." *Social Science and Medicine, 11*, 3–10.

Kleinman, A. M. (1978). Three faces of culture-bound syndromes: Their implications for cross-cultural research. *Culture, Medicine and Psychiatry, 2*, 207–208.

Kleinman, A. (1980). *Patients and healers in the context of culture*. Berkeley, CA: University of California Press.

Kleinman, A. (1982). Neurasthenia and depression: A study of somatization and culture in China. *Culture, Medicine and Psychiatry, 6*, 117–190.

Kleinman, A. (1986). *Social origins of distress and disease: Depression, neurasthenia and pain in modern China*. New Haven, CT: Yale University Press.

Kleinman, A. (1988). *The illness narratives: Suffering, healing and the human condition*. New York: Basic Books.

Kreuger, R. F., Markon, K. E., Chentsova–Dutton, Y. E., Goldberg, D., & Ormel, J. (2003). A cross-cultural study of the structure of comorbidity among common psychopathological syndromes in the general health setting. *Journal of Abnormal Psychology, 112*, 437–447.

Levine, R. E., & Gaw, A. C. (1995). Culture-bound syndromes. *The Psychiatric Clinics of North America, 18*, 523–536.

Lewis–Fernandez, R. (1994). Culture and dissociation: A comparison of ataque de nervios among Puerto Ricans and " 'possession syndrome' " in India. In D. Speigel (Ed.), *Dissociation: Culture, mind and body*. Washington, DC: American Psychiatric Press.

Lewis–Fernandez, R. (1996). Diagnosis and treatment of nervios and ataques in a female Puerto Rican migrant. *Culture, Medicine and Psychiatry, 20*, 155–163.

Lewis–Fernandez, R. (1998). "Eso no estaba en mí . . . no pude controlarme": El control, la identidad y las emociones en Puerto Rico. *Revista de Ciencias Sociales, 4*, 268–299.

Lewis–Fernandez, R., Guarnaccia, P. J., Martinez, I. E., Salman, E., Schmidt, A., & Liebowitz, M. (2002). Comparative phenomenology of *ataques de nervios*, panic attacks, and panic disorder. *Culture, Medicine and Psychiatry, 26*, 199–223.

Lewis–Fernandez, R., & Kleinman, A. (1995). Cultural psychiatry: Theoretical, clinical and research issues. *The Psychiatric Clinics of North America, 18*, 433–448.

Liebowitz, M. R., Salman, E., Jusino, C. J., Garfinkel, R., Street, L., Cardenas, D. L., Silvestre, J., Fyer, A., Carrasco, J. L., Davies, S., Guarnaccia, P., & Klein, D. F. (1994). Ataque de nervios and panic disorder. *American Journal of Psychiatry, 151*, 871–875.

Like, R. C. (2005). Culturally competent family medicine: Transforming clinical practice and ourselves. *American Family Physician* [Online], 72. Available: http://www.aafp.org/afp/20051201/editorials.html

Manson, S. M., Shore, J. H., & Bloom, J. D.(1985). The depressive experience in American Indian communities: A challenge for psychiatric theory and diagnosis. In A. Kleinman & B. Good (Eds.), *Culture and depression: Studies in the anthropology and cross-cultural psychiatry of affect and disorder.* (331–368). Berkeley, CA: University of California Press.

Mezzich, J. E., Kirmayer, L. J., Kleinman, A., Fabrega, H., Jr., Parron, D. L., Good, B. J., et al. (1999a). The place of culture in DSM-IV. *The Journal of Nervous and Mental Disease, 187,* 457–464.

Mezzich, J. E., Kleinman, A., Fabrega, H., & Parron, D. L. (1999b). *Culture and psychiatric diagnosis.* Washington, DC: American Psychiatric Press.

Morris, W. (Ed.). (1981). *The American heritage dictionary of the English language.* Boston, MA: Houghton Mifflin.

Nichter, M. (1981). Idioms of distress: Alternatives in the expression of psychological distress. *Culture, Medicine and Psychiatry, 5,* 5–24.

Prince, R., & Tcheng–Laroche, F. (1987). Culture-bound syndromes and international disease classifications. *Culture, Medicine and Psychiatry, 11,* 3–19.

Rogler, L. H. (1997). Making sense of historical changes in the *Diagnostic and Statistical Manual of Mental Disorders:* Five propositions. *Journal of Health and Social Behavior, 38,* 9–20.

Rubel, A., O'Nell, C. W., & Collado–Ardon, R. (1984). *Susto: A folk illness.* Berkeley, CA: University of California Press.

Salman, E., Liebowitz, M. R., Guarnaccia, P. J., Jusino, C. M., Garfinkel, R., Street, L., et al. (1998). Subtypes of ataques de nervios: The influence of coexisting psychiatric diagnoses. *Culture, Medicine and Psychiatry, 22,* 231–244.

Simons, R. C. (1985). Sorting the culture-bound syndromes. In R. C. Simons & C. C. Hughes (Eds.), *The culture-bound syndromes: Folk illnesses of psychiatric and anthropological interest* (pp. 25–38). Dordrecht, Holland: Reidel.

Taub, B. (1992). *Calling the soul back to the heart: Soul loss, depression and healing among indigenous Mexicans* [Online]. UCLA doctoral dissertation. Available: wwwlib.umi.com/dxweb/results, #9310870

Weller, S. C., Baer, R. D., Garcia de Alba Garcia, J., Glazer, M., Trotter, R., Pachter, L., et al. (2002). Regional variations in Latino descriptions of *susto. Culture, Medicine and Psychiatry, 26,* 449–472.

Weller, S. C., Baer, R. D., Garcia de Alba Garcia, J., Salcedo Rocha, A. L. (December 2005). *Folk illness as an indicator for mental health comorbidities.* Paper presented at the annual meeting of the American Anthropological Association, Washington, DC.

World Health Organization. (1992). *The ICD-10 classification of mental and behavior disorders: Clinical descriptions and diagnostic guidelines.* Geneva: World Health Organization. [Online: http://www.who.int/classification/apps/icd/icd10online/gf40.htm]

Yap, P. M. (1969). The culture-bound reactive syndromes. In W. Caudill & T.-Y. Lin (Eds.), *Mental health research in Asia and the Pacific.* (33–53)Honolulu: East-West Center.

Yap, P.M. (1974). *Comparative psychiatry: A theoretical framework.* Toronto: University of Toronto Press.

Zheng, Y. P, Lin, K. M., Takeuchi, D., Kurasaki, K. S., Wang, Y., & Cheung, F. (1997). An epidemiological study of neurasthenia in Chinese-Americans in Los Angeles. *Comprehensive Psychiatry, 38,* 249–259.

Zinbarg, R. E., Barlow, D. H., Liebowitz, M., Street, L., Broadhead, E., Katon, W., Roy–Byrne, P., Lepine, J.- P., Teherani, M., Richards, J., Brantley, P. J., & Kraemer, H. (1994). The DSM-IV field trial for mixed anxiety–depression. *American Journal of Psychiatry, 151,* 1153–1162.

4

The Epidemiology of Mood Disorders Among U.S. Minority Populations

SANA LOUE

This chapter provides an overview of the epidemiology of mood disorders among U.S. minority populations. The literature relating to the incidence and prevalence of these disorders is reviewed, followed by a discussion of the risk and protective factors for these illnesses.

Prior to embarking on any discussion of the epidemiology of mental illness among minority populations, however, it is important to highlight the challenges that are inherent in such an examination. These include, but are not limited to, the validity and reliability of the criteria used to assess the occurrence of a mood disorder and the sampling strategy utilized in conducting the study.

Issues related to the validity and reliability of diagnostic criteria and instruments are discussed in detail elsewhere in this book and are only briefly reviewed here. What we know is, to a large degree, shaped by what we permit ourselves to see. If we do not know or understand, for instance, how symptom presentation and expression vary across cultures or language, we will not know what to look for and, as a consequence, we will underestimate the occurrence of illness. As an example, physicians have been found less likely to detect mental health problems, including depression, among their African American patients compared with their white patients (Borowsky, Rubenstein, Meredith, Camp, Jackson–Triche, & Wells, 2000). Accordingly, epidemiological investigations utilizing existing clinical records may seriously underestimate the incidence and prevalence of mood disorders in some groups.

Conversely, if we disregard what we do see as irrelevant, we are likely to underestimate disease occurrence. For instance, psychological problems are commonly somatized within some ethnic minority groups (Kleinman, 1986). If these symptoms are eliminated from consideration in assessing mental health and

54

illness because they are "physical," we may fail to recognize depression or other disorders.

The large epidemiological studies of mental illness that have included minority populations have reported their findings as they relate to large ethnic/racial groups, such as African Americans or Asians and Pacific Islanders. However, each such large groups comprise numerous smaller groups that are widely diverse in terms of their culture, language, religion, and historical experience. Consequently, the prevalence and incidence rates that are reported for these larger groups may not accurately reflect the experience of the various subgroups comprised within them.

Many studies report prevalence, rather than incidence rates, of mood disorders. Prevalence rates are based on the identification of individuals who possess the disease or illness during a defined period of time, which may vary in length depending upon the goals of the particular study. In contrast, incidence rates are derived from the number of individuals who are experiencing the onset of their illness. A study of incident cases offers many advantages, because it becomes easier to distinguish between those factors that may instigate disease development and initiation, and those that are related to its maintenance and/or progression. However, the ascertainment of incident cases is particularly difficult because of the unreliability of self-reports of symptoms, the significant lapse of time that may occur between the first experience of symptoms and the diagnosis of the illness, and disagreements concerning diagnostic classification of symptoms and criteria for illness diagnosis (American Psychiatric Association, 2000).

INCIDENCE AND PREVALENCE RATES
OF MOOD DISORDERS

General Findings

Data from epidemiological studies throughout the world indicate that the prevalence rate of major depression ranges from 2.6% to 5.5% for men and is between 6.0% and 11.8% for women (Lehtinen & Joukamaa, 1994). The prevalence of depressive symptoms, rather than a diagnosis of major depression is, however, much higher, with rates ranging from 10% to 19% in men and 18% to 34% in women.

The lifetime risk of bipolar disorder has been found to range from 0.6% to 0.9% in industrialized countries. The annual incidence of bipolar disorder ranges from 0.009% to 0.015% among men, which translates to between 9 and 15 new cases per 100,000 per year; and 0.007% to 0.03% among women, or 7 to 30 new cases per 100,000 per year (Goodwin & Redfield Jamison, 1990). Rates differ across specific studies as a result of variations in sampling strategies and location, diagnostic criteria, and assessment methodologies.

Several major psychiatric epidemiological studies have been conducted in the United States. The Epidemiologic Catchment Area (ECA) studies, conducted during the 1980s, sampled residents of Baltimore, St. Louis, Durham–Piedmont, Los Angeles, and New Haven. The sample of 4638 African Americans, 12,944 whites, and 1600 Hispanics included both individuals living in the community at large and residents of institutions (mental hospitals, jails, drug and alcohol treatment facilities, and nursing homes) (Robins & Regier, 1991). Across four of the five sites, the annual incidence of major depression was found to be 1.6% (Eaton et al., 1989). One-year prevalence rates of depression were found to be higher among women compared with men of the same age group, with the prevalence decreasing in both groups as age increased. Rates of depression were found to be highest among those ages 18 to 44 years, with a prevalence of 1.6% among men and 4.8% among women (Weissman, Leaf, Tischler, Blazer, Karno, Bruce, et al., 1988). The ECA found a one-year prevalence rate of bipolar disorder per 100 persons of 0.9% among men and 1.1% among women (Weissman et al., 1988).

The more recent NCS utilized a representative sample consisting of 666 African Americans, 4498 whites, and 713 additional U.S. residents (Kessler, McGonagle, Zhao, Nelson, Hughes, Eshleman, et al., 1994).

Research findings suggest that the prevalence rates for major depression have consistently increased since World War II. The Cross-National Collaborative Group (1992) reported not only higher rates of depression among women in comparison with men, but also increasing rates among young adults. These increases have been variously attributed to increasing urbanization, changes in family structures, exposure to toxic substances, increased life expectancy, the availability of more effective treatments, increased access to diagnostic and treatment services, and variations over time in the definition of major depression (Cross-National Collaborative Group, 1992; Gastpar, 1986). A study of the changes in the prevalence rates of major depression between 1991–1992 and 2001–2002 in large representative samples of the U.S. population found that the prevalence rate among adults increased from 3.33% to 7.06% during this 10-year period (Compton, Conway, Stinson, & Grant, 2006). The increase observed among young African American males was attributable to a concomitant increase in substance use. Patterns in the United States appear to parallel what is occurring on a global level. World Health Organization (WHO) investigators noted a higher prevalence of mental disorders in urban areas compared with rural areas; and low socioeconomic status, frequently seen among minority groups, is known to be associated with mood and psychotic disorders, substance abuse, and personality disorders (WHO International Consortium on Psychiatric Epidemiology, 2000).

African Americans

The ECA study found a prevalence of major depression in the preceding 12-month period of 2.2% among African Americans and 2.8% among whites. The lifetime prevalence of major depression was found to be 3.1% among African Americans and 5.1% among whites (Weissman, Bruce, Leaf, Florio, & Holzer, 1991). The lifetime prevalence of dysthymia was found to be 4.0% among African Americans compared with 6.3% among whites (Robins & Regier, 1991).

Findings from the NCS were similar to those from the ECA. The prevalence of major depression during the preceding 12-month period was 8.2% among African Americans compared with 9.9% among whites, whereas the lifetime prevalence was 11.6% among African Americans and 17.7% among whites. The lifetime prevalence of dysthymia was also found to be lower among African Americans than among whites (5.4% and 6.7%, respectively). Both studies reported higher rates of depression among African American women compared with African American men.

The ECA and other relatively more recent studies reported similar rates of bipolar disorder among African Americans compared with non-Hispanic whites (Blazer, George, Landerman, et al., 1985; Helzer, 1975; Weissman & Myers, 1978). This finding stands in contrast to the conclusions of earlier studies that reported higher annual incidence rates of bipolar disorder among African Americans (Pollock, 1931; Wagner, 1938). These earlier reports may reflect significant diagnostic bias as a result of racial insensitivity and misdiagnosis resulting from the nonrecognition of manic or hypomanic symptoms (Horgan, 1981; Lewis & Hubbard, 1931). As an example, a significant body of literature exists that documents the inappropriate diagnosis of schizophrenia among African Americans with bipolar disorder (Strakowski, Keck, Arnold, Collins, Wilson, Fleck, Corey, Amicone, & Adebimpe, 2003).

Relatively few data are available relating to the mental health of older African Americans. Several studies of African American elders residing in the community suggest that there are few differences in the depressive symptoms between African Americans and whites (Blazer, Landerman, Hays, Simonsick, & Saunders, 1998; Gallo, Cooper–Patrick, & Lesikar, 1998; Husaini, 1997). Elevated symptoms of depression among both African American and white older adults have been found to be associated with physical health problems (Okwumabua, Baker, Wong, & Pilgrim, 1997).

Hispanics/Latinos

Data from large epidemiological studies, including the ECA, suggest that Latinos and European Americans experience similar rates of mental illness (Burnam, Hough, Escobar, Karno, Timers, Telles, et al., 1987; Golding & Karno, 1988; Karno, Hough, Burnam, et al., 1987; Kessler et al., 1994, Robins & Regier, 1991). Data from the ECA indicate that Mexican American individuals born in the United States experience higher rates of depression than those born in Mexico (Burnam et al., 1987). Several other studies also indicate that foreign-born Hispanics/Latinos experience lower rates of depression than those born in the United States. Puerto Ricans from the island have been found to have lower rates of lifetime depression than Puerto Ricans in New York (Canino, Bird, Shrout, Rubio–Stipec, Bravo, Martinez, et al., 1987; Moscicki, Rae, Regier, & Locke, 1987). An investigation of the mental health of Mexicans and Mexican Americans in family practice settings in two towns that were equidistant from the Mexico border reported that 8% of the Mexican Americans had had a lifetime episode of depression, compared with only 4% of those in Mexico (Hoppe, Garza–Elizondo, Leal–Isla, & Leon,, 1991).

The NCS found that the rate of major depression for Hispanics was much greater than for non-Hispanics during a 30-day period (Blazer et al., 1994).

Slightly more than 8% of Hispanics, compared with 4.7% of non-Hispanic whites, experienced major depression during a 30-day period. The lifetime prevalence of major depression was approximately 18% in both groups. It should be noted, however, that the NCS was conducted only in English and, consequently, monolingual Spanish-speaking Hispanics/Latinos were not included.

Among adolescents, Mexican Americans have reported more depressive symptoms (Roberts & Chen, 1995; Roberts & Sobhan, 1992) and appear to experience higher rates of depression (Roberts, Roberts, & Chen, 1997) compared with white adolescents. Similar to the findings related to adults, studies of Hispanic/Latino adolescents indicate that Mexican American youths residing in the United States are at higher risk of experiencing depressive symptoms than their counterparts living in Mexico (Swanson, Linskey, Quintero–Salinas, Pumariega, & Holzer, 1992).

Among Latinos, women have been found to experience more psychological disorders than men and are more likely to be depressed (Frerichs, Aneshensel, & Clark, 1981; Mosicki, Locke, Rae, & Boyd, 1989). Based on ECA data, it appears that the lifetime prevalence of dysthymia is higher among Mexican American women older than 40 years compared with all other groups (Burnam et al., 1987; Karno et al., 1987). Among Latino/Hispanic immigrants, research suggests that adult Latinas are at higher risk of depression than are younger male and female immigrants (Golding & Karno, 1988; Salgado de Snyder, 1987; Vega, Kolody, Valle, & Hough, 1986).

Data from the ECA also indicate that the risk of suicide attempts is higher for Hispanics suffering from major depression than in those with other psychiatric diagnoses. In the Los Angeles ECA study, it was found that the rate of suicidal ideation among Hispanics was less than half that reported by non-Hispanic whites (8.8% and 18.9%, respectively), and the rate of suicide attempts by Hispanics was approximately two thirds that of non-Hispanic whites (Sorenson & Golding, 1988b), a finding that is consistent with other reports (Sorenson & Golding, 1988a). Reports from the ECA data also indicate that (a) compared with Hispanic and non-Hispanic white men, women of both groups reported more suicide attempts; (b) Hispanics with lower educational levels were at lower risk of suicidal ideation and suicide than Hispanics of higher educational level; (c) Hispanic and non-Hispanic whites who were divorced or separated were at increased risk of suicidal ideation and suicide; and (d) the presence of a psychiatric disorder, particularly major depression, resulted in a sevenfold increase in the risk of suicide attempts (Sorenson & Golding, 1988b).

Variation in the prevalence of mood disorders has been noted across Hispanic/Latino subgroups. Compared with Cuban Americans and Mexican Americans, Puerto Ricans have been found to have higher rates of depressive symptoms even after controlling for socioeconomic differences (Moscicki et al., 1989). Among both island and mainland Puerto Ricans, however, the occurrence of depressive disorders has been found to be more than twice as prevalent in women as in men, whereas the prevalence of dysthymia is almost four times higher in women than in men (Canino et al., 1987; Moscicki et al., 1989).

Asians and Pacific Islanders

The national ECA and the ECA in Los Angeles included relatively small samples of Asian and Pacific Islander individuals (242 and 161, respectively). The lifetime prevalence rates for depression, dysthymia, and manic episodes in both the national ECA and Los Angeles ECA samples of Asians were lower than those reported for the general ECA sample (Robins & Regier, 1991; Zhang & Snowden, 1999).

However, the Chinese American Psychiatric Epidemiological Study (CAPES), designed to investigate the prevalence of specified psychiatric disorders as defined by the *DSM-III-R* (American Psychiatric Association, 1987) included more than 1700 Chinese Americans living in Los Angeles county. Investigators found that 3.4% had been depressed during the preceding year, and 6.9% of the respondents reported depression during their lifetimes (Sue, Sue, Sue, & Takeuchi, 1995; Takeuchi, Chung, Lin, Shen, Kurasaki, Chun, et al., 1998). This compares with a 12-month prevalence of 10.0% and a lifetime prevalence of 16.9% in the national NCS sample of adults (Kessler et al., 1994). Slightly less than 1% of the participants in the CAPES reported dysthymia during the preceding 12 months, compared with 2.5% of NCS participants. The lifetime prevalence of dysthymia among CAPES participants was 5.2%, compared with 6.4% among NCS respondents. The lifetime prevalence of manic episodes among CAPES respondents was also much lower (0.1%) than the lifetime prevalence among NCS respondents (1.6%) (Kessler et al., 1994; Takeuchi et al., 1998; Zheng, Lin, Takeuchi, Kurasaki, Wong, & Cheung, 1997).

Native Americans and Alaskan Natives

There is a notable dearth of research relating to the incidence and prevalence of mood disorders among Native Americans and Alaskan natives (U.S. Department of Health and Human Services, 2001). One clinic-based study reported that more than 30% of the older Native Americans receiving services experienced significant depressive symptoms (Manson, 1992). The high rates of suicide among Native Americans and Alaskan natives may reflect high underlying rates of mental illness, including mood disorders. The suicide rate among Native American males age 15 to 24 years is between two to three times the national rate (Kettle & Bixler, 1991). In fact, Alaskan native males have one of the highest rates of suicide in the world (U.S. Department of Health and Human Services, 2001).

RISK AND PROTECTIVE FACTORS

Familial Patterns

Reports from twin and adoption studies have been inconsistent in their findings of a link between genetic factors and the occurrence of depression. A number of studies have found genetic effects (Kendler, Neale, Kessler, Heath, & Eaves,

1993; Wender, Kety, Rosenthal, Schulsinger, Ortman, & Lunder, 1986), whereas others have concluded that environmental factors predominate (Cadoret, O'Gorman, Heywood, & Troughton, 1985; Von Knorring, Cloninger, Bohman, & Sigvardsson, 1983).

Some investigators have concluded that bipolar disorder has a high degree of heritability, based on the consistency of lifetime prevalence rates of bipolar disorder across countries and findings from family and molecular genetic studies (National Institute of Mental Health, 1998), and that cultural and societal factors play a secondary role in its causation (U.S. Department of Health and Human Services, 2001). First-degree biological relatives of persons diagnosed with bipolar I disorder have been found to have elevated rates of bipolar I disorder (4% to 24%), bipolar II disorder (1% to 5%), and major depression (4% to 24%). They are also more likely to experience the onset of the mood disorder at a younger age.

Age

The mean age of onset of major depressive disorders in the United States is between the ages of 40 and 50 years. In contrast to depression, bipolar disorder has been found to have a mean age of onset of 30 years. Among young adults, individuals at increased risk of major depression include those who are female, who have had multiple major depressive episodes in adolescence, who have a higher proportion of family members with recurrent major depressive disorder, who have elevated symptoms of borderline personality disorder, and, in females, who are in conflict with their parents (Lewinsohn, Rhode, Seeley, Klein, & Gotlib, 2000).

Epidemiologic Catchment Area data indicate that the lifetime prevalence of major depression appears to be higher among younger age groups, with the lowest prevalence observed among those 65 years of age or older (Weissman et al., 1991). Other studies have reached similar conclusions (Brown, Ahmed, Gary, & Milburn, 1993; Brown, Gary, Greene, & Milburn, 1992; Jones–Webb & Snowden, 1993). This appears to be counterintuitive, in view of the increased likelihood among the aging population of chronic illness, physical disability, loss of family and friends as a result of aging and illness, and the loss of income and social and professional status (Klerman, 1988).

Several theories have been proffered in an effort to understand this finding. The decreased prevalence of depression that has been observed among elderly persons may be attributable to (a) nonresponse by potential study participants resulting from infirmity, depression, or frailty; (b) the exclusion from study of individuals whose depressive symptoms are potentially attributable to physical illness or medication, which could disproportionately affect the participation of the elderly; (c) a higher mortality rate among depressed elderly persons, leading to a finding of decreased prevalence; (d) a shorter duration of depression among elderly persons, leading to a finding of decreased prevalence; (e) stronger social supports among the elderly; (f) the reduced occurrence of adverse life events among the elderly; and (g) the development of a "resistance" to depression throughout the life span as a result of increased exposure to stress (Henderson,

1994). Lastly, culturally determined expectations of age-appropriate attitudes and orientation toward life may lead to underdetection of mood disorders in older adults, particularly those with medical comorbidities.

Sex

Sex has been found to be associated with the occurrence of mood disorders. The ratio of affective illness in females to males ranges from 1.3:1 to 3:1 (Goodwin & Redfield Jamison, 1990). Although the rate of major depression was greater for women than men in all age groups in the ECA, the rate of bipolar disorder was comparable between the groups (Weissman et al., 1988).

Data from the NCS also indicate that women suffer higher rates of depression. Researchers estimated the prevalence of current major depression to be 5.9% in women compared with 3.8% in men, and the lifetime prevalence to be 21.3% in women but 12.7% in men (Blazer et al., 1994).

The large difference in prevalence rates of major depression between men and women may be the result of a number of factors. First, women may report their symptoms more freely than men, and may be more likely to seek diagnosis and treatment. Second, it is possible that men may experience similar depressive feelings as women, but attempt to deal with them differently, such as through substance use and antisocial behavior, which are more prevalent in men than in women. Last, it is possible that women may be more susceptible to depression as a result of societal bias and devaluation.

Contrary to popular belief, menopause does not appear to be a risk factor for depression. Rather, it appears that women who seek care for menopause-related complaints have a greater number of co-occurring psychiatric disorders (Stewart & Boydell, 1993), which have been hypothesized to relate to life cycle developmental issues (Greene & Cooke, 1980). In contrast, postpartum depression has been associated with a number of factors, including thyroid hormone changes (Walfish, Meyerson, Provias, Vargas, & Papsin, 1992), estriol levels (O'Hara, Schlechte, Lewis, & Wright, 1991), family histories of depression, and stressful life events (O'Hara et al., 1991).

Social Class, Socioeconomic Status, and Educational Level

Data from the ECA revealed a higher one-year prevalence of major depression among unemployed individuals compared with those who were employed (3.4% vs. 2.2%, respectively). The prevalence was slightly higher among white collar workers compared with other employed individuals (2.5% vs. 1.7%), those with 12 or more years of education (2.8% vs. 2.6%), and those with annual incomes less than $15,000 (2.9% vs. 1.8%) (Weissman et al., 1991).

The NCS found that lower level of education and employment classification as a homemaker or "other," including unemployment, were significant risk factors for major depression, even after controlling for other possible confounding variables such as gender, sex, and age. Although the rates of major depression were higher among unemployed persons in the NCS study, NCS data did not indicate an association between socioeconomic status and major depression. Other studies have reported increased rates of depressive symptoms among unemployed persons and those with lower incomes (Brown et al., 1992; Dressler & Badger, 1985).

The literature suggests that there may be an association between the occurrence of bipolar disorder and higher social class (Goodwin & Redfield Jamison, 1990). However, the reported findings may reflect a diagnostic bias, in that middle- and upper class individuals are more likely to be diagnosed with bipolar disorder, whereas individual of a lower social class are more frequently diagnosed with schizophrenia. It has been suggested that the apparent association between social class and bipolar disorder may be the result of the similarity between features of bipolar disorder and characteristics associated with success. For instance, many of the features of hypomania are also characteristics that are associated with achievement and accomplishments. These include increased energy and productivity, and being outgoing (Bagley, 1973).

Racism and Discrimination

Racism and discrimination have been identified as risk factors for depression among minority groups. Racism, which has been defined as "beliefs, attitudes, institutional arrangements, and acts that tend to denigrate individuals or groups because of phenotypic characteristics or ethnic group affiliation" (Clark, Anderson, Clark, & Williams, 1999, p. 805) may be manifested at the individual, institutional, and/or cultural levels (Rollock & Gordon, 2000). Depression becomes an adaptive response to subordination, exploitation, and defeat, which may occur as the result of a loss of or scarce resources, internal and external sources of attack, and social depreciation (Gilbert, 2000). Increased prevalence of depression has been found, for instance, among Latinos who experience high levels of discrimination (Alderete, Vega, Kolody, & Aguilar-Axiola, 1999).

Social Affiliation

Marital status has been found, in a number of studies, to be associated with the rate of depression. Divorced and separated men and women were found, in the ECA study, to have the highest rates of major depression (Weissman et al., 1991). For example, in relation to current marital status, the one-year prevalence of major depression was found to be 2.1% among those currently married, 2.1% among widowed persons, 6.3% among those who were separated or divorced, and 2.8% among those who had never married (Weissman et al., 1991). It is possible, then, that the social support received through marriage may act as a protective factor against the onset of depression. However, it is also possible that a partner's depression may precipitate or exacerbate marital strain and lead to separation or divorce.

Bipolar disorder has been found to be more prevalent among single and divorced individuals compared with those who are married (Boyd & Weissman, 1985; Jones et al., 1981, 1983; Weeke et al., 1975). It is unclear, however, whether being single or divorced constitutes a risk factor for the disorder, or whether the symptoms of the disorder bring about sufficient marital discord and stress that result in divorce.

Other family ties, religious involvement, and voluntary associations may be associated with depression. Brown and colleagues (1992) found in their study of 927 African American adults in Norfolk, Virginia, that family ties, religious involvement, and voluntary associations were inversely related to the occurrence of depression.

The Norwood–Montefiore Aging Study involved the sampling of approximately 2480 Medicare households from the Norwood section of the North Bronx. A total of 1855 randomly selected individuals from these households participated in the baseline interview. Catholics ($n = 1075$) were significantly less likely to report a significant level of depressive symptoms, whereas Jews ($n = 900$) were more than twice as likely to evidence symptoms (Kennedy, Kelman, Thomas, & Chen, 1996). Almost three fourths of the Catholic participants reported having attended religious services during the preceding month, compared with 20% of the Jewish participants and 38% of those classified as "other" (no religious preference, no specified religious preference, and preference other than Catholic, Jewish, or Protestant). Two of the seven factors identified that explained the variance in the prevalence of depression related to social affiliation: nonattendance at religious services and the receipt of formal and informal social support services (Kennedy, 1998).

Immigration Status

Studies have consistently found a higher rate of depression and bipolar disorder among immigrants compared with native-born individuals (Gershon & Liebowitz, 1975; Rowitz & Levy, 1968; Westermeyer, 1988). The apparent increased rates among immigrants may be attributable to the stress associated with the immigration process itself and/or the process of acculturation, a higher incidence of mental illness in the immigrants' native countries; and/or the preexisting health status of the immigrants themselves (Westermeyer, 1988).

REFERENCES

Alderete, E., Vega, W. A., Kolody, B., & Aguilar–Axiola, S. (1999). Depressive symptomatology: Prevalence and psychosocial risk factors among Mexican migrant farmworkers. *Journal of Community Psychology, 27,* 457–471.

American Psychiatric Association. (1987). *Diagnostic and statistical manual of mental disorders* (3rd ed. rev., DSM-III-R), Washington, D.C.: American Psychiatric Association.

American Psychiatric Association. (2000). *Diagnostic and statistical manual of mental disorders* (4th ed., DSM-IV-TR). Washington, DC: American Psychiatric Association.

Bagley, C. (1973). Occupational class and symptoms of depression. *Social Science and Medicine, 7,* 327–340.

Blazer, D. G., George, L. K., Landerman, R., et al. (1985). Psychiatric disorders: A rural/urban comparison. *Archives of General Psychiatry, 42,* 651–656.

Blazer, D. G., Kessler, R. C., McConaggle, K. A., et al. (1994). The prevalence and distribution of major depression in a national community sample: The National Comorbidity Survey. *American Journal of Psychiatry, 151,* 979–986.

Blazer, D. G., Landerman, L. R., Hays, J. C., Simonsick, E. M., & Saunders, W. B. (1998). Symptoms of depression among community-dwelling elderly African-American adults. *Psychological Medicine, 28,* 1311–1320.

Borwosky, S. J., Rubenstein, L. V., Meredith, L. S., Camp, P., Jackson–Triche, M., & Wells, K. B. (2000). Who is at risk of nondetection of mental health problems in primary care? *Journal of General Internal Medicine, 15,* 381–388.

Boyd, J. H., & Weissman, M. M. (1985). Epidemiology of major affective disorders. In R. Michels, J. O. Cavenar, H. K. H. Brodie, et al. (Eds.), *Psychiatry* (Vol. 3, pp. 1–16). Philadelphia: J.B. Lippincott.

Brown, D. R., Ahmed, F., Gary, L. E., & Milburn, N. G. (1993). Major depression in a community sample of African Americans. *American Journal of Psychiatry, 152,* 373–378.

Brown, D. R., Gary, L. E., Greene, A. D., & Milburn, N. G. (1992). Patterns of social affiliation as predictors of depressive symptoms among urban blacks. *Journal of Health and Social Behavior, 33,* 242–253.

Burnam, M. A., Hough, R. L., Escobar, J. I., Karno, M., Timbers, D. M., Telles, C. A., et al. (1987). Six-month prevalence of specific psychiatric disorders among Mexican Americans and non-Hispanic whites in Los Angeles. *Archives of General Psychiatry, 44,* 687–694.

Cadoret, R. J., O'Gorman, T. W., Heywood, E., & Troughton, E. (1985). Genetic and environmental factors in major depression. *Journal of Affective Disorders, 9,* 155–164.

Canino, G. J., Bird, H. R., Shrout, P. E., Rubio–Stipec, M., Bravo, M., Martinez, R., et al. (1987). The prevalence of specific psychiatric disorders in Puerto Rico. *Archives of General Psychiatry, 44,* 727–735.

Clark, R., Anderson, N. B., Clark, V. R., & Williams, D. R. (1999). Racism as a stressor for African Americans: A biopsychosocial model. *American Psychologist, 54,* 805–816.

Compton, W. M., Conway, K. P., Stinson, F. S., & Grant, B. F. (2006). Changes in the prevalence of major depression and comorbid substance use disorders in the United States between 1991–1992 and 2001–2002. *American Journal of Psychiatry, 163,* 2141–2147.

Cross-National Collaborative Group. (1992). The changing rate of major depression: Cross-national comparisons. *Journal of the American Medical Association, 268,* 3098–3105.

Dressler, W. W., & Badger, L. W. (1985). Epidemiology of depressive symptoms in black communities: A comparative analysis. *Journal of Nervous and Mental Disease, 173,* 212–220.

Eaton, W.W., Kramer, M., Anthony, J.C., Dryman, A., Shapiro, S., & Locke, B.Z. (1989). The incidence of specific DIS/DSM-III mental disorders: Data from the NIMH epidemiologic Catchment Area Program. *Acta Psychiatrica Scandinavica, 79,* 163–168.

Frerichs, R. R., Aneshensel, C. S., & Clark, V. A. (1981). Prevalence of depression in Los Angeles county. *American Journal of Epidemiology, 113,* 691–699.

Gallo, J. J., Cooper–Patrick, L., & Lesikar, S. (1998). Depressive symptoms of whites and African Americans aged 60 years and older. *Journal of Gerontology: Psychological Sciences, 53B,* P277–P286.

Gastpar, M. (1986). Epidemiology of depression (Europe and North America). *Psycho-pathology, 19*, 17–21.

Gershon, E. S., & Liebowitz, J. H. (1975). Sociocultural and demographic correlates of affective disorders in Jerusalem. *Journal of Psychiatric Research, 12*, 37–50.

Gilbert, P. (2000). Varieties of submissive behavior as forms of social defense: Their evolution and role in depression. In L. Sloman & P. Gilbert (Eds.), *Subordination and defeat: An evolutionary approach to mood disorders and their therapy* (pp. 3–45). Englewood Cliffs, NJ: Lawrence Erlbaum.

Golding, J. M., & Karno, M. (1988). Gender differences in depressive symptoms among Mexican Americans and non-Hispanic whites. *Hispanic Journal of Behavioral Sciences, 10*, 1–19.

Goodwin, F. K., & Redfield Jamison, K. (1990). *Manic-depressive illness*. New York: Oxford University Press.

Greene, J.G. & Cooke, D.J. (1980). Life stress and symptoms at climacterium. *British Journal of Psychiatry, 136*, 486–491.

Helzer, J. E. (1975). Bipolar affective disorder in black and white men: A comparison of symptoms and familial illness. *Archives of General Psychiatry, 32*, 1140–1143.

Henderson, A. S. (1994). Does aging protect against depression? *Social Psychiatry and Psychiatric Epidemiology, 29*, 107–109.

Hoppe, S. K., Garza–Elizondo, T., Leal–Isla, C., & Leon, R. I. (1991). Mental disorders among family practice patients in the United States–Mexico border region. *Social Psychiatry and Psychiatric Epidemiology, 26*(4), 178–182.

Horgan, D. (1981). Change of diagnosis to manic-depressive illness. *Psychological Medicine, 11*, 517–523.

Husaini, B. A. (1997). Predictors of depression among the elderly: Racial differences over time. *American Journal of Orthopsychiatry, 67*, 48–58.

Jones, B.E., Gray, B.A., & Parson, E.B. (1981). Manic-depressive illness among poor urban blacks. *American Journal of Psychiatry, 138*, 654–657.

Jones, B.E., Gray, B.A., & Parson, E.B. (1983). Manic-depressive illness among poor urban blacks. *American Journal of Psychiatry, 140*, 1208–1210.

Jones–Webb, R. J., & Snowden, L. R. (1993). Symptoms of depression among blacks and whites. *American Journal of Public Health, 83*, 240–244.

Karno, M., Hough, R. L., Burnam, M. A., et al. (1987). Lifetime prevalence of specific psychiatric disorders among Mexican Americans and non-Hispanic whites in Los Angeles. *Archives of General Psychiatry, 44*, 695–701.

Kendler, K. S., Neale, M. C., Kessler, R. C., Heath, A. C., & Eaves, L. J. (1993). A longitudinal twin study of 1-year prevalence of major depression in women. *Archives of General Psychiatry, 50*, 863–870.

Kennedy, G. J. (1998). Religion and depression. In H. G. Koening (Ed.), *Handbook of religion and mental health* (pp. 129–145). San Diego, CA: Academic Press.

Kennedy, G. J., Kelman, H. R., Thomas, C., & Chen, J. (1996). Religious preference, practice, and the prevalence of depression among 1855 older community residents. *Journals of Gerontology: Psychological Sciences, 51B*, 301–308.

Kessler, R. C., McGonagle, K. A., Zhao, S., Nelson, C. B., Hughes, M., Eshleman, S., et al. (1994). Lifetime and 12-month prevalence of *DSM-III-R* psychiatric disorders in the United States. *Archives of General Psychiatry, 51*, 8–19.

Kettle, P. A., & Bixler, E. O. (1991). Suicide in Alaskan natives, 1979–1984. *Psychiatry, 54*, 55–63.

Kleinman, A. (1986). *Social origins of distress and disease: Depression, neurasthenia, and pain in modern China*. New Haven, CT: Yale University Press.

Klerman, G. L. (1988). The current age of youthful melancholia: Evidence for increase in depression among adolescents and young adults. *British Journal of Psychiatry, 152,* 4–14.

Lehtinen, V. & Joukamaa, M. (1994). Epidemiology of depression: Prevalence, risk factors and treatment situation. *Acta Psychiatrica Scandinavica, 377,* 7–10.

Lewinsohn, P. M., Rhode, P., Seeley, J. R., Klein, D. N., & Gotlib, I. H. (2000). Natural course of adolescent major depressive disorder in a community sample: Predictors of recurrence in young adults. *American Journal of Psychiatry, 157,* 1584–1591.

Lewis, N. D., & Hubbard, L. D. (1931). Manic-depressive reactions in negroes. *Research Publications of the Association for Research in Nervous & Mental Diseases, 11,* 779–817.

Manson, S. M. (1992).Long-term care of older American Indians: Challenges in the development of institutional services. In C. Barresi & D. E. Stull (Eds.), *Ethnicity and long-term care* (pp. 130–143). New York: Springer.

Moscicki, E. K., Locke, B. Z., Rae, D. S., & Boyd, J. H. (1989). Depressive symptoms among Mexican Americans: The Hispanic Health and Nutrition Examination Survey. *American Journal of Epidemiology, 130,* 348–360.

Moscicki, E. K., Rae, D., Regier, D. A., & Locke, B. Z. (1987). The Hispanic Health and Nutrition Examination Survey: Depression among Mexican Americans, Cuban Americans, Puerto Ricans. In M. Gaviria & J. D. Arana (Eds.), *Health and behavior: Research agenda for Hispanics (pp. 145–159).* Chicago: University of Illinois.

National Institute of Mental Health. (1998). *Genetics and mental disorders: Report of the National Institute of Mental Health's Genetics Workgroup.* Rockville, MD: National Institute of Mental Health.

O'Hara, M.W., Schlechte, J.A., Lewis, D.A. & Wright, E.J. (1991). Prospective study of postpartum blues. Biologic and psychosocial factors. *Archives of General Psychiatry, 48(9),* 801–806.

Okwumabua, J. O., Baker, F. M., Wong, S. P., & Pilgrim, B. O. (1997). Characteristics of depressive symptoms in elderly urban and rural African American residents. *Journal of Gerontology: Medical Sciences, 52,* M241–M246.

Pollock, H. M. (1931). Recurrence of attacks in manic-depressive psychoses. *American Journal of Psychiatry, 11,* 568–573.

Roberts, R. E., & Chen, Y. (1995). Depressive symptoms and suicidal ideation among Mexican-origin and Anglo adolescents. *Journal of the American Academy of Child and Adolescent Psychiatry, 34,* 81–90.

Roberts, R. E., Roberts, C., & Chen, Y. R. (1997). Ethnocultural differences in prevalence of adolescent depression. *American Journal of Community Psychology, 25,* 95–110.

Roberts, R. E., & Sobhan, M. (1992). Symptoms of depression in adolescence: A comparison of Anglo, African, and Hispanic Americans. *Journal of Youth and Adolescence, 21,* 639–651.

Robins, L., & Regier, D. A. (1991). *Psychiatric disorders in America: The Epidemiologic Catchment Area Study.* New York: Free Press.

Rollock, D., & Gordon, E. X. (2000). Racism and mental health into the 21st century: Perspectives and parameters. *American Journal of Orthopsychiatry, 70,* 5–13.

Rowitz, L., & Levy, L. (1968). Ecological analysis of treated mental disorders in Chicago. *Archives of General Psychiatry, 19,* 571–579.

Salgado de Snyder, V. N. (1987). Factors associated with acculturative stress and depressive symptomatology among married Mexican immigrant women. *Psychology of Women Quarterly, 11,* 475–488.

Sorenson, S. B., & Golding, J. M. (1988a). Prevalence of suicide attempts in a Mexican-American population: Prevention implications of immigration and cultural issues. *Suicide and Life-threatening Behavior 18*, 322–333.

Sorenson, S. B., & Golding, J. M. (1988b). Suicidal ideation and attempts in Hispanics and non-Hispanic whites: Demographic and psychiatric disorder issues. *Suicide and Life-threatening Behavior 18*, 205–218.

Stewart, D.E. & Boydell, K. (1993). Psychological distress during menopause: Associations across the reproductive life cycle. *International Journal of Psychiatry in Medicine, 23*, 157–162.

Strakowski, S. M., Keck, P. E., Arnold, L. M., Collins, J., Wilson, R. M., Fleck, D. E., Corey, K. B., Amicone, J., & Adebimpe, V. R. (2003). Ethnicity and diagnosis in patients with affective disorders. *Journal of Clinical Psychiatry, 64*, 747–754.

Sue, S., Sue, D. W, Sue, L., & Takeuchi, D. T. (1995). Psychopathology among Asian Americans: A model minority? *Cultural Diversity and Mental Health, 1*(1), 39–54.

Swanson, J. W., Linskey, A. O., Quintero–Salinas, R., Pumariega, A. J., & Holzer, C. E., III. (1992). A binational school survey of depressive symptoms, drug use, and suicidal ideation. *Journal of the American Academy of Child and Adolescent Psychiatry, 31*, 669–678.

Takeuchi, D. T., Chung, R. C., Lin, K. M., Shen, H., Kurasaki, K., Chun, C., et al. (1998). Lifetime and twelve-month prevalence rates of major depressive episodes and dysthymia among Chinese Americans in Los Angeles. *American Journal of Psychiatry, 155*, 1407–1414.

U.S. Department of Health and Human Services. (2001). *Mental health: Culture, race, and ethnicity. A supplement to mental health: A report of the Surgeon General.* Rockville, MD: U.S. Department of Health and Human Services, Substance Abuse and Mental Health Services Administration, Center for Mental Health Services.

Vega, W. A., Kolody, B., Valle, V. R., & Hough, R. L. (1986). Depressive symptoms and their correlates among immigrant women in the United States. *Social Science and Medicine, 22*, 648–652.

Von Knorring, A. L., Cloninger, C. R., Bohman, M., & Sigvardsson, S. (1983). An adoption study of depressive disorders and substance abuse. *Archives of General Psychiatry, 40*, 943–950.

Wagner, P. S. (1938). A comparative study of negro and white admissions to the Psychiatric Pavilion of the Cincinnati General Hospital. *American Journal of Psychotherapy, 95*, 167–183.

Walfish, P. G., Meyerson, J., Provias, J. P., Vargas, M. T., & Papsin, F. R. (1992). Prevalence and characteristics of post-partum thyroid dysfunction: Results of a survey from Toronto, Canada. *Journal of Endocrinologic Investigation, 15*, 265–272.

Weeke, A., Bille, M., Videbech, T., Dupont, A., & Juel-Nielsen, N. (1975). Incidence of depressive syndromes in a Danish county. The Arhaus County investigation. *Acta Psychiatrica Scandinavica, 51*, 28–41.

Weissman, M. M., Bruce, M., Leaf, P., Florio, L., & Holzer, C. (1991). Affective disorders. In L. Robins & E. Regier (Eds.), *Psychiatric disorders in America* (pp. 53–80). New York: Free Press.

Weissman, M. M., Leaf, P. J., Tischler, G. L., Blazer, D. G., Karno, M., Bruce, M. L., et al. (1988). Affective disorders in five United States communities. *Psychological Medicine, 18*, 141–153.

Weissman, M. M., & Myers, J. K. (1978). Affective disorders in a US urban community: The use of research diagnostic criteria in an epidemiological survey. *Archives of General Psychiatry, 35*, 1304–1311.

Wender, P. H., Kety, S. S., Rosenthal, D., Schulsinger, F., Ortman, J., & Lunder, I. (1986). Psychiatric disorders in the biological and adoptive families of adopted individuals with affective disorders. *Journal of Neurology, Neurosurgery and Psychiatry, 52,* 940–948.

Westermeyer, J. (1988). Resuming social approaches to psychiatric disorder: A critical contemporary need. *Journal of Nervous and Mental Diseases, 176,* 703–706.

WHO International Consortium on Psychiatric Epidemiology. (2000). Cross-national comparisons of the prevalence and correlates of mental disorders. *Bulletin of the World Health Organization, 78,* 413–426.

Zhang, A. Y., & Snowden, L. R. (1999). Ethnic characteristics of mental disorders in five U.S. communities. *Cultural Diversity and Ethnic Minority Psychology, 5*(2), 134–146.

Zheng, Y.- P., Lin, K.- M., Takeuchi, D., Kurasaki, K., Wong, Y., & Cheung, F. (1997). An epidemiological study of neurasthenia in Chinese-Americans in Los Angeles. *Comprehensive Psychiatry, 38*(5), 249–259.

5

Treatment Modalities and Culture

JOSEPH J. WESTERMEYER

CULTURAL INFLUENCES ON TREATMENT MODALITIES

Culture can affect treatment modalities in numerous ways. If people in a society understand a treatment modality and accept its application, they are more likely to accept and comply with the treatment. If the treatment is not familiar, or conflicts with cultural notions regarding treatment, acceptance and adherence will suffer (Moore & Boehnlein, 1991, p. 1029). Cultural familiarity and approval serve as a critical first step toward family acceptance, societal access to and availability of the modality, and the support of other societal institutions for the modality. Society endorses treatment alternatives through such institutions as education, religion, health care, health law, industrial production, and courts.

Concepts regarding etiology prevalent in a culture drive treatment seeking, but can also foster treatment avoidance. For example, acceptance of biological models for disturbed or disturbing behavior would support biomedical interventions, such as medications or other somatotherapies (Koss, 1990, p. 5). Psychosocial theories lend themselves to a variety of psychotherapies and learning strategies, family therapies, and social system interventions. Spiritual–religious causation buttress religious ceremonies, shamanistic rituals, prayer, and confession (Lukoff, Lu, & Turner, 1995).

Models of treatment at large in the culture influence the acceptance of a modality (Westermeyer, 1982, p. 709). For example, use of herbal compounds paves the way for biomedical interventions. Acceptance of advice and counseling for personal problem resolution would foster use of the psychotherapies. Societies recognizing that cultural beliefs or social structures can be pathogenic are more apt to accept social interventions or change (Johnson, Feldman, Lubin, & Southwick, 1995, p. 283).

Culture can affect treatment via indirect mechanisms. Diet, prevalence of obesity, and even climate can affect the pharmacokinetics, and hence the efficacy per dose, of a medication. Culture-related symbolism associated with particular side effects can affect adherence with medications and other forms of care. Development of a strong transferential relationship with a clinician can threaten a tight-knit clan system.

Adjustment problems related to culture can pose the major clinical challenge for a clinician treating a migrant. Among migrants, failure to acculturate to the prevailing culture can precipitate psychiatric disorders or complicate clinical care. Special therapeutic modalities must evolve to address the failure to adjust to a new culture (Szapocnik, Santisteban, Kurtines, Perez–Vidal, & Hervis, 1984, p. 317).

INFLUENCE OF TREATMENT MODALITIES ON CULTURE

Just as culture can affect treatment, treatment can affect cultural beliefs and practices (Littlewood & Lipsedge, 1987, p. 289). For example, the efficacy of medications and other somatotherapies can undermine belief in spiritual or moral contributions to mental, emotional, or behavioral conditions. Success of therapies previously deemed inappropriate or worthless can pave the way for acceptance of new concepts and models of behavior. For much of the 20th century, psychoanalytic concepts affected social and political theory, language/communication studies, child-raising practices, and even legal principles (Grinberg & Grinberg, 1984, p. 13).

An example of treatment influence on culture (and vice versa) lies in the modern approaches to addictive disorder (Westermeyer, 1996, p. 110). Social theory during past centuries categorized alcoholism and drug addiction as sinful behaviors, so that interventions were largely punitive or spiritual. As various treatment modalities proved successful in ameliorating cases of addiction, social theories supported the involuntary treatment commitment of addicted persons, who were viewed as unable to rid themselves of addictive behaviors. More recently, in a time when social entities have not wanted to assume responsibilities for addictive disorders, those refusing to seek and comply with treatment are viewed as irresponsible, and thus again morally responsible for reprehensible behavior.

IMPORTANCE OF LABELS, DIAGNOSIS, AND EXPLANATORY MODELS

Diagnosis: Labeling the Disorder

Labeling comprises a first step in the identification of disturbed or disturbing behavior as a health condition (Fabrega, 1987). Many of our current diagnoses owe their etymology to theories common at the time of recognizing syndromal similarities in a set of signs and symptoms. For example, melancholia refers to the Greco-Roman theory implicating "black bile" in the cause of persisting, disabling depression. Other terms are more descriptive, such as *alcoholism, schizophrenia (split mind)*, or *panic disorder*.

Labeling serves the purpose of concentrating and distilling human experience with a condition or syndrome, so that observers (and sufferers themselves) can study the course, associated characteristics, and presumed causes of a condition (Lu, Lim, & Mezzich, 1995). Ultimately, labeling lends itself to the evolution of treatment, as clinicians seek effective and culturally acceptable ways of ameliorating, controlling, or curing a disorder. Without the development of reliable (and, hopefully, valid) diagnostic conditions, the accretion of knowledge, understanding, and effective therapy for a condition is extremely difficult. One might even say impossible, although serendipitous discoveries have sometimes allowed a therapeutic breakthrough even when prevalent theory did not favor treatment advances. The serendipitous observations that chlorpromazine, imipramine, and lithium relieved certain psychiatric conditions occurred despite widely held theories about mental disorder. In turn, these serendipitous discoveries changed the way in which many societies viewed psychiatric disorder.

From the simplest to the most advanced societies, sufferers and their families expect that their clinicians will accurately label their condition before launching into treatment. Inherent in this widespread expectation is the general human awareness that (a) signs and symptoms do not equal disorders, (b) treatment of signs and symptoms alone may relieve the symptoms but not relieve the disorder, and (c) treatment of the underlying disorder may alleviate the resulting signs and symptoms (Westermeyer, 1985, p. 798).

Even in simple cultures, the average person can name a number of conditions with mental, emotional, or behavioral manifestations. However, the folk healers in these societies can name a much larger number of such conditions than laypeople. Thus, the reliance on specialists to label or diagnose these confusing conditions is virtually universal (Westermeyer, 1979, p. 301).

The Patient's Explanatory Model

The explanatory model involves more than labeling or diagnosis. It involves the perceived causes that the patient (or family) uses to explain the illness. This model usually bears a relationship to popular sources of care in the culture, including the patient's preferences or expectations for care of the current episode. It is important in any case, but especially so in cross-cultural care, to ascertain the patient's (and family's) diagnosis and cause for the illness. These lay diagnoses or explanations, sometimes known as *explanatory models*, are described in Appendix I of the *DSM-IV* (American Psychiatric Association, 1994) (see Table 5.1).

Family (and sometimes neighbors and friends) have often tried their hand at initially labeling and treating psychiatric conditions—much as they might a sore muscle, headache, or cough. If the condition improves, no further treatment

Table 5.1 Outline for Cultural Formulation (Appendix I)

Cultural Identity of the Individual: patient's ethnic or cultural reference group(s), along with language abilities, use, and preference

Cultural Explanations of the Individual's Illness: predominant idioms of distress, meaning and perceived severity of symptoms, any local illness category, perceived causes, and preferred source of care

Cultural Factors Related to Psychosocial Environment and Levels of Functioning: social stressors, support, levels of function and disability, role of religion and kin network in providing support

Cultural Elements of the Relationship between the Individual and the Clinician: differences in culture and social status, along with problems that these differences may cause in diagnosis and treatment

Overall Cultural Assessment for Diagnosis and Care: how cultural considerations influence comprehensive diagnosis and care (in the instance of this particular patient and clinician)

Source: American Psychiatric Association. (1994). *Diagnostic and statistical manual of mental disorders, fourth edition.* Washington, DC: American Psychiatric Association.

seeking may ensue. If the condition persists or worsens, the individual and/or family may eventually seek treatment (Westermeyer & Wintrob, 1979a, p. 755). By the time they seek treatment, they may have lost faith in their own explanatory model. Nonetheless, this model may have relevance to the case or its treatment. Thus, it is important for the clinician to determine this model. Learning the nature of the patient's explanatory model comprises an important first step in formulating and implementing a treatment plan (Figure 5.1). The family may also have a cogent explanatory model, which may differ from that of the patient. In order for clinician, patient, and family to develop a coherent plan, knowledge all around regarding one another's model is an important first step.

Conveying the Diagnosis: Integrating Patient and Clinician Explanatory Models

Awareness of the patient's or family's explanatory model comprises a key first step in discussing and negotiating treatment. For example, a patient who believes that a deceased relative has cursed him or her may not perceive medications as a logical form of treatment. Or a patient who believes that loss of the soul has produced the condition may not see the utility of marital counseling. After the patient's model is known, the next step consists of the clinician providing a label (diagnosis) and a psychiatric explanatory model (Figure 5.1).

Being aware of the patient's explanatory model can guide the clinician in how to convey the diagnosis and psychiatric/psychological model appropriately to the patient and family (Weiss, Doongaji, Siddhartha, Wypij, Pathare, Bhatawdekar, et al., 1992, p. 819; Westermeyer & Wintrob, 1979b, p. 901). At times, the clinician and patient models may align closely, facilitating a course of treatment accepted by all, as in the following case.

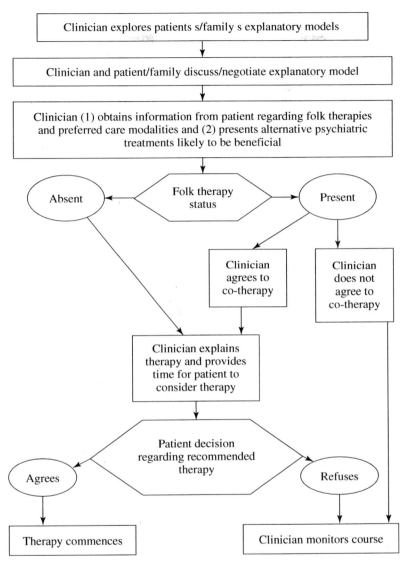

Figure 5.1 Algorithm for cross-cultural care.

Blood Crazy

A 28-year-old Southeast Asian immigrant presented to a psychiatry clinic with insomnia, weight loss, racing thoughts, grandiose delusions, irritability, and poor judgment, consistent with manic–depressive disorder, manic phase, with mood congruent psychotic features. His family diagnosed him as "blood crazy," a folk condition marked by these same symptoms and so labeled because such patients tended to have a flush faced, indicating (in the folk cosmology based on body humors) an excess of blood (Westermeyer, 1979). The patient and family concurred that medications would be the proper intervention for this disorder. Moreover, they concurred that the patient's condition warranted a brief period of hospitalization while the proper medications and doses could be achieved. Adherence with treatment was excellent, and the clinical outcome was optimal.

In other cases, the patient and clinician explanatory models may not parallel each other. One reason for this could be that no folk diagnostic entity comes even close to the clinician's diagnosis. In such cases, it is often possible to create a term that describes the condition in terms comprehensible to the patient.

Creating a Label

In a psychiatry clinic serving a large number of Southeast Asian refugees, major depressive disorder was the most common condition. The ethnic groups attending this clinic had no one folk entity that encompassed the signs and symptoms of this condition. Although they had terms for various degrees of sadness, they recognized that this condition was not like the ordinary time-limited sadness that one experienced after a loss. This sadness entailed frustration, loss of self-confidence, failure to remit naturally with time, and unrelenting misery. After discussion with several people who had the condition or were recovering from it, the term *a sickness of the soul, mind, and heart* was created. Clinicians, patients, and bilingual workers participated in developing this label, which suffering patients related to as describing their condition. In addition, it allowed clan elders, folk healers, and other indigenous gatekeepers to identify others with the same condition. Furthermore, it permitted sufferers to tell their family and friends the name of the condition for which they were receiving care.

Negotiating the Diagnosis

As in the case just described, at times it may not be feasible to agree on a diagnosis. This could be the result of the clinician's inability to accept the patient's or family's label or the patient's or family's inability to accept the clinician's diagnosis. Or the clinician's diagnosis may be tentative or not fully integrated (Davidson & Strauss, 1995, p. 44). This creates a problem that the clinician must surmount in some way. Fortunately, it is often feasible to find a way around or through this type of dilemma.

Ghost Disease

A 38-year-old widowed Hmong refugee woman, employed and mother of five children, developed a major depressive disorder in the weeks after being robbed in a grocery store parking lot. She soon developed a recurring dream in which her deceased mother was walking toward her. When a short distance away, her mother would stop, look at her for a time, and then disappear. The patient interpreted the dream as an omen that she would soon die (consistent with her culture, in which such dreams could be a harbinger of death). In the patient's view, her mother wanted her to join her in the afterworld, and had sent this illness as a means of ending her life. The clinician told the patient that, although she might be correct, another explanation for her illness was possible. The recent robbery may have produced this illness through its damaging effect on her morale and through its replicating in several ways the insecurities that had led her (and her deceased husband, who died in the flight) to flee their homeland. Her mother might be making the long and difficult journey from the next world to offer her solace and support in her misery. Because the patient's mother needed her grandchildren to offer respect and continuity to the family ancients, it was in her mother's best interests to help the patient survive and raise her children. Finally, it was suggested that the clinic might help her by treating this illness with a combination of medications and weekly visits over a period of time, aided by the mother's benign support through the patient's dreams. An appointment was made for two days later, so the patient would have time to consider this alternative. The next appointment would permit discussion regarding whether she would be willing to take medication and commit herself to a clinic visit weekly throughout the coming few months. The patient returned a few days later, stating that her mother had smiled in her most recent dream, signaling to the patient that her mother did indeed want her to live and care for her children. The patient adhered closely to the medication regimen and visits.

Early on in the previous case, the patient and clinician did not agree on the cause of her condition. She perceived her condition as being supernatural and not amenable to natural or medication intervention. However, she had failed to improve after preternatural interventions in her community. Subsequently, she perceived her condition as hopeless. On the recommendation of a friend, who had been treated for (and recovered from) a similar condition, she came to the clinic. She had sufficient doubt about her own label, as well as hopeful wishes for her eventual recovery, to abide the gap between her diagnosis and that of the clinician. A common course of treatment was feasible despite the patient and clinician having two quite different explanatory models.

SETTING THE STAGE FOR EFFECTIVE TREATMENT

Negotiating Treatment

After the diagnosis and explanatory models have been negotiated, the next step lies in negotiating treatment. The step between recommending and then implementing treatment is a large one. Even if clinician and patient share ethnic identity, they may not share beliefs regarding the causes for the patient's mood disorder or the means of ameliorating it. If treatment occurs across cultural boundaries, this "step" can be very large indeed — perhaps more like a trek than a step.

It is helpful at this juncture for the clinician to set priorities. For example, the ultimate recovery of the patient is a major priority, considerably more important than whether the patient accepts a particular treatment modality today. With this greater good in mind, the clinician may be willing to negotiate an interim plan that is less than ideal from the clinician's perspective, as in the following case.

Lupus Case

A 52-year-old European American woman with lupus erythematosus (LE) was referred to a psychiatry clinic with "depression." She had never been depressed previously. Other than her starting to take cortisone prior to her depressive symptoms, as well as physical limitations imposed by her LE, she had experienced no losses or major life reversals. A diagnosis of organic mood disorder secondary to LE and cortisone was made; antidepressant medication and supportive psychotherapy were recommended for her moderately severe symptoms. She agreed with her clinician's diagnosis, but indicated that she had recently started an herbal medication, had begun to feel somewhat better, and wanted to remain on that regimen for now. Her clinician agreed to her plan, but suggested that they meet briefly in a month to monitor her course, because failure to recover could have severe consequences for her personal and occupational life. She agreed readily to the plan. During a period of a few months, her symptoms continued to worsen. At that point she agreed to discontinue the herbal compound and initiate formal psychotherapy and pharmacotherapy for her depressive disorder. She made an uneventful recovery.

In this case, coadministration of the herbal compound and the medication was risky, because the herbal compound affected enzyme systems shared by antidepressants. It could thus adversely affect the blood level, worsen the side effects, and impede therapeutic benefit.

In another case, the clinician deemed that cotherapy with folk care and psychiatric treatment would be safe. However, this can lead to political or ethnic considerations, as in the following case.

Confrontation by a Clergyman

During the course of treating a Southeast Asian woman in Asia, a European American clergyman paid the European American clinician a visit. The clergyman indicated that he knew the women was being treated, emphazing her husband's leadership status in the community and the importance of this case. Then he expressed his concern that the clinician was treating the woman at the same time that she was undergoing spirit-based ceremonies to relieve her condition. The clergyman's concern was that, as the woman was the improving, the credit for her "cure" would fall to "demons," thereby undermining the credibility of the clergyman's god and sect. Thus, he asked that the clinician immediately cease treating the women, because the clinician would be doing the work of the devil, undermining community belief in the true god, and impeding the eternal salvation of many people.

The clergyman's intervention raises a serious point. Treatment, especially if successful, can change a person's worldview, reinforce a traditional worldview, or perhaps both concurrently. The clergyman feared that a traditional cosmology would gain at the expense of the new order he was proposing, including converts to his sect. The clinician's view was that the patient, her husband, and family had found a means of both trusting to a traditional intervention while utilizing an unfamiliar approach that had benefited others in their community—a most reasonable strategy. A potential political consequence was that the clergyman, as a gatekeeper for similar conditions, might not refer cases for psychiatric care, given the gap between the two worldviews. In this case, the clinician decided that care should not change as a result of the clergyman's plea, regardless of the effects on the clergyman's future referrals.

Addressing Treatment Expectations: A Clinical Plan

For many patients coming to psychiatric care from other cultural settings, their working models of pharmacotherapy may involve rapidly acting medications, such as analgesics and antibiotics (Blendon, Scheck, Donelan, Hill, Smith, Beatrice, & Altman, 1995, p. 341; Pelz, Merskey, Brant, Patterson, & Heseltine, 1981, p. 345). In their experience, these and similar nostrums have had fairly rapid results. Analgesics can relieve pain within minutes or a few hours. Antibiotics can produce a near-miraculous reprieve from lethal infections, such as pneumonia, in days. Thus, patients with mood disorders may rationally believe that their conditions will remit in hours to days with treatment. When their condition fails to remit during this time frame, they may stop their therapy and return to the clinician, declaring the treatment to be ineffective.

An effective antidote to these unrealistic expectations, nonadherence, and premature treatment dropout does exist (Figure 5.1). It consists of, first, thorough education of the patient and family regarding the course of the disorder with and without treatment, likely duration of the treatment, and any side effects or complications apt to occur. Second, the clinician then asks the patient (and, as appropriate, the family) to consider the alternatives after their meeting and return to discuss them. An appointment is arranged to see the patient and family in a few days to hear their decision and decide on the next steps. Depending on the circumstances (e.g., acuity of the case, distance to travel for the appointment, and so on), the return visit may occur that day, in a few days, or the following week. Third, if the patient and family decide not to engage in the recommended treatment, the clinician may offer a follow-up appointment to monitor the course over time. Fourth, if they decide to engage in the treatment, the clinician may request that they commit to an adequate time on the regimen before the clinician and patient/family together (and patient and family alone) declare it to be ineffective.

The longer time required by this process might seem to be a liability, in that it delays treatment by a short period of time. It also requires some additional clinical time during which the full therapeutic regimen is realized (in addition to the assessment and support already provided). Clinicians may worry the delayed treatment also could increase the time during which the patient is exposed to a variety of untoward events (e.g., changed behavior in the family, suicide, additional weight loss or insomnia, secondary somatic health problems), but major complications such as these occur rarely, if at all, within such a brief period. The following advantages accrue from this approach:

- It actively involves the patient (and usually the family as well) in the process of judging, learning about, and selecting treatment from among alternatives. This more active role in the treatment process can enhance self-esteem and self-confidence.
- Simply learning more about the disorder and realizing that recovery is possible can produce clinical improvement. Especially if stressors have been great or the course has been short-lived, this level of improvement may encourage patient and clinician to opt for "watchful waiting" or less intrusive treatment alternatives.
- Patients and families can more realistically assess the nature of their current problem and the likely courses associated with treatment. This step can effectively undermine the "magical thinking" that patients and families often pursue in their desire for immediate relief.
- During this period, patients and families can gird themselves for the difficult weeks and months ahead, because psychiatric treatments usually involve the kind of crises, anxieties, and temporary worsening that accompany many (if not most) medical and surgical interventions.
- A cautious hope often surfaces as patients and families begin to appreciate the capacity for change, perhaps even renewal, emerging from the treatment process. This step can reverse the demoralization that so commonly accompanies a mood disorder.

Some patients choose their own therapeutic course, such as the LE patient mentioned earlier. Most often, they choose the treatment, despite its inconveniences, cost, or added symptoms. The small extra time spent in fostering commitment to a difficult and unexpected course of care has been worthwhile in the majority of instances. It usually saves time in various therapeutic misadventures based on misunderstanding and miscommunication.

Concurrent Psychiatric and Folk Therapies

In one case study presented earlier, the clinician chose not to cotreat the patient taking the herbal compound. On the contrary, the clinician did treat the patient who was undergoing spiritual healing. What was the thinking behind these two apparently inconsistent decisions? Behind this discrepancy lies a principle for proceeding with cotherapy in some instances and not proceeding in other instances. The decision hinges on the dictum, "First, cause no harm." See Figure 5.1 for the locus of this decision in the treatment process.

If the clinician discerns that cotherapy may cause harm, the clinician should not collude in it. In the case of medications, certain herbal compounds are apt to produce untoward interactions with prescribed medications, ranging from increased metabolism of the therapeutic agent, to decreased metabolism of the agent, to increased side effects, to toxic or life-threatening interactions or complications (Muskin, 2000). St. John's wort is apt to inhibit cytochrome P450 enzymatic action, thereby leading to potential toxicity from prescribed medications. Certain psychotherapies may also conflict with folk therapies, for example if the psychotherapy instills increasing self-responsibility while the folk therapy is recommending external blame.

On the other hand, if the combined therapies are apt to have no mutually detrimental effect, to be neutral or, ideally, to be mutually reinforcing, the clinician would support their utilization. An example might consist of a patient who engages in daily medication and weekly psychotherapy while also praying for deliverance several times a day.

Demon Possession

A Cree holy man had come to the United States to preach and conduct services. While in the United States, he became suddenly catatonic in the midst of service. His hosts perceived him as being possessed by the devil, and provided him with care as best they could. When he had not taken food or water for two days, they became alarmed and brought him to the hospital. Admitted to a psychiatry inpatient unit, he began to improve with intravenous fluids and antipsychotic medication. With the agreement of the patient, his hosts also conducted a healing exorcism ceremony on the inpatient ward. After several days in the hospital, he was able to return to Canada.

Although this man had been treated for psychosis in the past, he had not been in an inpatient hospital unit. The intravenous fluids and injections were frightening to him. At the same time, the presence of his hosts at the hospital and the conduct of a familiar ceremony was comforting and reassuring to him. Both psychiatric and traditional modalities were mutually beneficial and hastened his safe return home.

Patients' families may request folk modalities that the clinician has approved, but the patient may decline the traditional modality, as in the following case.

The Chippewa College Student

A 22-year-old Anishinabe (Chippewa) college student had been episodically drinking heavily throughout his teenage and early college years. During the previous year he had undergone treatment, achieving one year of sobriety. During that period he had grown progressively depressed. His mother, a hospital worker, referred him for care. He was severely depressed, had lost 30 pounds, had severe insomnia, and could no longer continue his studies. His mother and father wanted him to seek care with a shaman, but he refused. In addition to not believing that a shaman could help him, he feared that the family would blame him in the event that a cure was not forthcoming. He was also concerned that the cost of arranging a shamanistic ritual would be more than his parents could afford. However, he was willing to enter psychiatric care for his major depressive disorder.

Some healers (perhaps like some clinicians) blame their patients for the lack of therapeutic benefit. Common rationales include "not believing" in the healer, not surrendering one's will or destiny to the healer, or not collaborating with one or another taboo or stricture associated with the ritual healing. People whose cultures use these modalities know this, thus resulting in their occasional preference for "foreign" modalities in which peer, self-, or family blame is not an issue.

Although many people perceive traditional healing as costing little, it can be very expensive. The expense is greater if the healer must be transported from a distance, if the ritual must go on for several days, of if the healer is well-known and commands a large fee.

PSYCHOTHERAPY IN CULTURAL CONTEXT

Cultural Transference

Patients can have attitudes toward their clinicians based on their beliefs, experiences, or even historical relationships between the patients' and the clinicians' cultural groups. These attitudes may enhance trust in the clinician as well as treatment adherence. On the contrary, these attitudes can undermine trust and undermine treatment (Spiegel, 1976, p. 447).

Although the clinician may have notions about cultural transference with a patient, these attitudes cannot be assumed. They must be explored with the patient. Therein lies a double bind. Approaching this topic requires a good deal of mutual trust, or the patient is unlikely to express his or her true feelings toward the clinician on whom they must rely for compassionate, competent care.

One entrée to this information can occur through a third person. During a 15-year period, I supervised psychiatry residents and psychology postdoctoral students in providing care in a weekly cultural psychiatry clinic. Patients were predominantly refugees, but also included large numbers of immigrants, foreign students, foreign workers, and other foreign visitors as well as American minority groups with ethnic origins that were well away from the societal mainstream. The following case exemplifies an instance in which the burgeoning clinician feared negative transference.

Palestinian Patient

A Palestinian patient presented to a university psychiatry clinic with major depressive disorder persisting despite two months of abstinence after treatment for drug dependence. An American Jewish psychiatrist received this patient in the day's random assignments of residents to patients. After a competent evaluation and a discussion of the case, the third-year resident expressed concern that this patient could not possibly trust him. The supervisor returned to the patient alone and inquired about the patient's willingness to work with this resident under supervision. The patient reported that a Jewish psychiatrist had treated him some years earlier in Israel with good results. He reported feeling that the psychiatric resident had been thorough and sensitive in his evaluation, he liked the resident, and he would trust his care to him.

At times, patients prefer clinicians with backgrounds other than their own. In one community, despite several highly competent Korean American psychiatrists, patients from this group often resisted referral to a Korean American psychiatrist because of the close-knit nature of this community through church affiliations, Saturday morning school for children, and other ethnic associations.

It is possible to ask about cultural transference after a trusting, continuous relationship has been established with the patient, as seen in the following case.

Blue-Eyed Devil

During the course of several months, a clinician provided pharmacotherapy and psychodynamic psychotherapy to an African American graduate student who developed a major depressive disorder soon after starting graduate school. This was his first experience outside of settings that were predominantly African American—a situation that he found, at times, confusing and often stressful. He had considerable difficulty trusting his European American peers and faculty, whom he referred to as "blue-eyed devils." Over time he was able to establish relationships with several peers and a few faculty members who were European Americans, with considerable benefit in his depressive symptoms. However, he continued to refer to others he didn't trust as blue-eyed devils. At a point when there was reliable trust in the therapeutic relationship, the clinician asked the patient what color his eyes were. Without looking at the clinician, he responded, "They're brown, of course." When the clinician asked him to look again, the patient said with some surprise, "They're blue."

In this instance, the patient, early during therapy, had the strength to define the clinician as someone he could trust, even if that meant changing the perceived nature of the clinician's physiognomy. In the following case, the patient changed the clinician's entire ethnic identity.

Lao Doctor

A 16-year-old Lao patient newly arrived in the United States required hospitalization for her first acute psychotic episode of manic–depressive disorder, manic phase. In light of her inability to speak English and the clinician's moderate skills in her language, the European American clinician spoke to her in Lao during their daily visits. After two weeks in the hospital her parents were able to travel from their town to visit her. After the visit they went to the nurses' station, asking to talk to the "Lao doctor" who was providing care for their daughter. The nurse introduced them to the European American psychiatrist. They said this couldn't be, because their daughter had indicated that a Lao and not an "American" doctor was treating her.

In this case, this young, confused, frightened patient found comfort in perceiving the clinician as a member of her own ethnic group, especially in the context of her becoming mentally ill in a foreign land.

In sum, cultural transference cannot be assumed or easily predicted. It may have a factual basis or may be entirely fanciful. In some instances, it may be blatantly wrong or even delusional. Beneficial cultural transference need not have a connection to reality.

A kind of "familial transference" may also occur. In some cultural groups, in which ongoing personal relationships with a clinician are unknown, the patient's regular visits and reliance on the clinician may pose a threat to the family. The family may fear the foreign influences being introduced into the family from the foreign physician. Including the family in every third or fourth visit can prevent the development of negative family transference.

Other kinds of cultural transference may intrude even if physician and patient share ethnicity. Cross-religion care or cross-gender treatment can also threaten family stability in some cultural groups. However, even these impediments can sometimes be creatively addressed.

Islamic Wife

A 34-year-old Islamic woman from Southeast Asia, college educated, developed moderately severe depressive symptoms. Her husband, ambivalent about her seeking psychiatric care, told her that she had to have a female relative of her husband in the room during the entire time of her visit. The clinician and patient arranged for her to have a relative who knew no English in the room throughout her treatment. This arrangement was acceptable to all, and the treatment proceeded as usual.

Cultural Countertransference

Clinician feelings related to feelings regarding the patient's culture can also intrude on the clinical relationship. In the case of the Palestinian patient described earlier, the resident did not feel that he could cope with his own hostile feelings toward the patient's culture and he demurred from assuming responsibility for the Palestinian man's care. Although most of us like to believe that we can manage our own cultural countertransference, we should be alert to the possibility of not being able to do so (Comas–Diaz & Jacobsen, 1991, p. 392).

It probably requires a level of experience and maturation to transcend our ethnocentrifugal feelings toward historical enemies of those people with whom we identify. A psychiatrist of ethnic Jewish origin provided care for the incarcerated Nazi Germans being tried at Nuremberg for crimes against Jews and others during World War II. Around age 30 at the time, he accomplished this by focusing on their current clinical conditions, the task at hand (to provide health care to enable them to participate in the trial), his role in the larger scene, and his Hippocratic oath. In this setting he was able to make recommendations that improved the clinical condition of those under his charge, enhancing the fairness of the trial process.

Acceptability and Utility of Diverse Psychotherapies

Some clinicians aver that psychotherapy is only possible with Western patients or patients who share ethnicity or at least a worldview with the clinician. On the contrary, Cooper and colleagues (2003, p. 479) observed that depressed African and Hispanic Americans were more apt to accept "counseling" compared with Caucasians. It is possible to provide a wide variety of therapies, and probably all psychotherapies, across cultural boundaries. Perhaps the difference is that the average American patient assumes that psychotherapy can help and is usually (although not always) willing to join in the endeavor. On the contrary, the typical refugee or immigrant patient (as well as some minority patients) may not accept automatically the premise that thinking, acting upon, or talking about distressing topics may have therapeutic advantages.

Many patients in cross-cultural settings are not apt to disagree with the clinician or require additional rationale before proceeding. More often they will simply stop coming for care, or come for care but not comply with treatment. To counteract this outcome, the clinician should explain the psychotherapeutic modality to the patient. This account may include a mechanism by which the therapy may help, provided within the patient's terms and worldview. This can be a challenge, given the fact that the patient may conceive of the disorder as involving a ghost, a curse, or an ongoing relationship with someone who is deceased.

Attacking Ghosts of Lost Comrades

A 34-year-old Asian refugee developed a major depressive disorder in the several weeks after having been laid off from his job. In addition to weight loss, insomnia, fatigue, and thoughts of impending death, he was preoccupied by two worries: his inability to support his wife and two children, and a recurring nightmare in which the ghosts of his former army squad members were chasing him. Although he preferred not to speak about either worry, because it distressed him to do so, he agreed to four meetings during which he and the clinician would discuss them. While discussing the ghosts, the clinician discovered that they were the souls of men who died in his squad during a battle in Asia. At the time, the patient was 18 or 19 years old; the squad members were slightly younger. During this particular battle, the patient was wounded early during the fight and was removed to a safe place. The rest of his squad all died when their position was overrun. Although the patient felt guilty about it at the time, he did not agonize over it. The loss of his job recently rekindled and magnified this earlier guilt, because he feared that he would harm his family in the same fashion as he "harmed" his squad years earlier. Access to this information allowed the clinician and patient to engage in cognitive–behavioral therapy focused on his "catastrophizing" his temporary employment setback and the "survival" of his family as related to his employment. Although his condition improved notably, his nightmares continued. The clinician suggested that the patient cease running from his deceased colleagues during one of these recurring dreams, let them catch up, and ask them what they wanted of him. At the next session, the patient reported that they told him, "Don't forget us!" The clinician then discussed ritual and ceremonial ways in which the patient could keep their memory and their sacrifice alive. The nightmare faded in the following weeks as he implemented these "remember us" plans.

Therapeutic paradigms that involve learning apply readily across cultures and languages in most cases. Examples include desensitization and cognitive–behavioral therapy. Dialectical–behavioral therapy requires greater explanation and rationale, because it must persist over a long period of time and follow certain rules to show benefit.

Psychodynamic interpretations can be as beneficial in cross-cultural as in iso-cultural contexts. The key lies in using analogies that tap into the proverbs, myths, literature, and song of the patient's culture. This step involves learning these aspects of the patient's culture, and they may be written or also verbal.

Riding the Tiger

A 28-year old patient, a survivor of the Pol Pat regime in Cambodia, repeatedly got herself into double-bind situations. These binds involved especially her relationships with men and with employers. After another failed liaison with a man who abused her, she first developed a major depressive disorder and comorbid PTSD soon thereafter. Early during therapy, she could not see the link between decisions that she made early in a relationship and the ultimate victimization that she experienced. In seeking for a cognate that she might be able to use, the European American clinician used the Asian proverb about "riding the tiger's back" to portray the patient's recurrent dilemmas. This proverb captured the concept of one entering into a risky or potentially aversive situation and then ending up in a double bind in which either "riding the tiger" or "getting off the tiger" had unpleasant, perhaps even dire, consequences. Over time she was able to utilize this cognate, which she knew from early childhood, in a variety of circumstances to understand herself, her motivations, and the ultimate consequences of earlier flawed decisions. This permitted her to change her worldview from one in which she was repeatedly victimized to one in which she could more effectively influence her destiny.

Marital and Family Therapy

Perhaps the most sensitive therapy to cultural influences is couples/family therapy. To conduct marital therapy, the clinician should know the ideal and actual nature of marital relationships in the couple's culture. Regardless of the nature of their particular partnership, each member of the couple carries beliefs about the ideal nature of marriage. Marital therapy can be more difficult when the couple do not share a common belief or expectation of marriage.

Marriage Gone Wrong

A 52-year-old European American artist presented with a major depressive disorder that had been developing during the previous few years in association with menopause and her children leaving home. She was coping well with both these changes in her life (and even welcomed both changes). The notable loss in her life was the decreasing time that she had with her husband, a Native American and also an artist, with whom she had experienced an exceptional marriage. He was spending increasing amounts of time on his home reservation mentoring young people with artistic talents and serving as an elder in his clan and in the tribe at large. As he was winding down his successful artistic career, her artistic career was just burgeoning as she was freed from child-raising and domestic responsibilities. She had planned that this era in their lives would involve more time together, painting together, visiting married children, and enjoying the fruits of their many years of labor. On the other hand, he conceived this time as a "giving back" to the many people who had helped him when he was young, and taking advantage of his maturity and resources to benefit his clan and tribe. After they became aware of their separate concepts regarding this phase of their lives, they looked for opportunities to meld their separate destinies, while also recognizing their separate culture-driven life courses. The wife managed this phase by first surrendering her righteous anger, then grieving for her lost expectations, and finally recommitting herself to her art. The husband looked for opportunities to bring his cultural duties and his wife's career into apposition (such as art festivals that included Native American art).

Martial therapy may involve the extended clan in cultures that conceive of marriage as involving the intersection of two clans in the not-so-private lives of the married couple. Native American psychologist Attneave, working with Speck, has described "social network" therapy for these situations (Speck & Attneave, 1974). This approach often requires sessions that last at least one and a half hours, and possibly twice that long. The advantage lies in that such sessions need to occur less often, because the extended family can serve as a therapeutic milieu in which continued benefit may accrue.

Extended family therapy across cultures can involve polygamous families, as in the following case study.

Depression in a Polygynous Family

An 18-year-old refugee woman was referred for severe postpartum depression after the delivery of her first-born child. Her 35-year-old husband, who accompanied her to the intake, volunteered that he had developed the same condition since their arrival in the United States six months earlier. The common theme in their two stories was the loss of the "major wife" and several children from their family. The younger, second wife, orphaned during the flight out of her homeland, had been married to her husband in the refugee camp as a way of ensuring her a proper role in her culture. Prior to resettlement, American officials informed them that they could not relocate as a polygynous family. It was decided that the younger woman should become the "legal wife," because she was young, immature, and pregnant. The major wife would separate on her own, because she was able to run a household and look after the needs of their four children. Upon reaching the United States, the husband became depressed in association with missing his children and major wife. The younger wife also became depressed, because she had married anticipating that the major wife would be a mentor, guide, and comother in raising her child. Resolution of the couple's major depressive disorders involved addressing alternatives for reconstituting the family in an American context.

The hierarchical nature of family organization in some cultures may require interventions that resemble "shuttle diplomacy" more than therapy. The prevailing family system may not permit direct confrontation, but may abide meditation when families prove unable to settle an issue. Although village elders or religious leaders would have mediated these issues in the culture of origin, separation from these cultural resources may entail the therapist playing this role.

This role may require several separate meetings before the clinician can convene a meeting of all family members to address the family problem.

Group Therapy

This venue of care can offer an excellent entrée to understanding the day-to-day struggles experienced by those recovering from psychiatric disorders in a multi-cultural context. The works of Speck and Attneave (1974), Pattison and colleagues (Pattison, 1973, p. 396; 1977, p. 25), and Berne (1961) all impart valuable concepts for conducting cross-cultural group therapy. A key element is the language to be used in the group, because translation after each person speaks would slow down the communication considerably.

Several advantages accrue to conducting group therapy sessions with members from the same or similar ethnic groups. For one thing, they can often help one another to identify common challenges. As an example, a group of Hmong refugee women were having difficulty with transplanting a culturally important relationship—the mother-in-law/daughter-in-law dyad—into American society. In addition, group members can help one another find ways of coping with acculturation issues, including such mundane matters as transportation around town or survival issues such as obtaining a job.

Certain liabilities may limit the utility of this approach. Members of a small community, such as an urban ethnic group or a rural town or reservation, may demur from confiding highly personal or potentially embarrassing material to their neighbors and relatives. At times, patients may actually obtain more benefit in addressing such material by joining a group with whom they do not share ethnic affiliation.

PHARMACOTHERAPY ACROSS CULTURES

Patient Expectations

As indicated in chapter 12, "Psychopharmacology and Culture," numerous factors besides pharmacology guide pharmacotherapy in a cultural context. In some cases, ethnic factors may augur against medication. For example, depressed African Americans may be less likely to accept pharmacotherapy compared with Caucasians and Hispanic Americans (Cooper et al., 2003, p. 479). This reluctance among people of African descent could be the result of one or more of the following:

- Greater prevalence of side effects from medication (Fleck, Hendricks, DelBello, & Strakowski, 2002, p. 658; Taylor, 2004, p. 241)
- Fear of becoming dependent upon or addicted to medication (Fleck et al., 2002, p. 658)
- Propensity of clinicians in some studies to treat African Americans with higher doses or stronger medications (Fleck et al., 2002, p. 658)
- Higher symptoms when presenting for treatment, which could result in clinicians prescribing higher doses or stronger compounds, in turn causing some

African-American patients to avoid pharmacotherapy (Emsley, Roberts, Ratae-mane, Pretorius, Oosthuizen, Turner, Niehaus, Heyter, & Stein, 2002, p. 9), although the latter finding has not been universal (Barrio, Yamada, Atuel, Hough, Yee, Berthot, & Russo, 2003, p. 259)
- Therapeutic response to lower doses of some medications, such as antidepressants, compared with other groups (Varner, Ruiz, & Small, 1998, p. 117)

On the other hand, refugee and immigrant patients from other societies are often primed by previous experience to believe that a physician will provide them with medication. Failure to do so may suggest to the patient that the physician does not want to treat the patient (Lin, Anderson, & Poland, 1995, p. 635).

Adherence and Negotiated Treatment

Patients in cross-cultural situations may be reluctant to tell the physician that they do not want to take prescribed medication, or that they have discontinued a medication as a result of side effects, cost, or other factors. They may not want to disappoint the physician, or may fear a negative reaction when they want the physician's help. A more likely consequence is that the patient may simply stop the medication and not inform the clinician. Kinzie (1991) has reported that a large number of his refugee patients from Southeast Asia had negative tests for antidepressant medication despite their reporting that they were taking medication.

A potent antidote lies in the process of negotiated treatment described earlier (see also Figure 5.1). This process accomplishes the following therapeutic ends:

- The patient and family learn the clinician's rationale for recommending alternative treatments.
- The patient (and sometimes family) becomes an active partner in choosing and implementing treatment, thereby sharing in the success (or failure) of the treatment venture.
- The entire process of treatment is presented as a topic for open discussion and negotiation between patient, clinician, and (oftentimes) family, so that secret decisions regarding treatment nonadherence do not have an opportunity to drive a wedge into the patient–clinician collaboration.

Diet, Culture, and Pharmacotherapy

Diet can affect pharmacotherapy in several ways. A high-protein diet can increase serum albumin, which can in turn affect the level of protein-bound medication. If serum protein is low, the levels of unbound medication are higher. The unbound form of the drug is more apt to be biologically active (e.g., passing across the blood–brain barrier) as well as more available for metabolism and excretion. Small differences in serum albumin can exert large differences in both the pharmacokinetics and pharmacodynamics of a given drug.

With medications involving protein binding (most psychotropic medications, with exceptions such as lithium), lower serum albumin will result in high unbound serum levels (with possible toxic effects). However, lower serum albumin may favor a shorter duration of action, depending upon how the drug is metabolized and excreted. In dosing patients with lower serum albumin, the clinician should consider starting with lower doses and building up to a steady-state dosage more gradually.

Diet may also induce or increase certain enzyme activity, which can hasten medication metabolism and reduce blood levels and duration of medication effect (Lim, 2006). Other substances can inhibit enzyme activity, thereby retarding medication metabolism and leading to increased blood levels and duration of medication effect. These substances may exist in food stuffs, herbs added for taste, and herbal compounds consumed for therapeutic or recreational effects (Edie & Dewan, 2005, p. 17; Michalets, 1998, p. 84).

Hospitalization

Hospitals are located in all corners of the world, so people everywhere are familiar with them. At times people's images of hospitals are positive, so that inpatient admission may be quite acceptable to patients unfamiliar with American psychiatry. Hospitalization may offer solace, social approval for the sick role, relief of environmental stressors, and relief of suicidal impulses. It can signal the patient's and family's willingness to seek outside help for an overwhelming problem or crisis.

In other cases, hospitalization may not be acceptable. The patient or family may perceive hospitals as a place where "people go to die," or they may believe that psychiatric hospitalization inevitably involves long-term stays and institutionalization. Patients may fear loss of control, absence from family, abandonment by family, or being locked up. Even in these latter cases, the patient and family may be willing to negotiate hospitalization under certain circumstances.

Foreign Student With Paranoid Psychosis

A 26-year-old man developed a paranoid psychosis, with delusions focused on his sponsor, whom he planned to kill in reprisal for presumed offenses. The patient was unwilling to enter the hospital, because he feared he might be harmed. In recent days, he had relied on his wife to "protect" him from dangers that he perceived lurked everywhere. His wife told him she would be willing to stay with him and help him in assessing dangers. It was arranged for the wife to stay with him in his room. After the first 24 hours on the ward, the patient felt much safer and was willing to have her return home. He complied with care and was able to return to his studies.

At times, other arrangements can be negotiated with extended family members, as in the following case:

Urgently Suicidal Patient

A 43-year-old refugee man was urgently suicidal, in association with severe melancholic depression. He had previously been a prisoner of war in his homeland and could not willingly enter a locked inpatient unit. The assessment team informed the family of the urgent risk involved and the need for around-the-clock supervision for weeks, if a suicide were to be averted. The patient and family agreed to inpatient care if the patient were not much improved and no longer suicidal at the end of two weeks. During that time, the patient (with several relatives in tow) came to the outpatient center for reevaluation. Although this plan required the combined efforts of 20 relatives, it was successful and hospitalization was avoided.

Extended families are often familiar with organizing a contingent of relatives to provide around-the-clock help in crisis. However, even with this tradition, families can find the burden of this approach quite burdensome. In some cases, patients and families have agreed to hospitalization after a few days on this regimen. In many cases, it has also proved beneficial. It is important that the clinician understand the risk that he or she is assuming in such cases. Patient and family should sign a "memo of understanding" regarding the risk and benefit of this method.

Electroconvulsive Therapy (ECT)

Although many people from other cultures have not heard of ECT, nonetheless a general aversion exists toward the therapeutic use of electricity. Awareness of electricity and its painful, even lethal, effects prevails everywhere. Added to this is the general aversion to convulsions, which patients must appreciate to give informed consent. Despite these obstacles, ECT may be the only viable therapeutic alternative in longstanding cases of chronic affective psychosis. The following case exemplifies common themes in negotiating ECT in extreme cases.

Pol Pot Survivor

More than a decade before presentation, a 54-year-old Cambodian woman observed her husband and a son killed in front of her. To save herself and her other children, she could not show emotion at their violent deaths. During subsequent months, she received word that her parents, two siblings, and several other relatives had died of starvation or execution. She began to manifest signs of depression, with crying spells and insomnia. However, she continued to work to help her family. Two years later, as her relatives were recovering from their ordeal in a refugee camp, her condition worsened. She became socially isolated, could not regain weight, and was unable to cook, garden, or perform other familiar tasks. Her condition worsened in the United States, where she began sleeping all day and staying up at night, talking to herself, and complaining of seeing ghosts at night. She became convinced that she had been cursed and was dying of an incurable disease. Her behaviors become nonadaptive and even dangerous. On one occasion she started a fire in the family residence after putting a pot on the stove to boil water for tea and then forgetting about it. On another occasion she sustained an injury when she wondered out into traffic. On psychiatric evaluation she manifested somatic and nihilistic delusions, and both auditory and visual hallucinations. Electroconvulsive therapy was recommended but refused. During the subsequent year, several pharmacotherapy regimens were tried without effect. Eventually agreeing to ECT, she fully recovered and was able to resume household duties and even care of her new grandchild within a few weeks of her last ECT treatment.

This patient and her family became a source of education for other refugee families who were considering ECT for severe, refractory mood disorder.

SUMMARY

Care for mood disorder in a cross-cultural context does not differ fundamentally from care in which patient and clinician share a culture. On the contrary, competent cross-cultural care builds on the knowledge, skill, and experience that the clinician already possesses regarding mood disorders on one hand, and the nature of culture on the other. The key lies in the following few steps:

1. Considering those cultural beliefs, attitudes, and experiences that the patient and clinician do not share, especially with regard to the patient's clinical condition
2. Making these differing beliefs and attitudes explicit, especially as they involve the patient's clinical condition and its treatment
3. Discussing and negotiating these differing opinions and expectations so that the treatment outcome for both patient and clinician are salutary

ACKNOWLEDGMENT

David Johnson, MD, MPH, provided valuable critique and recommendations for this chapter.

REFERENCES

American Psychiatric Association. (1994). *Diagnostic and statistical manual of mental disorders* (4th ed.). Washington, DC: American Psychiatric Association.

Barrio, C., Yamada, A. M., Atuel, H., Hough, R. L., Yee, S., Berthot, B., & Russo, P. A. (2003). A tri-ethnic examination of symptom expression on the Positive and Negative Syndrome Scale in schizophrenia spectrum disorders. *Schizophrenia Research, 60*(2–3), 259–269.

Berne, E. (1961). *Transactional analysis in psychotherapy*. New York: Grove Press.

Blendon, R. J., Scheck, A. C., Donelan, K., Hill, C. A., Smith, M., Beatrice, D., & Altman, D. (1995). How white and African Americans view their health and social problems: Different experiences, different expectations. *Journal of the American Medical Association, 273*(4), 341–346.

Comas–Diaz, L., & Jacobsen, F. M. (1991). Ethno-cultural transference and countertransference in the therapeutic dyad. *American Journal Orthopsychiatry, 61*(3), 392–402.

Cooper, L. A., Gonzales, J. J., Gallo, J. J., Rost, K. M., Meredith, L. S., Rubenstein, L. V., Wang, N.-Y., & Ford, D. E. (2003). The acceptability of treatment for depression among African-American, Hispanic, and white primary care patients. *Medical Care, 41*(4), 479–489.

Davidson, L., & Strauss, J. J. (1995). Beyond the biopsychosocial model: Integrating disorder, health and recovery. *Psychiatry, 58*, 44–55.

Edie, C. F., & Dewan, N. (2005). Which psychotropics interact with four common supplements? *Current Psychiatry, 4*(1), 17–30.

Emsley, R. A., Roberts, M. C., Rataemane, S., Pretorius, J., Oosthuizen, P. P., Turner, J., Niehaus, D. J. H., Keyter, N., & Stein, D. J. (2002). Ethnicity and treatment response in schizophrenia: A comparison of 3 ethnic groups. *Journal Clinical Psychiatry, 63*, 9–14.

Fabrega, H. (1987). Psychiatric diagnosis: A cultural perspective. *Journal Nervous Mental Disorder, 175*, 383–394.

Fleck, D. E., Hendricks, W. L., DelBello, M. P., & Strakowski, S. M. (2002). Differential prescription of maintenance antipsychotics to African American and white patients with new-onset bipolar disorder. *Journal Clinical Psychiatry, 63*(8), 658–664.

Grinberg, L., & Grinberg, R. (1984). A psychoanalytic study of migration: Its normal and pathological aspects. *Journal American Psychoanalytic Association, 32*, 13–38.

Johnson, D. R., Feldman, S. C., Lubin, H., & Southwick, S. M. (1995). The therapeutic use of ritual and ceremony in the treatment of post-traumatic stress disorder. *Journal Traumatic Stress, 8*(2), 283–298.

Kinzie, J. D. (1991). Development, staffing, and structure of psychiatric services. In J. Westermeyer, C. L. Williams, & A. N. Nguyen (Eds.), *Mental health services for refugees*. Washington, DC: Government Printing Office.

Koss, J. D. (1990). Somatization and somatic complaint syndromes among Hispanics: Overview and ethnopsychological perspectives. *Transcultural Psychiatric Research Review, 27*, 5–29.

Lim, R. F. (2006). *Clinical manual of cultural psychiatry*. Washington, DC: American Psychiatric Publishing, 146–156.

Lin, K.-M., Anderson, D., & Poland, R. E. (1995). Ethnicity and psychopharmacology: Bridging the gap. *Psychiatric Clinics of North America, 18*, 635–647.

Littlewood, R., & Lipsedge, M. (1987). The butterfly and the serpent: Culture, psychopathology and biomedicine. *Culture, Medicine and Psychiatry, 11*, 289–335.

Lu, F., Lim, R. F., & Mezzich, J. E. (1995). Issues in the assessment and diagnosis of culturally diverse individuals. In P. Ruiz (Ed.), *Annual review of psychiatry* (Vol. 14). Washington, DC: American Psychiatric Press.

Lukoff, D., Lu, F., & Turner, R. P. (1995). Cultural considerations in the assessment and treatment of religious and spiritual problems. *Psychiatric Clinics of North America, 18*, 467–485.

Michalets, E. L. (1998). Clinical significant cytochrome P450 drug interactions. *Pharmacotherapy, 18*(1), 84–112.

Moore, L. J., & Boehnlein, J. K. (1991). Treating psychiatric disorders among Mien refugees from highland Laos. *Social Science Medicine*, 32(9), 1029–1036.

Muskin, P. R. (Ed.). (2000). *Complementary and alternative medicine and psychiatry* (Vol. 19). Washington, DC: American Psychiatric Press.

Pattison, E. M. (1973). Social system psychotherapy. *American Journal of Psychotherapy*, 27, 396–409.

Pattison, E. M. (1977). Clinical social systems interventions. *Psychiatry Digest*, 38, 25–33.

Pelz, M., Merskey, H., Brant, C., Patterson, P. G., & Heseltine, G. F. (1981). Clinical data from a psychiatric service to a group of native people. *Canadian Journal of Psychiatry*, 26(5), 345–348.

Speck, R. W., & Attneave, C. (1974). *Family networks*. New York: Vintage Books.

Spiegel, J. P. (1976). Cultural aspects of transference and countertransference revisited. *Journal of the American Academy of Psychoanalysis*, 4, 447–467.

Szapocnik, J., Santisteban, D., Kurtines, W. M., Perez–Vidal, A., & Hervis, O. E. (1984). Bicultural effectiveness training: A treatment intervention for enhancing intercultural adjustment in Cuban American families. *Hispanic Journal of Behavioral Sciences*, 6(4), 317–344.

Taylor, D. M. (2004). Prescribing of clozapine and olanzapine: Dosage, polypharmacy, and patient ethnicity. *Psychiatric Bulletin*, 28, 241–243.

Varner, R. V., Ruiz, P., & Small, D. R. (1998). Black and white patients' response to antidepressant treatment for major depression. *Psychiatric Quarterly*, 69(2), 117–125.

Weiss, M. G., Doongaji, D. R., Siddhartha, S., Wypij, D., Pathare, S., Bhatawdekar, M., et al. (1992). The Explanatory Model Interview Catalogue (EMIC): Contribution to cross-cultural research methods from a study of leprosy and mental health. *British Journal of Psychiatry*, 160, 819–830.

Westermeyer, J. (1979). Folk concepts of mental disorder among the Lao: Continuities with similar concepts in other cultures and in psychiatry. *Culture, Medicine and Psychiatry*, 3(3), 301–317.

Westermeyer, J. (1982). Ethnic factors in treatment. In E. M. Pattison & E. Kaufman (Eds.), *The American encyclopedic handbook of alcoholism* (pp. 709–717). New York: Gardner Press.

Westermeyer, J. (1985). Psychiatric diagnosis across cultural boundaries. *American Journal of Psychiatry*, 142(7), 798–805.

Westermeyer, J. (1996). Alcoholism among New World peoples: A critique of history, methods, and findings. *American Journal of Addictions*, 5(2), 110–123.

Westermeyer, J., & Wintrob, R. W. (1979a). "Folk" criteria for the diagnosis of mental illness in rural Laos: On being insane in sane places. *American Journal of Psychiatry*, 136(6), 755–761.

Westermeyer, J., & Wintrob, R. W. (1979b.) "Folk" explanations of mental illness in rural Laos. *American Journal of Psychiatry*, 136(7), 901–905.

6

Health Care Seeking and Access

EARNESTINE WILLIS & SHERYL E. ALLEN

For centuries in the United States, mental health treatment and access to services have been influenced by an array of factors that includes ideologies of mental health reforms, reimbursement for mental health services, scientific advancements in treatment and technology, institutional response shifts, and the development of mental health professionals. This chapter focuses on mental health services, which are plagued with disparities in the availability of and access to effective services, according to *Mental Health: A Report of the Surgeon General* (U.S. Department of Health and Human Services, Substance Abuse and Mental Health Services Administration, Center for Mental Health Services, 1999). To reduce the burden of mental illness in our nation, it is imperative that we expand our knowledge and research about effective mental health services by examining health care-seeking preferences and utilization patterns, specifically for the common presenting conditions of mood disorders. As mental health services are designed and implemented, we must take into account existing challenges that patients face in the utilization of our mental health system, such as barriers and cultural factors in patients' selection processes. It has been well recognized that some populations experience major disparities in mental health services and those disparities span from access to care, appropriateness of care, insurance coverage and language, and cultural differences between providers and patients (Smedley, Stith, & Nelson, 2003).

HEALTH CARE SEEKING

In the overall U.S. population, the prevalence of any mental health disorders among children/adolescents and adults is 21% and 28%, respectively (Table 6.1). However, data from the Surgeon General's report on mental health referenced earlier reveals that in any one year, only 15% of children utilize mental health services (U.S. Department of Health and Human Services, Substance Abuse and Mental Health Services Administration, Center for Mental Health Services, 1999). Researchers have reported that within the same population that is diagnosed with mental health disorders within a one year period, approximately 11% of the children/adolescents and 20% of the adults receive no mental health services. For populations receiving mental health services, approximately 13.2% of children/adolescents and 9% of adults seek other mental health services from alternative sources, including social service agencies, schools, and religious or voluntary support such as self-help groups (Kessler, Nelson, McKinagle, Edlund, Frank, & Keaf, 1996; Regier, Narrow, Rae, Manderscheid, Locke, & Goodwin, 1993; Shaffer, Fisher, Dulcan, Davies, Piacentini, Schwab–Stone, & Lahey, 1996). It appears that for one fourth of the estimated 50 million Americans who experience a mental health disorder and seek mental health services, approximately 7.1% of American adults and 6.2% of children/adolescents suffer from mood disorders in any one year (U.S. Department of Health and Human Ser-

Table 6.1 U.S. One-Year Prevalence of Mental Health Disorders and Addictive Disorders, and Receiving Mental Health Services for Adults and Children/Adolescents

	Total Prevalence	Population with Mental/Addictive Disorders		Population Receiving MHS		Population with Treatment Overlapping MHS in the Human Sector
		Diagnosis + Treatment	Diagnosis + No Treatment	Treatment + Diagnosis	Treatment + No Diagnosis	
Any mental disorders for children/adolescents	21%	10%	11%	10%	11%	13.2%
Anxiety disorders	13.0%					
Mood disorders	6.2%					
Others	1.8%					
Any mental disorders for adults	28%	8%	20%	8%	7%	9%
Anxiety disorders	16.4%					
Mood disorders	7.1%					
Others	4.5%					

For those who use more than one sector of mental health services to include receiving general medical care, school services, human services, and voluntary support with preferential assignment given to the most specialized level of mental health treatment in the system.

Adapted from Shaffer and colleagues (1996), Regier and colleagues (1993) and U.S. Department of Health and Human Services, Substance Abuse and Mental Health Services Administration, Center for Mental Health Services (1999).

vices, Substance Abuse and Mental Health Services Administration, Center for Mental Health Services, 1999).

In most circumstances, seeking mental health services begins with a person or parent presenting with symptoms of functional impairment in thought processes, mood, or behaviors; someone interpreting the symptoms as treatable; someone deciding to seek medical assistance; someone deciding from whom to seek treatment; and someone receiving the mental health care and then someone deciding whether to sustain or continue with the recommended treatment plan (Kessler, Nelson, McKinagle, Edlund, Frank, & Keaf, 1996; Regier, Narrow, Rae, Manderscheid, Locke, & Goodwin, 1993). As an example, mothers with major affective disorders frequently have difficulties with tasks of day-to-day parenting and meeting their children's basic needs (Miller, 1997; Mowbray, Oyserman, & Bybee, 2000; Oyserman, Mowbray, Mears, et al., 2000). After adjusting for the type of treatment, race or ethnicity, and age, mothers with serious mental illness are almost three times more likely to have come to the attention of the child welfare system or to have lost custody of their children. This is an example of a concern that would provide a disincentive to obtain treatment among women with mental health needs. This suggests the need for greater awareness of these issues among mental health professionals, plus an urgent need for increased planning and coordination between child welfare and mental health systems (Park, Solomon, & Mandell, 2006).

Lin and colleagues (1982) examined the help-seeking processes in mental illnesses by analyzing the correlation of ethnicity with pathways to mental health services and the first contact and initiation of mental health treatments. Race and ethnicity were shown to be correlated with delays in seeking help for mental illnesses either in first contact or commitment to a treatment regimen. As illustrated in Table 6.2, Asians showed the longest mean delay and treatment (mean delay, 2.9 years for contact and 4.3 years for treatment) compared with African Americans (mean delay, 2.2 years for contact and 2.9 years for treatment) and whites (mean delay, 0.9 years for contact and 1.6 years for treatment). Asians and African Americans appear to have had more extended family involvement in their mental health interventions whereas only in Asian families were key family members more persistent and intensely involved. Additional studies are needed to determine how delay and pathway types are factors chosen in untreated populations with mental illnesses (Lin, Inui, Kleinman, & Womack, 1982).

Table 6.2 Mean Mental Health Services Delays in Years and Commitment to Treatment by Race/Ethnicity

Race/Ethnicity	First Signs and Symptoms	Commitment to Treatment Regimen
Asians	2.9	4.3
African Americans	2.2	2.9
Whites	0.9	1.6

Adapted from Lin et al. (1997).

Table 6.3 Reasons for Not Seeking Mental Health Services

Cost	Uninsured or underinsured status presents a significant barrier and results in disparities in access to mental services; represents 83% of the publically insured and 55% of the privately insured
Inability to obtain appointment	Few culturally identified providers for racial/ethnic populations, 59% of Medicaid users
Self-help and self-reliance for intervention	Reliance on traditional healers and other leaders more familiar with cultural practices
Mistrust	Based on historical experiences of segregation, racism, language barriers, immigration status, and discrimination
Clinician bias	Overdiagnosis of certain conditions or misdiagnosis of mental health disorders in certain racial/ethnic populations
Stigma and denial	Embarrassment and lack of awareness about the availability of mental health specialists

Adapted from Sussman (1987), Uba (1994), Snowden and Cheung (1990), Lawson (1994), Kessler and colleagues (1996), and Regier and colleagues (1993).

A national household telephone survey among those known to have a mental health disorder, sponsored by the Robert Wood Johnson Foundation, investigated the reasons people reported for not seeking mental health services (Table 6.3). Those with a perceived mental health or addictive disorder who did not seek care most frequently expressed concerns about cost. This is estimated to represent 83% of the uninsured and 55% of the privately insured population. Fifty-nine percent of the Medicaid population reported an inability to obtain an appointment, whereas many others believed that the problem would go away without intervention (Kessler, Nelson, McKinagle, Edlund, Frank, & Keaf, 1996; Regier, Narrow, Rae, Manderscheid, Locke, & Goodwin, 1993). The stigma and denial associated with being labeled as mentally ill may be associated with the lack of awareness of availability of mental health specialists. Clinician bias in the overdiagnosis of certain conditions or the misdiagnosis of others may contribute to an unwillingness to seek health services. Mistrust of providers from a different racial/ethnic background is grounded in a historical legacy of segregation, racism, discrimination, language barriers, and immigration status. Therefore, many racial/ethnic populations rely upon traditional healers and other leaders they feel are more familiar with their cultural practices.

UTILIZATION PATTERNS

Utilization of mental health services is complex and varies within populations (Table 6.4). Approximately 6% of the adult population uses specialty mental health care, 5% receives their mental health services from general medical,

Table 6.4 Utilization of Mental Health Services by
Different Sources for Children, Adolescents, and Adults

Children/adolescents (9–17 y)	21%
Specialty mental health providers	8%
General medical care	1.1%
School services	11%
Other human services and voluntary support	1.1%
Adults (18–54 y)	15%
Specialty mental health providers	6%
General medical care	5%
Other human services and voluntary support	4%

Overlap exists for those who use more than one sector of the service system.
Preferential assignment is given to the most specialized level of mental health
treatment in the system.
   Adapted from Shaffer and colleagues (1996), Regier and colleagues (1993),
Kessler and colleagues (1996), and the U.S. Office of Technology (1986).

providers and 4% receives services from human services providers or self-help groups (Kessler, Nelson, McKinagle, Edlund, Frank, & Keaf, 1996; Regier, Narrow, Rae, Manderscheid, Locke, & Goodwin, 1993). There is overlap in the latter two groups; more than half also seek services from mental health specialists for mental health and addictive disorders. This same survey estimated that during a one-year period, about 44 million adults have a diagnosable mental health disorder according to reliable and established diagnostic criteria, 3% have both mental health and addictive disorders, and 6% have an addictive disorder alone. However, only 15% of adults received mental health services and a majority, or more than two thirds of adults with mental health disorders, do not seek any type of treatment (Kessler, Nelson, McKinagle, Edlund, Frank, & Keaf, 1996).

Children/adolescents seeking mental health services can be grouped according to low-income or special needs using the Medicaid-eligible categories. When considering low-income programs, Zito and colleagues (2005) and Shone and associates (2003), examined computerized claims of children and youth continuously enrolled in a mid-Atlantic state, and many racial/ethnic groups were on Temporary Assistance to Needy Families (TANF) and the State Children's Heath Insurance Program (SCHIP). Since 1996, TANF has targeted families with income at or below the federal poverty level. Among near-poor families who qualify for SCHIP, typically they are living between 100% to 200% of the federal poverty threshold. The special-needs Medicaid-eligible categories include both children with documented disabilities (developmental or chronic physical and/or mentally disabling condition) who are entitled to Social Security Income (SSI) and children in out-of-home placement (foster care).

For one year, Zito and colleagues (2005) reviewed Medicaid claims for 189,486 youth, age 2 to 19 years old, who were continuously enrolled in the Medicaid program to determine how Medicaid eligibility categories contributed to disparities between African American and white youths in the prevalence of psychotropic medication. White youth were 2.17 times more likely than African American youth to have been given psychotropic medications. However, the disparity ratios between whites and African Americans were significantly lower for utilization of the psychotropic medications for children in the SSI and foster care groups (2.2 fold) than for children in TANF and SCHIP (3.8 and 3.2 fold, respectively). Psychotropic utilization in the SCHIP group was similar to that in the TANF group, although there was up to a sixfold lower difference in usage for the SCHIP group compared with the SSI and foster care groups. From this study it appears that Medicaid eligibility influences the use of psychotropic medication patterns among youth. This should be considered when examining access, culture, and undertreatment of children in racial/ethnic groups (Zito et al., 2005).

Shaffer and colleagues (1996) did a similar survey with children/adolescents and found that 21% of children/adolescents 9 to 17 years of age had some evidence of mental impairment associated with a specific diagnosis. Almost half of this group had some treatment in one or more sectors of the mental health service system, and the remainder (11%) received no treatment in any sector of the health care system. Clearly, the proportion of persons needing mental health services does not match the utilization of providers, but the mismatch is compounded by many factors such as sociocultural and economic factors, insurance plans, and reluctance by the populations experiencing the functional impairments to seek mental health services (Shaffer, Fisher, Dulcan, Davies, Piacentini, Schwab-Stone & Lahey, 1996).

Shaffer and colleagues (1996) also found that about 9% of the entire sample of children/adolescents received some mental health services within the health care delivery sector. The largest mental health providers for this population (11%) were the school systems exclusively, and another 5% of children/adolescents received school-based mental health services in addition to mental health services in the health care sector. One percent of the children/adolescents received their mental health service from human service professionals such as child welfare and juvenile justice system providers (Shaffer, Fisher, Dulcan, Davies, Piacentini, Schwab-Stone, & Lahey, 1996).

Since the 1980s, interventions for mental illnesses in children/adolescents have shifted from institutional to community-based services, with the range of services including case management, home-based services, therapeutic foster care, therapeutic group homes, and crisis services. These same models are being developed for older adults. Children and youth with emotional and behavioral disorders and severe emotional disorders are the most vulnerable populations. Children diagnosed with emotional and behavioral disorders and treated in residential and semiresidential mental health care settings showed a 4:1 boy-to-girl gender ratio (D'Oosterlinck, Broekaert, DeWilde, Bockaert, & Goethals, 2006). A similar gender proportion has been observed in the international literature. Girls are more frequently diagnosed with mental health problems related to abuse or neglect, separation anxiety, and reactive attachment disorders, whereas boys are more frequently diagnosed with attention deficit–hyperactivity disorder (ADHD), conduct disorders, and pervasive developmental disorders. Most European and

U.S. mainstream school systems are not well equipped to cope with the disruptive, aggressive behaviors of children with mental health disorders.

According to the U.S. Office of Technology Assessment (1986), about 70% of children/adolescents in need of mental health services do not get these services, and 75% to 80% of children do not receive health specialty services (U.S. Office of Technology Assessment, 1986). Researchers have reported that families are most likely to attribute underutilization to the demanding nature of the treatments, the stigma that is associated with mental illness, dissatisfaction with services, cost of treatment, and reluctance of the parents and/or children to seek treatment (Kazdin, Holland, & Crowley, 1997; Pavuluri, Luk, & McGee, 1996). According to Kazdin and colleagues (1997), about 40% to 60% of the families who begin treatment terminate it prematurely. The premature dropout rates may be the result, in part, of the arrangement/orchestration of the mental health appointments by the schools, courts, and other agencies for impoverished families, thereby increasing the probability of dropping out of services (Pavuluri, Luk & McGee,1996).

Even though we know that fewer children receive mental health services than those who need it, it is not known whether the utilization of services varies by race and ethnicity for children. Studies from California demonstrate that African American youths are overrepresented in arrests, detention, and incarceration in the juvenile justice system and also in public school classes for the severely mentally disturbed. Latino children are more likely to be detained than white children in the juvenile justice system and the child welfare system. This early involvement causes them to remain in the system longer (McCabe, Yeh, Hough, Landsverk, Hurlburt, Culver, & Reynolds, 1998). Both African American and Latino children drop out of mental health services more frequently than white children. Woodward and colleagues (1992) attributed the dropout patterns to the insensitivity of mental health providers to the culture of the children and their families. Specialized mental health programs with supports linked to the culture of the community being served have been found to be successful in promoting favorable patterns of service utilization for all age groups (Hu, Snowden, Jerrell, & Nguyen, 1991; Snowden & Cheung, 1990).

Chow and colleagues (2003) demonstrated differences in utilization rates, diagnoses, and patterns of mental health treatments for African Americans, Latinos, and Asian Americans. Racial/ethnic groups are underrepresented in outpatient mental health care and, for certain groups, are overrepresented in inpatient and emergency treatment (Hu, Snowden, Jerrell, & Nguyen, 1991; Snowden & Cheung, 1990). Although Asians are more likely to use emergency room services for mental disorders, they are less likely to be referred by the usual recognized sources (self-referral, family, friends, social service system, and criminal justice system), and they seek mental health services only as a last resort (Sue & Morishima, 1982; Uba, 1994). The survey by Swindle and colleagues (1997) of racial/ethnic populations revealed that these groups are more likely to cope with mental illnesses now by seeking informal social support such as self-help groups, whereas those who seek formal support increasingly show a preference for counselors, psychologists, and social workers.

CULTURAL CONSIDERATIONS
IN SELECTION OF PROVIDERS

The relationship between culture and mental illness can be summarized as resting on shared beliefs within cultural groups that reflect the ideal, "proper or normal" way for individuals to conduct their lives in relation to others. These shared beliefs and actions encompass relevant behaviors; appropriate dress, posture, and hairstyle; smell; facial gestures and expressions; language; and tone of voice. Because most cultures have a wide range of social norms that are acceptable for different age groups, genders, occupations, social ranks, and so forth, displays of behaviors that are temporarily "abnormal" must be weighed against the background of the cultures in which they appear.

For providers whose patients' demographics are predominantly among the high-risk racial/ethnic groups seeking mental health services, an understanding of the structural impediments, cultural characteristics, beliefs, values, and stressors that contribute to mental illnesses is necessary to provide effective treatment. The influence of cultural experiences on psychopathology is intertwined with interpersonal expectations, self-concepts, styles of communication, and coping mechanisms within different cultural groups. It is not clear whether culturally oriented life experiences increase vulnerability or protect against the development of psychopathology. In addition, it is also undetermined whether the DSM-IV-defined categories are culturally standardized for the general population or are adaptable to subethnic subgroups of a population, such as specific Asian subgroups or Native American tribes. It is imperative that mental health providers be able to recognize and deal with differences in cultural values and their effects — negative and positive — on countertransference. Understanding the importance of cultural factors, such as prescribed gender roles, immigration experiences, language, cultural explanations of illness, religious beliefs, customary dietary practices, and non-Western/nonmainstream treatments for the management of mental disorders is essential if health care providers are to be effective in their planned treatment regimens (Foulks, 2004).

For many patients of racial/ethnic backgrounds consistent with Africian Americans, Asian-Pacific Islanders, Latinos, Native Americans, etc., psychotherapy is a foreign and a strange experience. A fear of exposure to culturally insensitive mental health professionals and feelings of discomfort with the fundamental values and goals of Western psychotherapy can be a deterrent to prevent some people of color from accessing formal mental health treatments (Constantine, 2002; Nickerson, Helms, & Terrell, 1994). It is well recognized that mental health providers from racial/ethnic groups are more likely to treat patients from similar backgrounds, thus they have good success in retaining their patients in treatment plans. Mental health programs oriented to racial/ethnic populations have been reported to achieve greater representation from the racial/ethnic population than other mental health settings (Sue, Fujino, Hu, Takeuchi, & Zane, 1991). These programs seem to succeed by maintaining active and committed relationships with community institutions and leaders, having aggressive outreach efforts, and having an open, familiar, and welcoming environment for members of the targeted racial/ethnic group, which helps patients feel more comfortable expressing themselves. The challenge for these models and existing mental health programs for the majority population is to meet sociocultural needs for a more diverse client constituent (Yeh, Takeuchi, & Sue, 1994).

Most mental health disorders have a range of treatments with evidence-based efficacy. These include counseling, psychosocial, pharmacotherapy, rehabilitation, ECT, ethnopsychopharmacology, and interactive and play therapy. Even though the research is limited, multimodal therapies for children and adults have been shown to be more efficacious. The term *efficacious* is referred to when the evidence has been generated in a research-controlled setting, as opposed to when one refers to *effectiveness*, which is usually used to indicate that the treatment has been evaluated in an actual practice setting. All too frequently, persons who have mental health problems or who have been told that they have symptoms consistent with a mood disorder find that the availability of culturally compatible mental health care providers and/or accessibility to mental health services are quite limited.

For Native Americans, it is important to consider the large variability with respect to language, culture, beliefs, acculturation, and dual culture. It is not uncommon for intermarriage and cultural blending to influence families across multiple racial, tribal, and lingual groups. For example, Constantine (2002) notes that the traditional Navajo understanding of health and illness revolves around the concepts of balance or harmony and is rooted in the cosmology of Navajo spiritual belief. This concept is so deeply embedded within the Navajo culture that the physical, emotional, and spiritual facets of life are completely intertwined. Some psychological illnesses may be described as physical manifestations, such as describing depression as feeling more tired or not being able to do things the way one use to do. For some tribal members, it is culturally taboo to talk about health issues or illness. The act of speaking is considered to be powerful, and language does not just describe reality; language shapes reality (Carrese & Rhodes, 1995). Cultural identity communicates distinct beliefs and practices within racial/ethnic groups, and some of these are coping styles and linkages to family and community resources.

African Americans and Asian Americans place emphasis on having the willpower to minimize the significance of stress, and are encouraged to prevail and strive in the face of adversity. For African Americans, there is a tradition of extended families functioning within political, economic, social, and religious affiliations. Most racial/ethnic groups (African Americans, Asian Americans, and Latinos) believe that religion and spirituality favorably impact their lives, and that well-being, good health, and religion are integrally intertwined (Bacote, 1994; Pargament, 1997).

As research on health disparity evolves in clinical encounters, health care providers and patients must be examined to assess the impact that racial/ethnic bias might contribute to disparate health outcomes as appropriate targets for interventions (Smedley, Stith & Nelson, 2003). Professionals in mental health must practice nondiscriminatory approaches to care, and move both systems and individuals within the systems forward to address poor levels of cultural awareness when it comes to race, gender, and institutionalized discriminatory practices.

BARRIERS

Research indicates that many individuals from racial and ethnic populations fear or do not feel at ease within the mental health system. These groups refer to the mental health system as products of white European cultures, with their cultural values and beliefs consistent with those of Europeans, as well as having the biases, misconceptions, and stereotypes of other cultures (Lin, Inui, Kleinman & Womack 1982; Scheffler & Miller, 1991; Sussman, Robins, & Earls, 1987). Repeatedly, experts have attributed the gaps between those who have mental health disorders and those who seek mental health services to the stigma surrounding mental disorders, the discrimination that exists in the insurance companies, and a lack of access to and availability of health care providers with similar cultural beliefs and values to those seeking the services in communities. Patients may fear hospitalization, lack time, think they can handle the situation without interventions, and fear the stigmatization that is associated with having a mental disorder (Brown & Bradley, 2001).

In addition, barriers to seeking mental health services can go beyond previously stated variables to be inclusive of patient attitudes toward a service system that has a track record of neglecting the needs of racial and ethnic groups when it comes to financial, organizational, and geographic factors. Sussman and colleagues (1987) and Gallo and associates (1995) documented that compared with whites, African Americans, Latinos, and low-income women are least likely to seek mental health treatment. Even though many of the same populations have health insurance, they believe that existing mental health services will not consider their cultural and linguistic practices when addressing their mental health needs. Lack of trust of the white majority population can be put into a contextual perspective for most of the racial/ethnic groups who do not readily seek mental health services. Mistrust among African Americans may have its origins in their experience with segregation, racism, and discrimination. Undocumented immigrants are more likely to mistrust authorities because of a fear of being deported. People from South America may have witnessed imprisonment or government abuse or murder of family members, or may have been refugees themselves. Historically, Native Americans' mistrust may be similar to that of African Americans, in that it derives from forced control, segregation on reservations, and discrimination (Gallo, Marino, Ford & Anthony, 1995; Sussman, Robins & Earls, 1987).

Cost is another major deterrent to seeking mental health care. Health care plans often place limitations on the availability of and accessibility to mental health services through the imposition of copayments and deductibles. Other costs include time away from work, transportation to and from the health care setting, and possibly childcare arrangements. Organizational barriers include the fragmentation of services and the provision of few, if any, culturally similar health care providers in the area of mental health. However, one significant barrier for children and youth with mental health symptoms is the shortage of child psychiatrists, appropriately trained clinical child psychologists, or social workers to consult (Thomas & Holzer, 1999).

Shone and colleagues (2003) concluded that ensuring access to mental health services is not sufficient, in and of itself, to ensure utilization among nonwhite enrollees. Studies conducted by Bauer and colleagues (2005) examined barriers confronting patients in the Veteran Affairs (VA) medical system who sought mental health treatment and reached a similar conclusion. Investigators assessed a diagnostically heterogeneous population in the VA primary and mental health clinics to quantify the overall level of perceived barriers, determine whether barriers are greater in participants from vulnerable populations (mental health symptoms, disabled underserved minorities and elder individuals), explore the underlying conceptual structure of perceived barriers, and examine whether those from vulnerable populations experience specific subtypes of barriers. In general, they recognized that health care access constitutes a significant contributor to health outcomes. Those in treatment for mental health symptoms expressed greater perceived barriers in travel difficulties, communication, and system glitches within the health care system. System glitches were defined to reflect difficulties navigating the health care site, physically or bureaucratically. Surprisingly, racial/ethnic participants (African Americans, American Indians, Latinos, Asians/Pacific Islanders) perceived no specific barriers, and the elderly reported fewer barriers. Those with disabilities perceived greater barriers in communication and system glitches, whereas the younger group reported significant barriers in travel, communication, and lifetime goals. This study demonstrated that patients participating in care may perceive barriers to their care, even when insurance is not a significant concern. The underlying conceptual structure to perceived barriers appears multidimensional. For vulnerable populations, researchers have noted that the barriers are not necessarily the same for all subpopulations (Bauer, Williford, McBride, & Shea, 2005).

Increasingly, evidence supports the contribution of provider attitudes and discriminatory behaviors to the existence of health disparities (Smedley, Stith & Nelson, et al. 2003). In health care there is substantial evidence that patient categories such as race/ethnicity, gender, age, sexual orientation, and socioeconomic status influence providers' beliefs about and expectations of patients. For example, individual patients many times are perceived by providers in ways that are consistent with stereotypes, but may be inaccurate for those patients, even though information about patients and their levels of education was contained in the medical records (Revenson, 1989; Van Ryn & Burke, 2000). Although attending to and processing individual information requires considerable cognitive resources, extensive evidence supports that automatic, rather than conscious, effortful thoughts and feelings dominate when we are busy with other tasks, distracted, tired, or under time pressure and are anxious (Macrae, Milne, & Bodenhausen, 1994). Providers, like all humans, are more likely to rely on stereotypes for "out-of-group members" (people not belonging to the same racial or ethnic group), thereby treating them as homogeneous populations, drawing few distinctions between them and stereotyped characteristics, and paying less attention to their individual characteristics. The strongest evidence of provider bias has been documented for African Americans with schizophrenia and depression. Several studies found that African Americans were more likely than whites to be diagnosed with schizophrenia, yet less likely to be diagnosed with depression (Hu, Snowden, Jerrell, & Nguyen, 1991; Lawson, Hepler, Hooaday, & Cuffel, 1994; Snowden & Cheung, 1990).

Often individuals who have physical disabilities in addition to a mental illness diagnosis face specific problems in accessing health care services. Delayed or denied access to needed health services can lead to negative consequences for the individuals' health, well-being, independence, and quality of life. In medicine, discrimination on the grounds of race, gender, sexual orientation, low-income levels, and lack of health insurance is increasingly acknowledged, but discrimination against disabled individuals also persists despite the Americans with Disability Act. Disabled persons often identify inappropriate staff attitudes and behaviors as the biggest barrier to using health services. Barriers for this group result in a diverse set of consequences that include social, psychological, physical, economic, and independent lives of the individuals with disabilities. Greater disability literacy would provide people with disabilities with more appropriate care in that health care providers would recognize their need for timely services and referrals. Enhanced disability literacy in the health insurance plans would also offer adequate coverage for maintenance and rehabilitation therapies. Environmental barriers are beginning to be addressed as the federal government calls for reduction of physical barriers in homes, schools, workplaces, and other community settings, and continues to address accessibility for racial/ethnic groups to mental health care providers (Neri & Kroll, 2003).

TYPE AND QUALITY OF CARE

It has been well established that drug metabolism is influenced by genetic variations and cultural practices such as diet, medication adherence, placebo effect, and simultaneous use of traditional and alternative health methods. For example, approximately one third of African Americans and Asians are slow to metabolize several antipsychotic medications and antidepressants. Instead, these patients are started on lower doses, and typically they have not experienced extrapyramidal side effects (Lin, Anderson, & Poland, 1997). Psychosocial factors can complicate therapeutic approaches and hinder adherence to a prescription regimen, whereas reliance on alternative health methods like medicinal plants and herbs may interact with prescribed medications.

Researchers have suggested that if providers are made aware of particular situations in which racial and ethnic groups receive inferior care, they may be motivated to reexamine their initial clinical decision for the possibilities of bias and thus correct their decision. Other studies suggest that structural changes in the health care delivery system that would permit health care providers to spend more time with their mental health patients might help to reduce some of the disparities while at the same time allowing for providers to incorporate self-assessment interventions into the components of their sessions. In the social cognition literature, patient–provider relationships can benefit from interpersonal skills such as active listening, relationship building, and communication skills; however, although these skills are fundamental and necessary, they may not be sufficient to foster high-quality and equitable health care (Constantine & Kwan, 2003).

On the other hand, therapist self-disclosure may provide a modeling function to help demystify the therapeutic process for many racial/ethnic groups and encourage patients' self-disclosure. Appropriate therapist self-disclosure with racial/ethnic groups requires that therapists (a) be aware of their own and the patients' cultural values, along with an awareness of the interactive impact of these values in treatment; (b) be knowledgeable about the cultural experience of their racial/ethnic groups and the effects of these experiences on the patients' presenting issues and on the therapeutic relationship; and (c) skillfully, sensitively, and competently respond to racial/ethnic groups based on individual information (Constantine & Kwan, 2003).

Family ties and community resources play an essential role in providing support to individuals with mental health problems, especially immigrants of many racial/ethnic groups (Africans, Latinos, Asians, Native Americans, Mexican Americans, and Asian Americans). Serious emotional disturbances with children/adolescents are best addressed by using a system approach in which multiple service sectors work together to achieve positive functional outcomes for children. Families can be enlisted and appreciated as essential partners in the delivery of mental health services for children/adolescents to provide resources, to serve as decision makers, and to contribute to the welfare and growth of other members of the family.

REFERENCES

Bacote, J. C. (1994). Transcultural psychiatric nursing: Diagnostic and treatment issues. *Journal of Psychosocial Nursing, 32*, 42–46.

Bauer, M. S., Williford, W. O., McBride, K., & Shea. N. M. (2005). Perceived barriers to health care access in a treated population. *International Journal of Psychiatry in Medicine, 35*(1), 13–26.

Brown, K., & Bradley, L. J. (2001). Reducing the stigma of mental illness. *Journal of Mental Health Counseling, 24*(1), 81–87.

Carrese, J. A., & Rhodes, I. A. (1995). Western bioethics on the Navajo reservation: Benefit or harm? *Journal of the American Medical Association, 274*(10), 826–829.

Chow, J. C., Jaffee, K., & Snowden, L. (2003). Racial/ethnic disparities in the use of mental health services in poverty areas. *American Journal of Public Health, 93*(5), 792–797.

Constantine, M.G. (2002). Predictors of satisfaction with counseling: Racial and ethnic minority patients' attitude toward counseling and ratings of their counselors' general and multicultural counseling competence. *Journal of Counseling Psychology, 49*, 255–263.

Constantine, M. G., & Kwan, K. K. (2003). Cross-cultural considerations of therapist self disclosure. *Journal of Clinical Psychology, 59*(5), 581–588.

D'Oosterlinck, F., Broekaert, E., DeWilde, J., Bockaert, L. F., & Goethals, I. (2006). Characteristics and profile of boys and girls with emotional and behavioral disorders in Flanders mental health institutes: A quantitative study. *Child: Care, Health & Development, 34*(2), 213–224.

Foulks, E. F. (2004). Commentary: Racial bias in diagnosis and medication of mentally ill minorities in prisons and communities. *The Journal of the American Academy of Psychiatry and the Law, 32*(1), 46.

Gallo, J. J. S. D., Marino, S., Ford, D., & Anthony, J. C. (1995). Filters on the pathway to mental health care, II. Sociodemographic factors. *Psychological Medicine, 25,* 1149–1160.

Hu, T., Snowden, L., Jerrell, J., & Nguyen, T. (1991). Ethnic population in public mental health: Services choice and level of use. *American Journal of Public Health, 81,* 1429–1434.

Kazdin, A. E., Holland, L., & Crowley, M. (1997). Family experience of barriers to treatment and premature termination from child therapy. *Journal of Consulting and Clinical Psychology, 65,* 453–463.

Kessler, R. C., Nelson, C. B., McKinagle, K. A., Edlund, M. J., Frank, R. G., & Keaf, P. J. (1996). The epidemiology of co-occurring addictive and mental disorders: Implications for prevention and service utilization. *American Journal of Orthopsychiatry, 66*(1), 17–31.

Lawson, W. B., Hepler, N., Holladay, J., & Cuffel, B. (1994). Race as a factor in inpatient and outpatient admissions and diagnosis. *Hospital and Community Psychiatry, 45,* 72–74.

Lin, K., Anderson, M. D., & Poland, R. E. (1997). Ethnic and cultural considerations in psychopharmacology. In D. L. Dunner (Ed.), *Current psychiatric therapy II* (pp. 75–81). Philadelphia: WB Saunders.

Lin, K., Inui, T. S., Kleinman, A. M., & Womack, W. M. (1982). Sociocultural determinants of the help seeking behavior of patient with mental illness. *Journal of Nervous and Mental Disease, 170,* 78–85.

Macrae, C. N., Milne, A. B., & Bodenhausen, G. V. (1994). Stereotypes as energy-saving devices: A peek inside the cognitive toolbox. *Journal of Personal Social Psychology, 66*(1), 33–47.

McCabe, K., Yeh, M., Hough, R., Landsverk, J., Hurlburt, M., Culver, S., & Reynolds, B. (1998). *Racial/ethnic representation across five public sectors of care for youth.* San Diego, CA: Center for Research on Child and Adolescent Mental Health Services.

Miller, L. (1997). Sexuality, reproduction and family planning in women with schizophrenia. *Schizophrenia Bulletin, 23,* 623–635.

Mowbray, C. T. Oyserman, D., & Bybee, D. (2000). Mothers with serious mental illness. *New Directions for Mental Health Services, 88,* 73–91.

Neri, M. T., & Kroll, T. (2003). Understanding the consequences of access barriers to health care: Experiences of adults with disabilities. *Disability and Rehabilitation, 251*(2), 85–96.

Nickerson, K. J., Helms, J. E., & Terrell, F. (1994). Cultural mistrust, opinions about mental illness and African American students' attitude toward seeking psychological help from white counselors. *Journal of Counseling Psychology, 41*(3), 378–385.

Oyserman, D., Mowbray, C., Mears, P., et al. (2000). Parenting among mothers with a serious mental illness. *American Journal of Orthopsychiatry, 70,* 296–315.

Pargament, K. I. (1997). *The psychology of religion and coping: Theory, research, practice.* New York: Guilford Press.

Park, J. M., Solomon, P., & Mandell, D. S. (2006). Involvement in the child welfare system among mothers with serious mental illness. *Psychiatric Services, 57*, 493–497.

Pavuluri, M. N., Luk, S. L., & McGee, R. (1996). Help-seeking for behavior problems by parents of preschool children: A community study. *Journal of the American Academy of Child and Adolescent Psychiatry, 35*, 215–222.

Regier, D. A., Narrow, W. E., Rae, D. S., Manderscheid, R. W., Locke, B. Z., & Goodwin, F. K. (1993). The de facto US mental and addictive disorders service system: Epidemiologic catchment area perspective 1-year prevalence rates of disorders and services. *Archives of General Psychiatry, 50*, 85–94.

Revenson, T. A. (1989). Compassionate stereotyping of elderly by physicians: Revising the social contact hypothesis. *Psychological Aging, 4*, 230–234.

Scheffler, R. M., & Miller, A. B. (1991). Difference in mental health service utilization among ethnic subpopulations. *International Journal of Law and Psychiatry, 14*, 363–376.

Shaffer, D., Fisher, P., Dulcan, M. K., Davies, M., Piacentini, J., Schwab–Stone, M. E., Lahey, B. B., et al. (1996). The NIMH diagnostic interview schedule for children, version 2.3 (DISC 2.3): Description, acceptability, prevalence rates and performance in the MECA study. Methods for the epidemiology of child and adolescent mental disorders study. *Journal of the American Academy of Child and Adolescent Psychiatry, 35*, 865–877.

Shone, L. P., Dick, A. W., Brach, C., et al. (2003). The role of race and ethnicity in the State Children's Health Insurance Program (SCHIP) in four states: Are there baseline disparities and what do they mean for SCHIP? *Pediatrics, 112*(6), e521–e532.

Smedley, B. D., Stith, A. Y., & Nelson, A. R. (Eds.). (2003). *Unequal treatment: Confronting racial and ethnic disparities in healthcare.* Washington, DC: The National Academies Press.

Snowden, L., & Cheung, F. (1990). Use of inpatient mental health services by members of ethnic minority groups. *American Psychology, 45*, 347–355.

Sue, S., Fujino, D. C., Hu, L. T., Takeuchi, D. T., & Zane, N. W. (1991). Community mental health services for ethnic minority groups: A test of the cultural responsiveness hypothesis. *Journal of Consulting and Clinical Psychology, 59*(4), 533–540.

Sue, S., & Morishima, J. (1982). *The mental health of Asian Americans.* San Francisco, CA: Josey Bass.

Sussman, L. K., Robins, L. N., & Earls, F. (1987). Treatment-seeking for depression by African American and white Americans. *Social Science and Medicine, 24*, 187–196.

Swindle, R., Heller, K., & Pescosolido, B. (August 1997). *Response to "nervous breakdown": In America over a 40-year period: Mental health policy implications.* Paper presented at the meeting of American Sociological Association, Toronto, Ontario.

Thomas, C. R., & Holzer, C. E., III. (1999). National distribution of child and adolescent psychiatrist. *Journal of the American Academy of Child and Adolescent Psychiatry, 38*, 9–15.

Uba, L. (1994). *Asian Americans: Personality patterns identity and mental health.* New York: Guilford Press.

U.S. Department of Health and Human Services. *Mental Health: A Report of the Surgeon General-Executive Summary.* Rockville, MD: U.S. Department of Health and Human Services, Substance Abuse and Mental Health Services Administration, Center for Mental Health Services, National Institutes of Health, National Institute of Mental Health, Chapters 3 and 4, 1999.

U.S. Office of Technology Assessment. (1986). *Children's mental health: Problems and services: A background paper*. Washington, DC: U.S. Government Printing Office.

Van Ryn, M., & Burke, J. (2000). The effects of patient's race and socio-economic status on physicians' perception of patients. *Social Science & Medicine, 50*, 813–828.

Woodward, A. M., Dwinell, A. D., & Arons, B. S. (1992). Barrier to mental health care for Hispanic Americans: A literature review and discussion. *Journal of Mental Health Administration, 19*, 224–236.

Yeh, M., Takeuchi, D., & Sue, S. (1994). Asian American children in the mental health system: A comparison of parallel and mainstream outpatient services centers. *Journal of Clinical Child Psychology, 23*(1), 5–12.

Zito, J. M., Safer, D. J., Zuckerman, I. H., Gardner, J. F., &. Soeken, K. (2005). Effect of Medicaid eligibility category on racial disparities in the use of psychotropic medications among youths. *Psychiatric Services, 56*(2), 157–163.

7

The Scientific Status of Complementary and Alternative Medicines for Mood Disorders

A Review

DECLAN T. BARRY & MARK BEITEL

Alternative medicine is here to stay. It is no longer an option to ignore or treat it as something outside the normal processes of science and medicine. The challenge is to move forward carefully, using both reason and wisdom, as we attempt to separate the pearls from the mud.
—Jonas (1998, p. 1617)

In recent years, mental health professionals, medical providers, patients, and the general public have demonstrated much interest in using complementary and alternative medicines (CAMs) to treat a variety of physical and psychiatric problems and disorders, including depression (Astin, 1998; Barnes, Powell–Griner, McFann, & Nahin, 2004; Eisenberg, Davis, Ettner, Appel, Wilkey, Van Rompay, et al., 1998; Kessler, Soukup, Davis, Foster, Wilkey, Van Rompay, et al., 2001b; McLennan, Wilson, & Taylor, 1996; Rhee, Garg, & Hershey, 2004; Unützer, Klap, Sturm, Young, Marmon, Shatkin, et al., 2000). This chapter discusses issues related to CAM use and depression, including efficacy and safety. It reviews in detail specific CAMs that have been empirically examined for the treatment of depression (one example from each of the five classifications of CAMs designated by the National Center for Complementary and Alternative Medicine [NCCAM]) and offers CAM practice recommendations for clinicians and providers who work with depressed patients.

DEFINING COMPLEMENTARY, ALTERNATIVE, AND ALLOPATHIC MEDICINE

Although there is a burgeoning literature on CAMs, many authors do not operationalize the terms *complementary medicine* or *alternative medicine*, or they use the terms interchangeably. In fact, complementary medicine and alternative medicine are not synonymous. Complementary medicine refers to nonallopathic (i.e., nontraditional) treatment, which is used in conjunction with standard medical interventions, whereas alternative medicine comprises treatment interventions that are used in place of standard medical care (Kim, Lichtenstein, & Waalen, 2002). Alternative or unconventional medicine has also been defined as "medical interventions not taught widely at U.S. medical schools, not generally available at U.S. hospitals, and not generally reimbursable by health insurance" (Eisenberg, Kessler, Foster, Norlock, Calkins, & Delbanco, 1993, p. 247). In contrast, the term *allopathic medicine* is often used to characterize conventional medicine in the United States (i.e., standard medical interventions with demonstrated efficacy and safety). For example, a psychiatrist who prescribes 15 minutes of daily physical exercise to a depressed patient (in addition to an antidepressant) is using complementary (in addition to allopathic) medicines. Conversely, a homeopathic practitioner who recommends that the same patient only ingest St. John's wort may be viewed as using alternative medicine. (Homeopathy is a type of alternative medicine developed by Samuel Hahnemann [1755–1843] that purports that the treatment of ill patients should involve therapeutic agents [drugs, remedies] with effects that, when administered to a healthy individual, correspond to the manifestation of the disorder in the individual ill patient [Ernst, 2002].) Generally, in the treatment of depression, conventional medicine is practiced by psychologists, psychiatrists, other medical doctors, and registered nurses.

It is important to note that there is not unequivocal agreement about the use of the terms *conventional, complementary, alternative,* or *allopathic* (Berkenwald, 1998; Gundling, 1998). Moreover, interventions that are considered allopathic today may in the past have been viewed as alternative or complementary. For example, cognitive–behavioral therapy and interpersonal therapy have demonstrated comparable efficacy to antidepressant medications in the treatment of acute major depressive episodes (DeRubeis, Hollon, Amsterdam, Shelton, Young, Salomon, et al., 2005; Hollon, Jarrett, Nierenberg, Thase, Trivedi, & Rush, 2005); consequently, cognitive–behavioral therapy is often used as a frontline treatment for depression (to be supplemented with pharmacotherapy only if depressive symptoms are not alleviated by cognitive–behavioral therapy alone after a certain time period). Thus, although cognitive–behavioral therapy may have once been viewed as a complementary treatment, nowadays it may be characterized as an allopathic intervention. The hallmark of allopathic medicine in the United States is scientific evidence regarding efficacy and safety. Complementary and alternative medicine interventions that are scientifically demonstrated to be efficacious and safe for a specific medical condition or illness tend to be incorporated into conventional medicine and are subsequently termed *allopathic* in the context of the specific medical condition or illness.

The NCCAM at the National Institutes of Health (NIH) classifies CAM treatments into the following five categories:

1. *Biologically based therapies,* which refer to treatments using biological agents found in nature, including herbs, foods, and vitamins (e.g., herbal medicines, dietary agents, special diets)
2. *Mind–body interventions,* which consist of various techniques that attempt to magnify the mind's capacity to control bodily function and symptoms (e.g., meditation, hypnosis, dance, art and music therapy, prayer and spiritual healing)
3. *Manipulative and body-based methods,* which include methods that systematically manipulate or alter movement in one or more body parts (e.g., massage, chiropractic, and aspects of osteopathic medicine)
4. *Alternative medical systems,* which often predate conventional medicine used in the United States and are based on complete systems of theory and practice, some of which were developed in Eastern cultures (e.g., acupuncture, Ayurveda), and others in Western cultures (e.g., homeopathic medicine, naturopathic medicine)
5. *Energy therapies,* which comprise *biofield therapies* and *bioelectromagnetic-based therapies.* Biofield therapies refer to a system of therapies designed to affect putative energy fields enveloping the human body. Adherents attempt to effect change by placing their hands in or through these biofields (e.g., Reiki, therapeutic touch, Qi Gong). Bioelectromagnetic-based therapies comprise nonstandard use of electromagnetic fields, including magnetic fields, pulsed fields, or alternating-current or direct-current fields (National Center for Complementary and Alternative Medicine, 2002).

PREVALENCE, PATTERNS, AND MOTIVATION FOR USE

Although the development of scientific medicine in the 20th century (which heralded dramatic advances in understanding and treating diseases) was accompanied by a waning of CAM practice in the United States (Gevitz, 1988), the use of CAMs among the general public appears to be on the rise. Findings from nationally representative phone surveys demonstrated that the use of CAMs among American adults had increased from 33.8% in 1991 ($n = 1539$) to 42.1% in 1997 ($n = 2055$) (Eisenberg et al., 1993, 1998). Complementary and alternative medicine therapies that had increased the most between 1991 and 1997 were herbal medicine, massage, megavitamins, self-help groups, folk remedies, and homeopathy. Participants in both studies by Eisenberg and colleagues (1993, 1998) reported using CAMs most frequently for chronic conditions such as depression, back problems, and headaches.

Findings from 31,044 American adults who completed the 2002 NHIS (which included detailed questions on CAMs) indicate that alternative medical systems, mind–body interventions, biologically based therapies, manipulative and body-based methods, and energy therapies were used by 2.7%, 52.6%, 21.9%, 10.9%, and 0.5% of participants, respectively. When prayer, specific to health, was excluded from the definition of mind–body medicine, the proportion reporting use of this type of CAM decreased to 17% (Barnes et al., 2004).

Findings from other national household surveys suggest that the use of CAMs by a large portion of the U.S. population is not a temporary fad, but represents a steadily increasing and continuing pattern (Barnes et al., 2004; Kessler, Davis, Foster, Van Rompay, Walters, Wiley, et al., 2001a). Conservative estimated out-of-pocket expenditures for CAM professional services increased from $12.2 billion in 1990 to $21.1 billion in 1997 (Eisenberg et al., 1998). By 2005, the annual out-of-pocket expenditures for CAMs were estimated to exceed $27 billion (Institute of Medicine, 2005). In sum, many Americans use CAMs and are willing to pay for these services out-of-pocket.

A national study of 1035 individuals randomly selected from a panel found that dissatisfaction with conventional medicine was not the driving motivation for the 40% of respondents who used CAMs during the previous year. Instead, CAMs appeared to be compatible with participants' values, beliefs, and philosophical orientations toward life and health (Astin, 1998). Benefits of CAMs included perceived symptom relief or therapeutic effectiveness, better outcomes than allopathic medicine, and the focus on overall health promotion as opposed to singular focus on symptoms alleviation. We note that only a small minority of participants in this study (5%) reported a primary reliance on unconventional medicine; thus, the majority used unconventional medicine in conjunction with rather than as an alternative to allopathic medicine (Astin, 1998).

This pattern of complementary (as opposed to alternative) medicine use was also documented in another study that analyzed survey data from a probability sample of 16,068 noninstitutionalized civilian adults. A small minority (1.8%) exclusively used unconventional medical services (Druss & Rosenheck, 1999). Moreover, those who used unconventional medicine in addition to allopathic medicine had significantly more outpatient physician visits than those who relied exclusively on allopathic medical interventions. Additional factors that may account for the increased popularity of CAMs in the United States are the increase in prevalence of chronic medical conditions (e.g., chronic pain), increased access to health information (e.g., via the Internet), belief that scientific medicine will not discover a breakthrough treatment relevant to one's medical condition, and the general public's reduced tolerance for paternalistic attitudes associated with traditional allopathic medicine (Furnham & Forey, 1994; Starr, 1982). Individuals who had used CAMs as reported in the NHIS endorsed the following five reasons, from which they were required to select (respondents were allowed to select more than one reason): thought CAM in combination with allopathic medicine would be beneficial (55%), thought it would be interesting to try it (50%), thought allopathic medicine would not help (28%), intervention was recommended by a conventional medical provider (26%), and allopathic medicine was viewed as too expensive (13%).

It is estimated that CAM therapies (excluding megavitamin therapy and prayer for health) are used by approximately 43% of Asian Americans, 26% of African Americans, 28% of Hispanics, and 36% of whites (Barnes et al., 2004). Use of CAM tends to be greater among women, whites, and individuals who are middle-aged, have higher educational levels, or who have been hospitalized during the last 12 months (Baldwin, Long, Kroesen, Brooks, & Bell, 2002; Barnes et al., 2004; Eisenberg et al., 1993, 1998; Kelner & Wellman, 1997). In addition, individuals who use CAMs tend to have greater co-occurring physical and/or mental health problems such as chronic pain and depression (Astin, 1998; Bausel, Lee, & Berman, 2001; Eisenberg et al., 1998; Kelner & Wellman, 1997; Paramore, 1997, Unützer et al., 2000).

CAM Use and Primary Care

Studies on ambulatory patients have found high rates of CAM use among primary care patients. For example, a recent study of 371 ambulatory patients from a lower socioeconomic stratum found that 85.4% had used CAMs, including some form of diet, exercise, and prayer (Rhee et al., 2004). A review of 19 studies conducted between 1982 and 1995 on physicians' practices and beliefs concerning five CAMs (acupuncture, chiropractic, homeopathy, herbal medicine, and massage therapy) found high mean rates of referral for acupuncture (43%) and chiropractic (40%). Mean rates of referral for homeopathy, herbal medicine, and massage therapy were 15%, 4%, and 21%, respectively (Astin, Marie, Pelletier, Hansen, & Haskell, 1998). Physicians participating in the studies were "mainstream physicians," who were doctors of medicine with no known specific or vested interest in CAMs. In the same study, mean rates for physician practice of acupuncture, chiropractic, homeopathy, herbal medicine, and massage therapy were 17%, 19%, 9%, 16%, and 19%, respectively. Other studies have documented the apparent willingness of physicians to use CAMs themselves (Borkan, Neher, Anson, & Smoker, 1994; McLennan et al., 1996). In sum, CAM use is common among primary care patients, and many primary care physicians not only use CAMs themselves, they also use them with their patients and are willing to refer their patients for such services.

EFFICACY AND SAFETY

Although several authors have questioned the efficacy of a variety of CAMs for depression and other psychiatric disorders, concerns about CAM safety have centered on herbal agents and dietary supplements, including the lack of regulation or quality control surrounding their use (Cardellina, 2002; Fontanarosa & Lundberg, 1998; Jonas, 1998; National Center for Complementary and Alternative Medicine, 2005), possible interactions of some CAMs with prescribed medications (Curtis & Gaylord, 2005; Fugh–Berman, 2000; Izzo & Ernst, 2001), the side effects of some CAMs (De Smet, 2004; Ernst, Rand, Barnes, & Stevinson, 1998a; Hammerness, Basch, Ulbricht, Barrette, Foppa, Basch, et al., 2003; Markman, 2002; National Center for Complementary and Alternative Medicine, 2005), and the reluctance of some patients to disclose CAM use to their providers (Eisenberg et al., 1993, 1998; Hensrud, Engle, & Scheitel, 1999) (see also "Points to Consider" on p.118). It is important to note that most CAM products and treatments that are used in clinical practice have not been systematically investigated in terms of either efficacy of safety (Berman & Straus, 2004). Concerns about the lack of governmental regulation regarding herbal agents and dietary supplements are also shared by the general public (Blendon, DesRoches, Benson, Brodie, & Altman, 2001). In some respects, the current lack of federal regulation over herbal and dietary agents parallels the circumstances surrounding the use of patent medications during the early part of the 20th century in the United States. Prior to the Pure Food and Drug Act of 1906, manufacturers who transported proprietary medications across state lines were not required to disclose their contents. Within a couple of years of the act's passage, sales of patent medications decreased by approximately 30% and a large number of medications, which consumers had previously thought to be safe, were withdrawn from the market (Stoller & Bigelow, 2006).

In one nationally representative study that used a random-household telephone survey, among 507 respondents who provided reasons for not disclosing their CAM use to their physician, 61% indicated that they thought it was not important to do so, 60% reported that their physician did not ask them about CAM use, 31% claimed that their CAM use was none of their provider's business, 20% reported that their provider lacked CAM expertise, and 14% stated that their doctor would disapprove or discourage CAM use (Eisenberg, Kessler, Van Rompay, Kaptchuk, Wilkey, Appel, et al., 2001). A review study of 12 studies on patient CAM nondisclosure to medical providers published between 1993 and 2002 found that the main reasons for nondisclosure were anticipated negative physician response, belief that the medical doctor did not need to know such information, and the fact that their provider did not ask about patient CAM use (Robinson & McGrail, 2004).

Physicians may be reluctant to probe CAM use in their patients because of time restraints during clinical visits or inability to offer informed advice about CAM use as a result of a lack of appropriate knowledge (Hughes, 2001). However, they should consider augmenting their knowledge about CAMs, including their benefits and risks, so that they can better advise their patients about CAM use (Fontanarosa & Lundberg, 1998). To enhance patients' safety, those receiving psychiatric medications should be encouraged to discuss any herbs or dietary supplements (and other CAM use) with their medical providers (Brown & Gerbarg, 2001; National Center for Complementary and Alternative Medicine, 2005). This may be particularly important given that most patients who use CAMs do not inform their doctors (Druss & Rosenheck, 1999; Eisenberg et al., 1998).

Research on CAM

Efficacy and safety are the cornerstones of allopathic medicine. One of the main impediments to evaluating the efficacy and safety of CAM for medical and psychiatric disorders, including depression, has been the relative paucity of rigorously designed randomized clinical trials investigating CAMs (Fong, 2002; Jonas, 1998; Mehling, DiBlasi, & Hecht, 2005; Nahin & Straus, 2001). Prior to the 1990s, there was a relative paucity of empirical research published in the English language on CAM efficacy, safety, mechanisms of action, or cost effectiveness (Hughes, 2001). Many of the earlier studies of CAM have been subsequently criticized for poor methodological rigor, including inadequate operationalization (i.e., the absence of clear definitions), lack of adequate control groups, and insufficient statistical power resulting from relatively small sample sizes (Ernst, Rand, & Stevinson, 1998b; Field, 1998; Nahin & Straus, 2001).

The establishment of the NIH Office of Alternative Medicine (OAM) in 1992 with an annual budget of $2,000,000 was an important impetus in advancing a scientific evaluation of CAMs in the United States. In 1998, Congress afforded the OAM full NIH center status and boosted its annual funding to $70,000,000. The OAM is now called the National Center for Complementary and Alternative Medicine. It has funded more than 1200 scientific projects and its annual budget in fiscal year 2006 grew to $122,692,000 (National Center for Complementary and Alternative Medicine, 2006). The NCCAM has four primary areas of focus: advancement of CAM scientific research, training of CAM researchers, disseminating accurate information about CAMs, and supporting the integration of empirically supported CAMs (National Center for Complementary and Alternative Medicine, 2006). Although not without its critics (Marcus & Grollman, 2006; Sampson, 2005), the NCCAM has made important contributions in advancing research on the efficacy and safety of different CAMs (Straus & Chesney, 2006).

Use and Perceived Helpfulness of CAMs in Treating Depression

Kessler and colleagues (2001b) have conducted one of the most comprehensive studies to date that has examined the use of specific CAMs to treat depression in the United States. A nationally representative sample of 2055 respondents was recruited using random-digit dialing, and information was collected on the use of 24 CAMs for the treatment of a variety of chronic conditions, including depression. One hundred and forty-eight participants (7.2%) reported "severe depression" in the previous 12 months, 53.6% of whom reported the use of one or more CAMs to alleviate their symptoms. However, most of these CAMs were not used under the supervision of a CAM therapist. Only 19.3% of those with severe depression sought treatment from a CAM therapist (vs. 63.9% who sought treatment from a conventional professional). The most frequently endorsed CAMs used for depression were "cognitive feedback" (relaxation techniques, imagery, self-help groups, hypnosis, and biofeedback) and "other therapies" (spiritual healing by others, dietary modifications, lifestyle diet, special diet for losing or gaining weight, energy healing, aromatherapy, folk remedies, laughter, other therapy to treat pain, and other lifestyle intervention programs), which were used by 30.2% and 27.4% of the respondents, respectively. By way of comparison, the most frequently used CAMs for depression in the study by Astin (1998) were relaxation, exercise, and herbs. Of those who were treated for severe depression by a "conventional professional" (i.e., psychiatrist, other physician, psychologist, social worker, clergy, or other), 66.7% also used CAMs to treat their symptoms. The perceived helpfulness of CAMs and conventional therapies was similar. Another national survey with a sample size of 9585 telephone participants, conducted in 1997–1998, found that those with a diagnosis of major depression were significantly more likely than those without to use CAMs (Unützer et al., 2000). Furthermore, findings from the 2002 NHIS, based on a nationally representative sample of 31,044 adults, indicated that common reasons for CAM use were depression and pain (Barnes et al., 2004).

CAMS IN THE TREATMENT OF MOOD DISORDERS

St. John's Wort

St. John's wort (*Hypericum perforatum*) is a yellow-flowered hedgerow plant that is typically taken for medicinal purposes as a tea or in tablet form. Although St. John's wort has been used for centuries in folk medicine as an antiseptic, analgesic, and antidepressant, its most common current indication in the United States is for the treatment of depression, anxiety, and/or sleep disorders (National Center for Complementary and Alternative Medicine, 2005; Zahourek, 2000). St. John's wort may be classified as a biologically based therapy in CAM (National Center for Complementary and Alternative Medicine, 2002).

Linde and colleagues (1996, 2005) have published two meta-analyses of randomized trials of St. John's wort. The first meta-analysis comprised 23 trials with 1757 outpatients with mild to moderately severe depression and the second involved 37 trials with 4925 outpatients with depressive disorders. Both meta-analyses found support for the effectiveness of St. John's wort for alleviating symptoms of mild to moderate depression. Not only did St. John's wort alleviate symptoms of depression better than placebo, its efficacy was similar to that of standard antidepressant medications. However, most of the studies reviewed in these meta-analyses had methodological flaws; in particular, many of the studies had small sample sizes, did not use a placebo group, did not use standard measures for assessing symptoms of depression, and did not use *DSM-IV* criteria for major depression.

To date, two double-blind, randomized, controlled trials have been conducted to test the efficacy of St. John's wort in treating major depression as defined by *DSM-IV* criteria (American Psychiatric Association, 1994). In the first randomized, controlled trial, 340 adult outpatients diagnosed with major depression were randomly assigned to *H. perforatum* (St. John's wort), sertraline (Zoloft, a selective serotonin reuptake inhibitor [SSRI], which served as the active comparator), or placebo for eight weeks (Hypericum Depression Trial Study Group, 2002). Based on clinical response, daily dose ranges for *H. perforatum* and sertraline could range from 900 to 1500 mg and 50 to 100 mg, respectively. St. John's wort was no more effective in alleviating depressive symptoms than placebo. In the second randomized, controlled trial, 200 adult outpatients diagnosed with major depression were randomly assigned to St. John's wort or placebo for eight weeks (Shelton, Keller, Gelenberg, Dunner, Hirschfeld, Thase, et al., 2001). Those taking St. John's wort received 900 mg/day for the first four weeks, which was subsequently increased to 1200 mg/day in the absence of an adequate response. St. John's wort and placebo responses were comparable. Overall, the findings of both randomized, controlled trials indicate that St. John's wort is not effective in treating major depression. Thus, although St. John's wort may be effective in treating symptoms of mild depression, it does not appear to be effective as a stand-alone treatment for major depression.

Given the complexity of its compounds, the exact mechanism by which St. John's wort acts in the human brain remains unclear. Most studies have examined two potential active compounds—hypericin and hyperforin. The former may inhibit serotonin receptor expression and monoamine oxidase, and the latter may inhibit the uptake of serotonin (5-HT), dopamine, noradrenaline, γ-aminobutyric acid, and L-glutamate (Chatterjee, Bhattacharya, Wonnemann, Singer, & Muller, 1998; Zahourek, 2000).

Points to Consider

Consumers need to exert care when purchasing St. John's wort because it is unclear which of the plethora of the available brands are most efficacious (Brown & Gerbarg, 2001). St. John's wort may also have interaction effects with medications (Ernst, 1999; Fugh–Berman, 2000; Hammerness et al., 2003; Izzo & Ernst, 2001). Although many patients and providers may assume that St. John's wort is safe because it is an herb that has been used for centuries (Ernst et al., 1998a), providers should be familiar with potential side effects, including increased sensitivity to sunlight, gastrointestinal problems, sexual dysfunction, dizziness, and dry mouth (De Smet, 2004; Hammerness et al., 2003; National Center for Complementary and Alternative Medicine, 2005). Moreover, given that St. John's wort appears to be ineffective in treating individuals with clinical levels of depression (e.g., major depression as defined by the DSM-IV), and that symptoms of depression may become exacerbated when untreated, we recommend that providers prescribe evidence-based psychotherapy and/or pharmacotherapy for individuals who have been diagnosed as clinically depressed by mental health experts (i.e., clinical psychologists and psychiatrists).

Mindfulness

Mindfulness has been a cornerstone of Buddhist thought and practice for 2500 years and is regarded as one of the steps on the path toward freedom from suffering. Recently, researchers in the West have become interested in mindfulness, regarding it variously as a personality trait, a cognitive style, and/or an ability (Sternberg, 2000). Bishop and colleagues (2004) described the construct as a form of "nonelaborative, nonjudgmental, present-centered awareness in which each thought, feeling, or sensation that arises in the attentional field is acknowledged and accepted as it is . . . thoughts and feelings are observed as events in the mind, without overidentifying with them and without reacting to them . . ." (p.232). Mindfulness involves the self-regulation of attention, a sustained focus on the current moment (on bodily experience in particular), and an openness to experience (Bishop et al., 2004). Mindfulness is a cognitive mode antithetical to relapse-oriented rumination (Segal, Teasdale, & Williams, 2004, p. 53). Mindfulness may be classified as a mind–body CAM intervention (National Center for Complementary and Alternative Medicine, 2002).

Several self-report measures of mindfulness have been developed recently, such as the Mindfulness Attention Awareness Scale (MAAS) (Brown & Ryan, 2003). The MAAS has correlated positively with measures of emotional self-awareness: The Trait Meta-Mood Scale (TMMS) (Salovey, Mayer, Goldman, Turvey, & Palfai, 1995) measures attention to feelings, clarity of emotional experience, and repairing unpleasant mood states. The MAAS correlated with overall emotional awareness on the TMMS ($r = .46$, $p < .001$), attention ($r = .19$, $p < .001$), clarity ($r = .49$, $p < .0001$), and repair ($r = .37$, $p < .0001$) in one study (Brown & Ryan, 2003). The MAAS has been associated positively with a variety of well-being measures, such as positive affect ($r = .30$, $p < .0001$) on the Positive and Negative Affect Schedule (PANAS) (Watson, Clark, & Tellegen, 1988). In contrast, it was inversely related to negative affect ($r = -.39$, $p < .0001$) (Brown & Ryan, 2003).

Just as there are a variety of mindfulness practices in the Buddhist traditions (some involve formal, sitting meditation; others do not), there are a variety of formal psychological interventions that have incorporated mindfulness techniques. These include acceptance and commitment therapy (Hayes, Strosahl, & Wilson, 1999), dialectical behavior therapy (Linehan, 1993), mindfulness-based cognitive therapy (MBCT) (Segal, Williams, & Teasdale, 2002), and mindfulness-based stress reduction (Kabat–Zinn, 1990). We focus on MBCT for depression in this section because it has been shown to reduce relapse rates in formerly depressed patients in two randomized clinical trials (Ma & Teasdale, 2004; Teasdale, Segal, Williams, Ridgeway, Soulsby, & Lau, 2000), and therefore may be regarded as "probably efficacious" for this purpose by American Psychological Association criteria (American Psychological Association, 1995).

Mindfulness-based cognitive therapy for depression is an eight-session, group program that combines elements of cognitive–behavioral therapy (Beck, Rush, Shaw, & Emery, 1979) and mindfulness-based stress reduction (Kabat–Zinn, 1990). In MBCT, patients participate in experiential learning designed to (a) enhance awareness of, (b) change relationship to, and (c) change response to unwanted thoughts, feelings, and bodily sensations. One strength of MBCT is that it is administered in group format, which makes it cost-effective in terms of service delivery.

The first multisite, randomized clinical trial of MBCT (Teasdale et al., 2000) enrolled 145 patients in remission or in recovery from major depression (*DSM-IV* criteria). Patients were randomized to continue treatment as usual (TAU) or to MBCT plus TAU. For patients with three or more previous depressive episodes, the MBCT group relapse rate was nearly half the rate for the TAU group. Mindfulness-based cognitive therapy for depression did not have a significant effect on relapse for patients experiencing fewer than three previous depressive episodes.

The second randomized clinical trial of MBCT took place at one site (Ma & Teasdale, 2004). Seventy-five patients meeting the *DSM-IV* criteria for past depressive episodes participated. They were randomized to one of two conditions: TAU or TAU plus MBCT. Replicating the findings of the first trial, patients in the MBCT group with three or more previous depressive episodes experienced half as many relapses during a 60-week period as did the TAU group (10 participants out of 28 and 21 out of 27, respectively).

Points to Consider

Mindfulness-based cognitive therapy for depression seems to be effective in reducing the incidence of relapse in some types of formerly depressed patients. There are two important caveats to make here. First, MBCT is "probably efficacious" in reducing depressive relapse (in patients with more than three prior episodes) only as it was tested — in its "manualized" format. A related issue is that it is difficult to tell how much of the benefits are attributable to the mindfulness components or to the traditional cognitive–behavioral therapy components in this intervention. Therefore, clinicians who choose to incorporate mindfulness practices into their individual work with patients should do so cautiously. It is also necessary to be cautious about referring patients to community organizations for mindfulness training. It is important to note that the effects on depression and relapse for the vast majority of mindfulness training programs remain untested.

Massage Therapy

Massage therapy refers to the systematic manipulation of bodily soft tissues for therapeutic purposes (Field, 1998). Massage therapy belongs to a family of interventions called *touch therapies*, comprising energy methods, manipulative therapies, and amalgams (i.e., combinations of both), which practitioners have used for thousands of years (Field, 2002). Massage therapy is a manipulative and body-based CAM intervention (National Center for Complementary and Alternative Medicine, 2002) and is one of the most popular CAMs among the general public and physicians (Boutin, Buchwald, Robinson, & Collier, 2000; Eisenberg et al., 1998; Verhoef, 1998). Massage therapy, especially Swedish massage, has few documented adverse health effects (Ernst, 2003).

Although massage therapy is often viewed as a CAM in the United States, it is regarded as a conventional medical intervention in other countries, including China, Japan, and Germany, where it is covered under national health insurance (Field, 2002). An assortment of massage therapies comprising therapeutic techniques have emanated from several countries, including *friction massage* (also known as *connective tissue massage*), during which strong pressure is applied to subcutaneous tissues of the torso and extremities; *lymph drainage*, which entails gentle manipulation or stroking along lymph vessels and over lymph nodes; *rolfing*, developed in the United States, which comprises deep manipulation of soft tissues; *shiatsu*, involving strong manipulation of acupuncture points; and *Swedish massage*, a type of muscular massage (Ernst, 2003). Swedish massage is perhaps the most popular type of massage therapy in the United States and it has received the most research attention. It comprises five specialized types of strokes, which are typically described using French terminology: *effleurage* or gliding, *petrissage* or kneading, *vibration* or shaking, *tapotement* or pounding, and *friction* or rubbing (Ernst, 2003).

Massage therapy has been practiced in different forms for thousands of years. However, its credibility and esteem among Western medical doctors have vacillated considerably. Although massage therapy was widely used by physicians in Ancient Greece and Rome, its popularity among Western physicians declined during the Middle Ages (Fritz, 2000). Per Henrik Ling (1776–1839), a pioneering figure in the field of physical therapy, drew medical attention to massage, which he included as part of a regimen of physical exercises that he and his followers claimed had curative effects on disease. Later, Johann Metzger (1839–1909), a Dutch physician, promoted Swedish massage using a medical model, and enhanced its credibility as a legitimate area of Western scientific research (Fritz, 2000).

Although studies have examined massage therapy in the treatment of a variety of physical and mental disorders, most were not based on clinical trials and eschewed control groups and random assignment to treatment and control conditions (Ernst et al., 1998b; Field, 1998). In a review of nine studies of back effleurage, Labyak and Metzger (1997) concluded that this form of massage therapy was effective in enhancing relaxation. In a review of seven studies of massage therapy, Ernst (1998) tentatively concluded that postexercise massage may attenuate physical soreness. Moyer and associates (2004) conducted a meta-analysis of massage therapy involving 37 studies and 1802 participants, 795 of whom received massage therapy. The nonspecific overall mean effect was statistically significant ($g = 0.34$, $p < .01$), indicating that in comparison with those receiving a control treatment, the average participant who received massage therapy exhibited significantly greater beneficial change on outcome variables.

Similar to studies of psychotherapy and pharmacotherapy, Moyer and colleagues (2004) examined dose effects, including single-dose (i.e., the immediate effect of a single intervention episode on outcome variables) and multiple-dose (i.e., the effects of multiple interventions over a period of time on outcome variables) effects. With respect to the short-term or single-dose effects, the average massage therapy participant experienced a reduction of state anxiety, blood pressure, and heart rate that was greater than 64%, 60%, and 66% of the respective comparison group participants. Moyer and colleagues (2004) also found "multiple-dose effects" for depression, pain, and trait anxiety. Thus, in studies in which participants received either a course of massage therapy or a control treatment and were assessed days or weeks after treatment termination, massage therapy participants exhibited longer term reductions in depression, pain, and trait anxiety that were greater, on average, than 73%, 62%, and 77% of the respective control treatment participants. Although a single-session episode of massage therapy did not produce an immediate beneficial effect on feeling/affect or pain, significant reductions in depression and pain occurred after a course of massage therapy. Overall, this well-conducted meta-analysis provides support for both the short-term and long-term benefits of massage therapy.

Massage therapy is said to work by releasing bodily muscle tension, promoting the removal of the body's toxic metabolic waste products, enhancing oxygen and nutrient flow to body cells and tissues, releasing the body's natural pain killers, and improving immune function (Field, 2002). The ameliorative effect of massage therapy on depression may be linked to its stress-alleviating (in particular, decreased cortisol) and activation effects, particularly in its promotion of dopamine and serotonin production (Field, Hernandez–Reif, & Diego, 2005). Additional research is needed to examine further these putative therapeutic mechanisms of change (Moyer et al., 2004).

Points to Consider

Although research to date generally supports the efficacy and safety of Swedish massage therapy in treating depression, there are other types of massage therapy practiced in the United States that have not been adequately researched. Studies that have demonstrated empirical support for massage therapy have generally used licensed massage therapists. Currently, 37 states in the United States have massage therapy licensure requirements (Associated Bodywork & Massage Professionals, 2006). Thus, clinicians who advertise themselves as massage therapists but who do not meet licensure requirements may be operating outside their scope of practice (see Cohen, 2002).

Acupuncture

Acupuncture was developed in China more than 2000 years ago and refers to a group of therapeutic procedures that involve stimulation of different body sites via the insertion of one or more needles (Nasir, 2002). Acupuncture is an important component of traditional Chinese medicine (TCM) and may be classified as an alternative medical system (National Center for Complementary and Alternative Medicine, 2002). Although widely practiced in China, most Americans were unfamiliar with acupuncture prior to 1971. While covering President Nixon's visit to China that year, *New York Times* reporter James Reston published an account of the analgesic effects of needles being inserted into his body for postappendectomy pain (Reston, 1971). By 2002, an estimated 8.2 million U.S. adults had used acupuncture in their lifetime, whereas an estimated 2.1 million had used it in the previous 12 months (Barnes et al., 2004).

One cardinal concept in acupuncture and TCM is the maintenance of a balanced state between two opposing yet interdependent putative life forces that are said to permeate the universe: *yin* and *yang*. Yin is often symbolized by water and yang by fire. Although yin may be characterized as slow and passive, yang is described as quick and active. In TCM, equilibrium or a balanced state between yin and yang engenders health; disequilibrium begets illness. Specifically, disequilibrium is said to block the flow of *qi* (life energy) along *meridians* or bodily pathways (Wong, 1997). Acupuncturists typically work on acupuncture points along these meridians. However, scientific evidence to support the existence of meridians or acupuncture points is scant (Ramey, 2001). Instead, studies suggest that acupuncture may affect neurotransmitter and hormone levels. For example, acupuncture in animal experiments has been shown to alter immune responses and other involuntary bodily responses, including blood flow and blood pressure (Lee, LaRiccia, & Newberg, 2004; Takeshige, 1989). In humans, acupuncture may promote self-regulatory processes irrespective of the type of acupuncture treatment used (Moffet, 2006).

In a review of seven randomized, controlled trials with 509 patients, Mukaino and associates (2005) found that acupuncture for the treatment of depression was not superior to a waitlist control, but electroacupuncture (a procedure similar to regular acupuncture in which needles are attached to a machine that produces regular electrical pulses, the intensity and frequency of which can be adjusted) and antidepressants produced comparable reductions in depressive symptoms. Mukaino and colleagues (2005) concluded that there is currently insufficient data to decide whether acupuncture is effective in treating depression, and recommended further trials of electroacupuncture for the treatment of depression.

Another randomized, controlled trial involving 47 depressed patients who were randomly assigned to five weeks of either electroacupuncture or the tricyclic antidepressant (TCA) amitriptyline hydrochloride found a comparable reduction in depressive symptoms for both treatment groups (Luo, Jia, & Zhan, 1985). Researchers conducting a larger randomized, controlled trial involving 241 depressed patients who were randomly assigned to six weeks of either electroacupuncture or amitriptyline hydrochloride reported a similar decrease in depressive symptoms among both treatment groups (Luo, Meng, Jia, & Zhao, 1998). Currently, there is an active NCCAM-sponsored randomized, controlled trial being conducted at the University of Pittsburgh (ClinicalTrials.gov identifier, NCT00071110) that may inform whether electroacupuncture for major depression is effective.

Despite the relative paucity of research supporting the efficacy of acupuncture in treating depression, a recent study conducted in the states of Massachusetts and Washington found that approximately 10% of acupuncture visits in both states were related to depression and anxiety (Sherman, Cherkin, Eisenberg, Erro, Hrbek, & Deyo, 2005). With respect to other psychiatric and medical conditions, there is much debate concerning the efficacy of acupuncture. Some review studies have concluded that acupuncture is efficacious in general (e.g., Birch, Hesselink, Jonkman, Hekker, & Bos, 2004) or for specific medical conditions such as nausea associated with pregnancy and postsurgery emesis or vomiting (Kaptchuk, 2002) whereas others have concluded the opposite (e.g., Ramey & Sampson, 2001), and still others report mixed support (e.g., Ernst, 2006).

In 1996, the U.S. Food and Drug Administration (1996) approved the use of sterile, nontoxic acupuncture needles for single use by licensed practitioners. When administered by licensed or qualified practitioners, acupuncture is a safe procedure (Ernst, 2006; Vincent, 2001). However, serious adverse effects may occur from improper needle insertion and inadequate sterilization, including bruising, soreness, dizziness, infections, or punctured organs (Berman, Lao, Langenberg, Lee, Gilpin, & Hochberg, 2004; Yamashita, Tsukayama, Tanno, & Nishijo, 1998). With regard to training standards and licensing, the Accreditation Commission for Acupuncture and Oriental Medicine, a national accrediting agency recognized by the U.S. Department of Education to accredit Master's level programs in acupuncture and oriental medicine, has accredited 48 acupuncture schools in the United States and assigned candidacy status to 10 (Accreditation Commission for Acupuncture and Oriental Medicine, 2006).

Points to Consider

There is much debate concerning the placebo (vs. active) contribution of acupuncture and the use of sham needles that may serve as a comparison control for acupuncture needles (Ernst, 2006; Kaptchuk, Goldman, Stone, & Stason, 2000; Moffet, 2006). Currently, 42 states in the United States have statutes governing the practice of acupuncture and oriental medicine (Acupuncture and Oriental Medicine Alliance, 2006). Thus, clinicians in these states who advertise themselves as acupuncturists but who do not meet licensure requirements may be operating outside their scope of practice (see Cohen, 2002).

Light Therapy

Light therapy (or phototherapy) has gained considerable research support (Golden, Gaynes, Ekstrom, Hamer, Jacobsen, Suppes, et al., 2005; Terman & Terman, 2005) in recent years as a treatment for major depressive disorder with a seasonal (winter) pattern (see Sato [1997] for a critical review). (The seasonal specifier first appeared in the DSM-III-R [American Psychiatric Association, 1987].) Under DSM-IV criteria, the seasonal specifier may be applied to the pattern of major depressive episodes in major depressive disorder (recurrent), or bipolar I or bipolar II disorders. The following criteria must be met to assign the specifier: (a) the presence of an established temporal relationship between the onset of major depressive episodes and a particular time of year (in the absence of seasonal-related psychosocial stressors, such as predictable seasonal unemployment), (b) full remission at the end of the season, (c) two major depressive episodes in season and no such nonseasonal episodes within the last two years, and (d) seasonal episodes substantially outnumber lifetime nonseasonal episodes.

Light therapy involves the direct application of filtered light energy to an individual recipient. In this treatment, the patient is positioned in front of a light source, which might be a downward-tilted light box or a light-emitting visor. Light energy is absorbed through the eyes, although participants are directed to avoid staring directly at the light source (Terman & Terman, 2005). Application of bright light to the skin has been shown to be significantly less effective than direct ocular exposure (Wehr, Skwerer, Jacobsen, Sack, & Rosenthal, 1987). Fluorescent light is typically used in light therapy treatments. Both full-spectrum and cool-white lightbulbs have been used effectively (Bielski, Mayor, & Rice, 1992).

Numerous studies have helped to establish a therapeutic dose for bright light, which ranges in intensity from 2,500 to 10,000 lux. Exposure to dim light (100 lux) does not produce robust results and has, in fact, been used as a placebo condition in clinical trials (Lam, Levitt, Levitan, Enns, Morehouse, Michalak, & Tam,

2006). It has been recommended that light therapy be administered on a daily basis throughout the season (Rosenthal, 1988). The typical treatment duration ranges from 30 minutes to two hours. Thirty minutes of exposure to 10,000 lux light has produced therapeutic benefits (Terman, 1988; Terman & Terman, 2005), as has a two-hour exposure at a lower dose of 5,000 lux light (Martiny, Simonsen, Lunde, Clemmensen, & Bech, 2004). Although the results are mixed, some evidence suggests that morning light administrations are preferable (Terman & Terman, 2005).

In an open trial (Martiny et al., 2004) of bright light therapy for seasonal (winter) depression (*DSM-III-R* criteria), 61% of participants experienced a 50% reduction in depressive symptoms (as rated on the Hamilton Depression Rating Scale [HDRS] [Hamilton, 1967]) after one week of treatment involving daily (morning) exposure to 5000 lux full-spectrum light for 120 minutes.

In a recent double-blind, randomized, controlled trial (Lam et al., 2006), light therapy (30 minutes of morning exposure to 10,000 lux white fluorescent light with an ultraviolet (UV) filter for eight weeks) resulted in a significant decrease in depressive symptoms on the HDRS. In this design, light therapy was compared with the antidepressant medication fluoxetine (20 mg/day). Patients undergoing light therapy received a therapeutic dose of light therapy and a placebo pill whereas the fluoxetine group received a nontherapeutic dose of light (100 lux). Intent-to-treat analysis revealed that both groups (light and antidepressant) exhibited significant decreases in depressive symptoms from baseline, but did not reveal statistically significant differences between groups. The fluoxetine group reported significantly more adverse events in the following categories: agitation, sleep disturbance, and palpitations.

Overall, side effects associated with light therapy have been regarded as generally minor to moderate (Sato, 1997; Terman & Terman, 2005). Headache, nausea, feeling "wired," and visual complaints (eyestrain, blurred vision, seeing spots) have been described as side effects (Terman & Terman, 2005). An increased risk of hypomania as a consequence of light therapy may also be an infrequent possibility (Terman & Terman, 2005), although no instances of hypomanic response were observed in a recent controlled trial (Lam et al., 2006). Although it appears to be rare, there have been some reported cases of increased suicide risk associated with the receipt of light therapy (Haffmans, Lucius, & Ham, 1999; Praschak–Rieder, Neumeister, Hesselmann, Willeit, Barnas, & Kasper, 1997). Seventy-seven percent of patients in a recent trial (Lam et al., 2006) reported at least one treatment-emergent adverse event in the light treatment condition (compared with 75% of patients in the fluoxetine condition). The most frequently occurring light-related events were dry mouth (18%), headache (16%), decreased appetite (14%), and decreased sex drive (14%), and were comparable with fluoxetine treatment.

Ocular safety is an obvious concern with light therapy (Terman & Terman, 2005), because the light intensity experienced in treatment is far greater than typically experienced outdoors. Infrared and UV waves are clearly dangerous; consequently, experts recommend filtering the light used during treatment.

There has been one ophthalmologic investigation of bright-light treatment recipients (Gallin, Terman, Reme, Rafferty, Terman, & Burde, 1995), which failed to show "obvious acute light-induced pathology" in patients described as normal in oculoretinal status (Terman & Terman, 2005, p. 655).

Points to Consider

Light therapy has shown promising results in controlled trials as a treatment for major depressive disorder with a seasonal pattern. Side effects have been regarded as mild to moderate, comparable with antidepressant medication. One potential drawback to the use of light therapy is that relapse rates are high, as high as 75%. For this reason, it has been recommended that light therapy be administered daily for the duration of the season (Rosenthal, 1988), a recommendation that might be impractical or unfeasible for some patients, particularly those who are not treatment motivated. Therefore, adherence to a light therapy regimen must be carefully monitored by clinical staff.

INTEGRATING CAMS AND ALLOPATHIC MEDICINE

The integration of CAMs and allopathic or conventional medicine is becoming more popular (Jonas, 1998; Mann, Gaylord, & Norton, 2004). The majority (60%) of medical schools in the United States now offer courses involving CAMs (Wetzel, Eisenberg, & Kaptchuk, 1998). Studies suggest, however, that these may not be sufficient because the majority of medical students and residents believe that their training leaves them unprepared to address patients' questions about CAMs and are unsure about which CAM providers are reputable and appropriate as referrals for their patients (Devries, 1999; Wetzel, Kaptchuk, Haramati, & Eisenberg, 2003). Hospitals in the United States are increasingly offering CAM interventions, and more managed care and medical insurance packages now cover CAMs (McHughes & Timmermann, 2005; Pelletier, Marie, Krasner, & Haskell, 1997). Researchers have offered different models for integrating CAMs and conventional medicine (Frenkel & Borkan, 2003; Mann, Gaylord, & Norton, 2004). Not only is there integration at the consumer level, but integration of CAMs and conventional medicine also occurs at the health care provider level; the clinical, institutional, and professional regulatory level; and the health care policy and system level (Boon, Verhoef, O'Hara, Findlay, & Majid, 2004).

However, in some respects, models outlining the integration of CAM and conventional medicine may be premature. More research is needed to document the efficacy and safety of CAM interventions for specific medical conditions, such as depression. The integration of CAMs and conventional medical treatments should proceed with caution and necessitates clear guidelines to assess the quality of CAM products, practices, and research (Fontanarosa & Lundberg, 1998; Jonas, 1998; Nahin, Pontzer, & Chesney, 2005). In addition to attending to efficacy and safety, CAM and allopathic practitioners need to be cognizant of professional licensure, scope of practice, and malpractice issues (Cohen, 2002).

RECOMMENDATIONS AND CONCLUSIONS

Complementary and alternative medicine use is common among patients with depression and other psychiatric disorders. However, there is a relative dearth of well-designed clinical research studies examining the efficacy and safety of CAMs. Although each of the CAMs examined in this chapter has shown some promise in controlled trials, Swedish massage therapy, electroacupuncture, and light therapy have garnered the most empirical research support to date. "Manualized" MBCT is "probably efficacious" in reducing depressive relapse in patients with more than three prior depressive episodes. St. John's wort appears to be effective in treating mild levels of depression but not major depression. Electroacupuncture is a promising, but as yet unproven, treatment for major depression. Light therapy appears to be effective in reducing symptoms of major depression with a seasonal pattern; however, as with conventional therapy with antidepressants, discontinuation of treatment results in high relapse to depression rates. Future research on CAM efficacy and safety may inform the development of integrated interventions (i.e., a combination of CAM and allopathic medicine) for this population. Future research on CAMs as therapies for depression may benefit from adopting a psychotherapy development and evaluation model, including use of manualized interventions and adequate control conditions.

Key Points
- Although CAMs are commonly used by depressed patients, based on current knowledge, their usefulness in treating clinical levels of depression is limited.
- Patients' exclusive reliance on CAM therapies as a first-line treatment appears to be rare. Typically in the United States, CAMs are used in conjunction with allopathic or conventional medicine.
- Integrating CAMs into allopathic medicine is becoming more common; however, there is a paucity of research that supports or informs such integration for patients with depression.

Practice Recommendations
- Assess CAM use in your depressed patients.
- Consider increasing your knowledge about the efficacy of safety or different CAM therapies and their interactions with allopathic interventions.
- Discuss efficacy and safety issues with patients in a nonjudgmental, empathic manner.
- Unless you are licensed to provide the CAM in question, consider referring patients to an appropriately trained and licensed professional.

REFERENCES

Accreditation Commission for Acupuncture and Oriental Medicine. (2006, August). *Accredited and candidate programs* [Online]. Available: http://www.acaom.org/acc ProgAddress.asp

Acupuncture and Oriental Medicine Alliance. (2006). *List of states with statutes and regulations* [Online]. Available: http://www.aomalliance.org

American Psychiatric Association. (1987). *Diagnostic and statistical manual of mental disorders* (3rd rev. ed.). Washington, DC: American Psychiatric Association.

American Psychiatric Association. (1994). *Diagnostic and statistical manual of mental disorders* (4th ed.). Washington, DC: American Psychiatric Association.

American Psychological Association, Task Force on Promotion and Dissemination of Psychological Procedures. (1995). Training in and dissemination of empirically-validated psychological treatments: Report and recommendations. *The Clinical Psychologist*, 48(1), 3–23.

Associated Bodywork & Massage Professionals. (2006). *State boards and requirements* [Online]. Available: http://www.massagetherapy.com/careers/stateboards.php

Astin, J. A. (1998). Why patients use alternative medicine: Results of a national study. *Journal of the American Medical Association*, 279, 1548–1553.

Astin, J. A., Marie, A., Pelletier, K. R., Hansen, E., & Haskell, W. (1998). A review of the incorporation of complementary and alternative medicine by mainstream physicians. *Archives of Internal Medicine*, 158, 2303–2310.

Baldwin, C. M., Long, K., Kroesen, K., Brooks, A. J., & Bell, I. R. (2002). A profile of military veterans in the southwestern United States who use complementary and alternative medicine. *Archives of Internal Medicine*, 162, 1697–1704.

Barnes, P. M., Powell–Griner, E., McFann, K., & Nahin, R. L. (2004). Complementary and alternative medicine use among adults: United States, 2002. *Advance Data*, 343, 1–19.

Bausel, R. B., Lee, W. L., & Berman, B. M. (2001). Demographic and health-related correlates of visits to complementary and alternative medical providers. *Medical Care*, 39, 190–196.

Beck, A. T., Rush, A. J., Shaw, B. F., & Emery, G. (1979). *Cognitive therapy of depression*. New York: Guilford Press.

Berkenwald, A. D. (1998). In the name of medicine. *Annals of Internal Medicine*, 128, 246–250.

Berman, B. M., Lao, L., Langenberg, P., Lee, W. L., Gilpin, A. M. K., & Hochberg, M. C. (2004). Effectiveness of acupuncture as adjunctive therapy in osteoarthritis of the knee: A randomized, controlled trial. *Annals of Internal Medicine*, 141, 901–910.

Berman, J. D., & Straus, S. E. (2004). Implementing a research agenda for complementary and alternative medicine. *Annual Review of Medicine*, 55, 239–254.

Bielski, R. J., Mayor, J., & Rice, J. (1992). Phototherapy with broad spectrum white fluorescent light: A comparative study. *Psychiatry Research*, 43, 167–175.

Birch, S., Hesselink, J. K., Jonkman, F. A. M., Hekker, T. A. M., & Bos, A. A. T. (2004). Clinical research on acupuncture: Part 1. What have reviews of the efficacy and safety of acupuncture told us so far? *Journal of Alternative and Complementary Medicine*, 10, 468–480.

Bishop, S. R., Lau, M., Shapiro, S., Carlson, L., Anderson, N. D., Carmody, J., et al. (2004). Mindfulness: A proposed operational definition. *Clinical Psychology: Science and Practice*, 11, 230–241.

Blendon, R. J., DesRoches, C. M., Benson, J. M., Brodie, M., & Altman, D. E. (2001). Americans' views on the use and regulation of dietary supplements. *Archives of Internal Medicine*, 161, 805–810.

Boon, H., Verhoef, M., O'Hara, D., Findlay, B., & Majid, N. (2004). Integrative healthcare: Arriving at a working definition. *Alternative Therapies in Health and Medicine*, 10, 48–56.

Borkan, J., Neher, J. O., Anson, O., & Smoker, B. (1994). Referrals for alternative therapies. *Journal of Family Practice*, 39, 545–550.

Boutin, P. D., Buchwald, D., Robinson, L., & Collier, A. C. (2000). Use of and attitudes about alternative and complementary therapies among outpatients and physicians at a municipal hospital. *Journal of Alternative and Complementary Medicine, 6*, 335–343.

Brown, R. P., & Gerbarg, P. L. (2001). Herbs and nutrients in the treatment of depression, anxiety, insomnia, migraine, and obesity. *Journal of Psychiatric Practice, 7*, 75–91.

Brown, K. W., & Ryan, R. M. (2003). The benefits of being present: The role of mindfulness in psychological well-being. *Journal of Personality and Social Psychology, 84*, 822–848.

Cardellina, J. H. (2002). Challenges and opportunities confronting the botanical dietary supplement industry. *Journal of Natural Products, 65*, 1073–1084.

Chatterjee, S. S., Bhattacharya, S. K., Wonnemann, M., Singer, A., & Muller, W. E. (1998). Hyperforin as a possible antidepressant component of hypericum extracts. *Life Sciences, 63*, 499–510.

Cochrane CAM Field [Online]. Available: http://www.compmed.ummc.umaryland .edu/Compmed/Cochrane/Cochrane.htm

Cohen, M. H. (2002). Legal issues in complementary and integrative medicine: A guide for clinicians. *Medical Clinics of North America, 86*, 185–196.

Curtis, P., & Gaylord, S. (2005). Safety issues in the interaction of conventional, complementary, and alternative health care. *Complementary Health Practice Review, 10*, 3–31.

DeRubeis, R. J., Hollon, S. D., Amsterdam, J. D., Shelton, R. C., Young, P. R., Salomon, R. M., et al. (2005). Cognitive therapy vs medications in the treatment of moderate to severe depression. *Archives of General Psychiatry, 62*, 409–416.

De Smet, P. A. (2004). Health risks of herbal remedies: An update. *Clinical Pharmacology Therapeutics, 76*, 1–17.

Devries, J. M. (1999). Emerging education needs of an emerging discipline. *Journal of Alternative and Complementary Medicine, 5*, 269–271.

Druss, B. G., & Rosenheck, R. A. (1999). Associations between use of unconventional therapies and conventional medical therapies. *Journal of the American Medical Association, 282*, 651–656.

Eisenberg, D. M., Davis, R. B., Ettner, S. L., Appel, S., Wilkey, S., Van Rompay, M., et al. (1998). Trends in alternative medicine use in the United States, 1990–1997: Results of a follow-up national survey. *Journal of the American Medical Association, 280*, 1569–1575.

Eisenberg, D. M., Kessler, R. C., Foster, C., Norlock, F. E., Calkins, D. R., & Delbanco, T. L. (1993). Unconventional medicine in the United States: Prevalence, costs, and patterns of use. *New England Journal of Medicine, 328*, 246–252.

Eisenberg, D. M., Kessler, R. C., Van Rompay, M. I., Kaptchuk, T. J., Wilkey, S. A., Appel, S., et al. (2001). Perceptions about complementary therapies relative to conventional therapies among adults who use both: Results from a national survey. *Annals of Internal Medicine, 135*, 344–351.

Ernst, E. (1999). Second thoughts about safety of St. John's Wort. *Lancet, 354*, 2014–2015.

Ernst, E. (2002). A systematic review of systematic reviews of homeopathy. *British Journal of Clinical Pharmacology, 54*, 577–582.

Ernst, E. (2003). The safety of massage therapy. *Rheumatology, 42*, 1101–1106.

Ernst, E. (2006). Acupuncture: A critical analysis. *Journal of Internal Medicine, 259*, 125–137.

Ernst, E., Rand, J. I., Barnes, J., & Stevinson, C. (1998a). Adverse effects profile of the herbal antidepressant St. John's Wort (*Hypericum perforatum*). *European Journal of Clinical Pharmacology, 54*, 589–594.

Ernst, E., Rand, J. I., & Stevinson, C. (1998b). Complementary therapies for depression: An overview. *Archives of General Psychiatry, 55*¡ 1026–1032.

Field, T. (1998). Massage therapy effects. *American Psychologist, 53,* 1270–1281.

Field, T. (2002). Massage therapy. *Medical Clinics of North America, 86,* 163–171.

Field, T., Hernandez–Reif, M., & Diego, M. (2005). Cortisol decreases and serotonin and dopamine increase following massage therapy. *International Journal of Neuroscience, 115,* 1397–1413.

Fong, H. H. S. (2002). Integration of herbal medicine into modern medical practices: Issues and prospects. *Integrative Cancer Therapies, 1,* 287–293.

Fontanarosa, P. B., & Lundberg, G. D. (1998). Alternative medicine meets science. *Journal of the American Medical Association, 280,* 1618–1619.

Frenkel, M. A., & Borkan, J. M. (2003). An approach for integrating complementary–alternative medicine into primary care. *Family Practice, 20,* 324–332.

Fritz, S. (2000). *Mosby's fundamentals of therapeutic massage.* St. Louis, MO: Mosby Publishing.

Fugh–Berman, A. (2000). Herb–drug interactions. *Lancet, 355,* 134–138.

Furnham, A., & Forey, J. (1994). The attitudes, behaviors, and beliefs of patients of conventional vs complementary (alternative) medicine. *Journal of Clinical Psychology, 50,* 458–469.

Gallin, P. F., Terman, M., Reme, C. E., Rafferty, B., & Burde, R. M. (1995). Ophthalmologic examination of patients with seasonal affective disorder before, and after bright light therapy. *American Journal of Ophthalmology, 119,* 202–210.

Gevitz, N. (1988). *Other healers: Unorthodox medicine in America.* Baltimore, MD: The Johns Hopkins University Press.

Golden, R. N., Gaynes, B. N., Ekstrom, R. D., Hamer, R. M., Jacobsen, F. M., Suppes, T., et al. (2005). The efficacy of light therapy in the treatment of mood disorders: A review and meta-analysis of the evidence. *American Journal of Psychiatry, 162,* 656–662.

Gundling, K. E. (1998). When did I become an allopath? *Archives of Internal Medicine, 158,* 2185–2186.

Haffmans, J., Lucius, S., & Ham, N. (1998). Suicide after bright light treatment in seasonal affective disorder: A case report. *Journal of Clinical Psychiatry, 59,* 478.

Hamilton, M. (1967). Development of a rating scale for primary depressive illness. *British Journal of Social and Clinical Psychology, 6,* 278–296.

Hammerness, P., Basch, E., Ulbricht, C., Barrette, E. P., Foppa, I., Basch, S., et al. (2003). St. John's Wort: A systematic review of adverse effects and drug interactions for the consultation psychiatrist. *Psychosomatics, 44,* 271–282.

Hayes, S. C., Strosahl, K. D., & Wilson, K. G. (1999). *Acceptance and commitment therapy: An experiential approach to behavior change.* New York: Guilford Press.

Hensrud, D. D., Engle, D. D., & Scheitel, S. M. (1999). Underreporting the use of dietary supplements and nonprescription medications among patients undergoing a periodic health exam. *Mayo Clinic Proceedings, 74,* 443–447.

Hollon, S. D., Jarrett, R. B., Nierenberg, A. A., Thase, M. E., Trivedi, M., & Rush, A. J. (2005). Psychotherapy and medication in the treatment of adult and geriatric depression: Which monotherapy or combined treatment? *Journal of Clinical Psychiatry, 66,* 455–468.

Hughes, E. F. (2001). Overview of complementary, alternative, and integrative medicine. *Clinical Obstetrics and Gynecology, 44,* 774–779.

Hypericum Depression Trial Study Group. (2002). Effect of *Hypericum perforatum* (St. John's Wort) in major depressive disorder: A randomized controlled trial. *Journal of the American Medical Association, 287,* 1807–1814.

Institute of Medicine. (2005). *Complementary and alternative medicine in the United States* Washington, DC: The National Academies Press.

Izzo, A. A., & Ernst, E. (2001). Interactions between herbal medicines and prescribed drugs: A systematic review. *Drugs, 61,* 2163–2175.

Jonas, W. B. (1998). Alternative medicine: Learning from the past, examining the present, advancing to the future. *Journal of the American Medical Association, 280,* 1616–1618.

Kabat–Zinn, J. (1990). *Full catastrophe living: Using the wisdom of your mind to face stress, pain and illness.* New York: Dell.

Kaptchuk, T. J. (2002). Acupuncture: Theory, efficacy, and practice. *Annals of Internal Medicine, 136,* 374–383.

Kaptchuk, T. J., Goldman, P., Stone, D. A., & Stason, W. B. (2000). Do medical devices have enhanced placebo effects? *Journal of Clinical Epidemiology, 53,* 786–792.

Kelner, M., & Wellman, B. (1997). Health care and consumer choice: Medical and alternative therapies. *Social Science & Medicine, 45,* 203–212.

Kessler, R. C., Davis, R. B., Foster, D. F., Van Rompay, M. I., Walters, E. E., Wiley, S. A., et al. (2001a). Long-term trends in the use of complementary and alternative medical therapies in the United States. *Annals of Internal Medicine, 135,* 262–268.

Kessler, R. C., Soukup, J., Davis, R. B., Foster, D. F., Wilkey, S. A., Van Rompay, M. I., et al. (2001b). The use of complementary and alternative therapies to treat anxiety and depression in the United States. *American Journal of Psychiatry, 158,* 289–294.

Kim, Y. H., Lichtenstein, G., & Waalen, J. (2002). Distinguishing complementary medicine from alternative medicine [letter]. *Archives of Internal Medicine, 162,* 943.

Labyak, S. E., & Metzger, B. L. (1997). The effects of effleurage backrub on the physiological components of relaxation: A meta-analysis. *Nursing Research, 46,* 59–62.

Lam, R. W., Levitt, A. J., Levitan, R. D., Enns, M. W., Morehouse, R., Michalak, E. E., & Tam, E. M. (2006). The Can-SAD Study: A randomized controlled trial of the effectiveness of light therapy and fluoxetine in patients with winter seasonal affective disorder. *American Journal of Psychiatry, 163,* 805–812.

Lee, B. Y., LaRiccia, P. J., & Newberg, A. B. (2004). Acupuncture in theory and practice. *Hospital Physician, 40,* 11–18.

Linde, K., Mulrow, C. D., Berner, M., & Egger, M. (2005). St. John's wort for depression (review). *Cochrane Database of Systematic Reviews, 2,* art. no.: CD000448. DOI: 10.1002/14651858.CD000448.pub2.

Linde, K., Ramirez, G., Mulrow, C. D., Pauls, A., Weidenhammer, W., & Melchart, D. (1996). St. John's wort for depression: An overview and meta-analysis of randomized clinical trials. *British Medical Journal, 313,* 253–258.

Linehan, M. M. (1993). *Cognitive–behavioral treatment of borderline personality disorder.* New York: Guilford Press.

Luo, H., Jia, Y., Wu, X., & Dai, W. (1990). Electro-acupuncture in the treatment of depressive psychosis. *International Journal of Clinical Acupuncture, 1,* 7–13.

Luo, H., Jia, Y., & Zhan, L. (1985). Electro-acupuncture vs amitriptyline in the treatment of depressive states. *Journal of Traditional Chinese Medicine, 5,* 3–8.

Luo, H., Meng, F., Jia, Y., & Zhao, X. (1998). Clinical research on the therapeutic effect of the electro-acupuncture treatment in patients with depression. *Psychiatry and Clinical Neurosciences, 52(S),* S338–S340.

Ma, S. H., & Teasdale, J. D. (2004). Mindfulness-based cognitive therapy for depression: Replication and exploration of differential relapse prevention effects. *Journal of Consulting and Clinical Psychology, 72,* 31–40.

Mann, D., Gaylord, S., & Norton, S. (2004). Moving toward integrative care: Rationales, models, and steps for conventional-care providers. *Complementary Health Practice Review*, 9, 155–172.

Marcus, D. M., & Grollman, A. P. (2006). Review for NCCAM is overdue. *Science*, 313, 301–302.

Markman, M. (2002). Safety issues in using complementary and alternative medicine. *Journal of Clinical Oncology*, 20, 39–41.

Martiny, K., Simonsen, C., Lunde, M., Clemmensen, L., & Bech, P. (2004). Decreasing TSH levels in patients with seasonal affective disorder (SAD) responding to 1 week of bright light therapy. *Journal of Affective Disorders*, 79, 253–257.

McHughes, M., & Timmermann, B. N. (2005). A review of the use of CAM therapy and the sources of accurate and reliable information. *Journal of Managed Care Pharmacy*, 11, 695–703.

McLennan, A. H., Wilson, D. H., & Taylor, A. W. (1996). Prevalence and cost of alternative medicine in Australia. *Lancet*, 347, 569–573.

Mehling, W. F., DiBlasi, Z., & Hecht, F. (2005). Bias control in trials of bodywork: A review of methodological issues. *Journal of Alternative and Complementary Medicine*, 11, 333–342.

Moffet, H. H. (2006). How might acupuncture work? A systematic review of physiologic rationales from clinical trials. *BioMed Central Complementary and Alternative Medicine*, 6, 25.

Moyer, C. A., Rounds, J., & Hannum, J. W. (2004). A meta-analysis of massage therapy research. *Psychological Bulletin*, 130, 3–18.

Mukaino, Y., Park, J., White, A., & Ernst, E. (2005). Effectiveness of acupuncture for depression: A systematic review of randomised clinical trials. *Acupuncture in Medicine: Journal of the British Medical Acupuncture Society*, 23, 70–76.

Nahin, R. L., & Straus, S. E. (2001). Research into complementary and alternative medicine: Problems and potential. *British Medical Journal*, 322, 161–164.

Nahin, R. L., Pontzer, C. H., & Chesney, M. A. (2005). Racing toward the integration of complementary and alternative medicine: A marathon or a sprint? *Health Affairs*, 24, 991–993.

Nasir, L. S. (2002). Acupuncture. *Primary Care: Clinics in Office Practice*, 29, 393–405.

National Center for Complementary and Alternative Medicine. (2002, May). *What is complementary and alternative medicine (CAM)?* [Online]. Available: http://nccam.nih.gov/health/whatiscam

National Center for Complementary and Alternative Medicine. (2005). *St. John's wort and the treatment of depression* [Online]. Available: http://nccam.nih.gov/health/stjohnswort

National Center for Complementary and Alternative Medicine. (2006). *Five-year strategic plan* [Online]. Available: http://nccam.nih.gov

Paramore, L. C. (1997). Use of alternative therapies: Estimates from the 1994 Robert Wood Johnson Foundation National Access to Care Survey. *Journal of Pain and Symptom Management*, 13, 83–89.

Pelletier, K. R., Marie, A., Krasner, M., & Haskell, W. L. (1997). Current trends in the integration and reimbursement of complementary and alternative medicine by managed care, insurance carriers, and hospital providers. *American Journal of Health Promotion*, 12, 112–123.

Praschak–Rieder, N., Neumeister, A., Hesselmann, B., Willeit, M., Barnas, C., & Kasper, S. (1997). Suicidal tendencies as a complication of light therapy for seasonal affective disorder: A report of three cases. *Journal of Clinical Psychiatry*, 58, 389–392.

Ramey, D. W. (2001). Acupuncture points do not exist. *Scientific Review of Alternative Medicine, 5,* 140–145.

Ramey, D. W., & Sampson, W. (2001). Review of the evidence for the clinical efficacy of human acupuncture. *Scientific Review of Alternative Medicine, 5,* 195–201.

Reston, J. (1971, July 26). Now about my operation in Peking. *The New York Times,* p. A6.

Rhee, S. M., Garg, V. K., & Hershey, C. O. (2004). Use of complementary and alternative medicines by ambulatory patients. *Archives of Internal Medicine, 164,* 1004–1009.

Robinson, A., & McGrail, M. R. (2004). Disclosure of CAM use to medical practitioners: A review of qualitative and quantitative studies. *Complementary Therapies in Medicine, 12,* 90–98.

Rosenthal, N. E. (1988). *Light therapy and treatment of affective disorders.* National Institute of Mental Health. Unpublished manuscript.

Salovey, P., Mayer, J. D., Goldman, S. L., Turvey, C., & Palfai, T. F. (1995). Emotional attention, clarity, and repair: Exploring emotional intelligence using the Trait Meta-Mood Scale. In J. W. Pennebaker (Ed.), *Emotion, disclosure, and health* (pp. 125–154). Washington, DC: American Psychological Association.

Sampson, W. (2005). Studying herbal remedies. *New England Journal of Medicine, 353,* 337–339.

Sato, T. (1997). Seasonal affective disorder and phototherapy: A critical review. *Professional Psychology: Research and Practice, 28,*164–169.

Segal, Z. V., Teasdale, J. D., & Williams, J. M. G. (2004). Mindfulness-based cognitive therapy: Theoretical rationale and empirical status. In S. Hayes, V. M. Follette, & M. M. Linehan (Eds.), *Mindfulness and acceptance: Expanding the cognitive–behavioral tradition (pp. 45–65).* New York: Guilford Press.

Segal, Z. V., Williams, J. M. G., & Teasdale, J. D. (2002). *Mindfulness-based cognitive therapy for depression: A new approach to preventing relapse.* New York: Guilford Press.

Shelton, R. C., Keller, M. B., Gelenberg, A., Dunner, D. L., Hirschfeld, R., Thase, M. E., et al. (2001). Effectiveness of St. John's wort in major depression: A randomized controlled trial. *Journal of the American Medical Association, 285,* 1978–1986.

Sherman, K. J., Cherkin, D. C., Eisenberg, D. M., Erro, J., Hrbek, A., & Deyo, R. A. (2005). The practice of acupuncture: Who are the providers and what do they do? *Annals of Family Medicine, 3,* 151–158.

Starr, P. (1982). *The social transformation of American medicine.* San Francisco, CA: Harper Collins.

Sternberg, R. J. (2000). Images of mindfulness. *Journal of Social Issues, 56,* 11–26.

Stoller, K. B., & Bigelow, G. E. (2006). Introduction and historical overview. In E. C. Strain & M. L. Stitzer (Eds.), *The treatment of opioid dependence.* Baltimore, MD: Johns Hopkins University Press.

Straus, S. E., & Chesney, M. A. (2006). In defense of NCCAM. *Science, 313,* 303–304.

Takeshige, C. (1989). Mechanism of acupuncture analgesia based on animal experiments. In B. Pomerantz & G. Stux (Eds.), *Scientific bases of acupuncture* (pp. 53–78). Berlin: Springer-Verlag.

Teasdale, J. D., Segal, Z. V., Williams, J. M. G., Ridgeway, V. A., Soulsby, J. M., & Lau, M. A. (2000). Prevention of relapse/recurrence in major depression by mindfulness-based cognitive therapy. *Journal of Consulting and Clinical Psychology, 68,* 615–623.

Terman, M. (1988). On the question of mechanism in phototherapy: Considerations of clinical efficacy and epidemiology. *Journal of Biological Rhythms, 3,* 155–172.

Terman, M., & Terman, J. S. (2005). Light therapy for seasonal and nonseasonal depression: Efficacy, protocol, safety, and side effects. *CNS Spectrums, 10,* 647–663.

Unützer, J., Klap, R., Sturm, R., Young, A. S., Marmon, T., Shatkin, J., et al. (2000). Mental disorders and the use of alternative medicine: Results from a national survey. *American Journal of Psychiatry, 157,* 1851–1857.

U.S. Food and Drug Administration. (1996). Acupuncture needles no longer investigational [electronic version]. *FDA Consumer, 30*(5). Also available at http://www.fda.gov/fdac/departs/596_upd.html.

Verhoef, M. J. (1998). Physicians' perspectives on massage therapy. *Canadian Family Physician, 44,* 1018.

Vincent, C. (2001). The safety of acupuncture. *British Medical Journal, 323,* 467–368.

Watson, D., Clark, L. A., & Tellegen, A. (1988). Development and validation of brief measures of positive and negative affect: The PANAS scales. *Journal of Personality and Social Psychology, 54,* 1063–1070.

Wehr, T. A., Skwerer, R. G., Jacobsen, F. M., Sack, D. A., & Rosenthal, N. E. (1987). Eye versus skin phototherapy of seasonal affective disorder. *American Journal of Psychiatry, 144,* 753–757.

Wetzel, M. S., Eisenberg, D. M., & Kaptchuk, T. J. (1998). Courses involving complementary and alternative medicine at US medical schools. *Journal of the American Medical Association, 280,* 784–787.

Wetzel, M. S., Kaptchuk, T. J., Haramati, A., & Eisenberg, D. M. (2003). Complementary and alternative medicine: Implications for medical education. *Annals of Internal Medicine, 138,* 191–196.

Wong, E. (1997). *Harmonizing yin and yang.* Boston: Shambhala Publishing.

Yamashita, H., Tsukayama, H., Tanno, Y., & Nishijo, K. (1998). Adverse events related to acupuncture [letter to the editor]. *Journal of the American Medical Association, 280,* 1563–1564.

Zahourek, R. (2000). Alternative, complementary, or integrative approaches to treating depression. *Journal of the American Psychiatric Nurses Association, 6,* 77–86.

8

Loss in Translation

Considering the Critical Role of Interpreters and Language in the Psychiatric Evaluation of Non-English-Speaking Patients

CAREY JACKSON, DOUG ZATZICK,
RAYMOND HARRIS, & LORIN GARDINER

Language is recursive in character. It is simultaneously a tool or medium for producing human thought and culture, and a product of human thought and culture. Thus, paradigm shifts in culture and work are often attended by concomitant shifts in language. These changes reflect the new metaphors and forms of thought that allow concepts to be configured in new ways and then shared through language.

Yet language is invisible to most clinicians in their technical work. Although they are communicators by profession, physicians are not routinely trained in the operations of speech, one of the primary tools of their trade. They communicate in technical language with each other, then rapidly and almost unconsciously shift register to speak in the vernacular with patients. There are attempts to train physicians in lay communication with patients, and priority is placed on clear and efficient presentations of cases between professionals. Still, the mechanics of this fundamental tool for creating and propagating medical culture are rarely explored.

The recursive nature of language, therefore, has important implications for culturally competent health care that remain unexamined. To engage in such care, an understanding of the relationship of language and culture is essential, because the clinical encounter is fundamentally "talking." Clinical work becomes problematic when two or more languages are in use during a clinical encounter. Such encounters can become a special instance of paradigm shift for patients. When new concepts and new words are introduced into old frameworks, they must be inserted in a manner congruent with existing semantic structures. If this process includes introducing concepts that do not exist in the target language, or retrieving information from the target language that is unrecognizable in bio-medical frameworks, the potential for confusion is enormous.

Discussions of the causes and consequences of sadness and madness are the substance of many mental health visits. Such encounters are especially ripe for cross-cultural confusion, because most cultures have working models of emotional distress and bizarre behavior that draw on both Western and traditional concepts. During the past two decades, in recognition of the increasing diversity of the U.S. population, a series of commentaries and reports has emphasized the importance of developing culturally appropriate mental health services (Kleinman, 1988; U.S. Census Bureau, 2000; U.S. Department of Health and Human Services, 2001).

The first steps toward culturally competent mental health care involve making interpreter services available whenever they are needed, and training clinical staff to address linguistic and cultural issues whenever they arise. However, the linguistic needs of a busy medical center can be daunting. As an example, we recently conducted investigations at the level 1 trauma centers associated with the University of California–Davis (UC-Davis) and the University of Washington (UW). Trauma patients hospitalized on the inpatient surgical unit were randomly approached and asked which language they spoke at home, spoke best, and preferred to speak in medical encounters. Approximately 12% of patients approached were non-English speaking. At UC-Davis, 11 different languages were identified among non-English speaking patients, including Armenian, Cambodian, Cantonese, Korean, Laotian, Punjabi, Russian, Spanish, Swedish, and Vietnamese. At UW, 12 different languages were identified, including Arabic, Cantonese, Hindi, Laotian, Mandarin, Portuguese, Russian, Spanish, Tagalog, Thai, Ukrainian, and Vietnamese (Santos, Russo, & Zatzick, 2003). Between 50% and 75% of these trauma survivors endorsed high levels of depressive, posttraumatic stress, and/or substance abuse-related comorbidities (Zatzick, Jurkovich, Russo, Roy–Byrne, Katon, Wagner, et al., 2004).

In this chapter we consider the complex role of the professional medical interpreter during an interpreted psychiatric interview. The chapter is divided into two parts. The first explores for the medical professional the complex linguistic tasks that are performed by the interpreter. Through individual vignettes, we discuss the aspects of language that bear directly on effective clinical interpretation in mental health. During the process we explore the ways in which language use can be a sign of mental illness that interpreters can be taught to observe. We will see how a lack of familiarity with somatic expressions of mental illness can confuse both patients and interpreters, and block their understanding of the Western psychiatric diagnostic process. We then highlight examples in which non-Western experiences of illness, relationships, or bodily functions make agreement on diagnosis difficult. We also consider how language itself structures and defines the ways in which things are talked about and subsequently linked by metaphor to related concepts and implied actions. We attend to the formidable demands placed on interpreters, who must retrieve complaints, recognize the linkages of these complaints to culturally defined syndromes or symptoms, transform the complaints into recognizable biomedical symptoms, and find phrases to express them that are appropriate in clinical culture. These tasks require close collaboration between mental health professionals and interpreters.

The second part of this chapter addresses the professional training and development needed to interpret in mental health settings. We briefly review the professional standards expected of health interpreters in general as well as the special considerations that apply to mental health interpreting. We then review various aspects of the mental health system that constitute psychiatric culture in the United States and require understanding on the part of interpreters before they can adequately represent psychiatric culture to the patients with whom they work.

A PRELIMINARY OBSERVATION ABOUT PRACTICAL APPLICATIONS

In clinical medicine and psychiatry, practitioners need practical guidelines for fixing common problems. Unfortunately, as with certain chronic illnesses, there are no rote, routine, or predictable fixes for some of the linguistic mismatches and misunderstandings that are frequently encountered. What worked last time may not work this time; what works for one patient may not work for another. Some approaches can successfully manage confusion, and these will be identified as needed. The emphasis of the first part of this chapter is on insight—namely, on understanding some of the ways in which language operates and some of the varied problems that often arise in interpreted mental health encounters. With such insight comes awareness, the essential first step in identifying a repertoire of interventions.

THE SOCIOLINGUISTIC TASK OF INTERPRETING IN MENTAL HEALTH

Sorting Symptoms to Make a Diagnosis: A Case of Headache, Insomnia, and Confusion

There are very few clinical settings in which issues of language become more complex and nuanced than in discussions of mental and emotional illness—especially illnesses born of trauma and torture, and therefore of physical as well as psychic suffering. These are not everyday conversations, and it is sometimes difficult to find the words, not to mention the will, to explain the requisite historical conditions, perceptions, meanings, and actions. It is retraumatizing for the patient to be asked to describe such private events to a stranger, even in a clinical setting, especially if the conversation brings back painful recollections of shame, loss, and deep grief. Such encounters can become still more difficult when one of the people in the room is an interpreter, a member of the often small, local immigrant community who is known to the patient socially outside the clinic.

Somatization of psychological problems is extremely common among immigrants (Van Ommeren, Sharma, Sharma, Komproe, Cardena, & de Jong,

2002), and it presents a substantial challenge for interpreters, insofar as the provider sees the symptom presented by the patient as the central issue. This disconnection, and the need to ensure that any resulting confusion does not engender unnecessary disagreement, presents a potential quagmire to interpreter and provider alike.

Consider the case of Sylvie, a 58-year-old immigrant to the United States from Bosnia. When Sylvie first presented to her primary care doctor four years ago, she had a litany of complaints: urinary incontinence, headaches, joint pain, rashes, insomnia, fatigue, and confusion. Her husband was very worried about her and alerted the doctor to her sitting and crying at length, her restless sleep, and her memory lapses. During the ensuing months the doctor identified further problems of which Sylvie was unaware: diabetes, hypertension, and hyperlipidemia. Not long after the initial presentation, the conversation got around to her sleep, whereupon it became evident that Sylvie's sleep was severely disrupted by frequent urination and nightmares. The nightmares were related to an event she witnessed during the Kosovo war.

Sylvie and her family are ethnic Albanians who lived in an Albanian village in Kosovo, an autonomous province of former Yugoslavia. Her family once owned farms and substantial property in the region. Her grandfather had been a provincial governor in the 1950s during the presidency of Josip Tito. Because of their Albanian heritage, their resources, and their local fame, Sylvie's family was targeted by the Serbian government after the breakup of Yugoslavia in the 1990s, and her son was conscripted into the army. When he deserted, the authorities simply pursued him to his native village and conscripted him again. He deserted a second time and escaped first to Western Europe and then to the United States. The local military authority punished Sylvie's family by seizing their lands. They protested loudly and formally through the local media and through legal action, unaware how foolhardy and outdated these means of protest had become. One night, people from Sylvie's village, including 20 male family members, were herded together by a platoon of soldiers and marched out of town. Sylvie followed them at a distance into the forest and witnessed as they were executed by machine gun fire and dumped into an open pit. She remembers watching through the trees and shadows, terrified of being found, feeling like a coward, aghast at the carnage and the apparent insignificance of her neighbors and family to these soldiers.

In Sylvie's nightmares she feels the floor rolling beneath her, the windows rattling, the walls heaving. It is as if an earthquake is destroying the family home. She runs to the window and sees the forest and the pit full of her dead family and mangled friends. Sometimes she just feels the floor roll, other times she sees the entire scene. A part of the dream can stand for the whole memory. She awakens with her pulse racing; she feels ashamed, angry, heartbroken; she is sobbing.

Treatment for the nightmares and the diabetes improved Sylvie's sleep as well as many of her somatic complaints. Her confusion and anhedonia persist, but her depressive symptoms are much less severe than in the past. Certain anniversaries, family events, discussion of legal documents, and news from home can set her back, but she makes gradual progress.

To make sense of the chief complaint of traumatized immigrants involves a number of overlapping issues that must be considered when working through interpretation.

The first challenge during interpreted psychiatric encounters is the common distraction of exploring somatic symptoms — such as headache, insomnia, abdominal pain, and neck ache — without discovering the affective root of these symptoms. Although this distraction is a feature of somatized affective disorders in any primary care presentation, regardless of the need for interpretation, the presence of an interpreter complicates the discussion of somatic complaints. Each symptom under review is potentially tied to other diagnostic possibilities, so that each one prompts a lengthy translated discussion involving patient, provider, and interpreter. The interpreter tries to explain to the patient that the physical complaints are not being ignored, but rather are being considered as only one possible location of the problem. Because somatizing patients have many urgent complaints, a fruitless search through possible physical causes will be exhausting to all concerned. By the time the provider discards nonpsychiatric possibilities, the patient and interpreter are fatigued and perhaps skeptical of the provider's skills.

Tocher and Larson (1999) have reported that the average time spent in an interpreted primary care encounter was 17 minutes, not significantly different from the time spent in an English-only encounter. Because each sentence must be passed both ways through an interpreter, the time available to discuss and clarify symptoms is only one half to one third of the total time available during the encounter. Exploring the review of symptoms around headaches, insomnia, weight loss, fatigue, stomachache, and myalgias is lengthy, and each one is potentially linked to biomedical and cultural constructions of illness. The possibility of finding a common thread of depression or anxiety is limited by time constraints and by the confusion involved in interpreting these myriad complaints. Summary questions such as "Do you think you are depressed?" often do not translate, for reasons to be discussed shortly. Thus the clinician must suspect depression and then pursue it efficiently, sometimes against resistance, to establish a diagnosis before the patient is lost to follow-up.

From a primary care provider's perspective, Sylvie's presentation shows the multiple diagnostic and educational tasks necessary to sort through a complaint and discard certain physiological possibilities to focus on the symptoms resulting from a history of trauma (Waitzkin & Magana, 1997). For example, Sylvie's provider told her that her urinary frequency resulted from the stretching impact of several childbirths on her pelvic structures and from the glucose load in her urine caused by diabetes. From Sylvie's perspective, then, her frequent urination, while embarrassing, could happen to anyone with a similar history of pregnancy and diabetes. But the headaches and confusion; the nausea brought on by disrupted sleep; the nightmares linked to loss of family, home, lands, and heritage; the murder of friends; the exile in America; the isolation and hopelessness; the thoughts of suicide — these symptoms were different. They did not go away with treatment of diabetes and incontinence. They emerged and persisted because of Sylvie's unique positioning historically, socially, and culturally. Like a terminal diagnosis, these symptoms did not just change Sylvie's life; they had the potential to stop meaningful life.

Therapy for depression or PTSD can stop the images of terror, restore life, and make it worth living (Ursano, Bell, Eth, Friedman, Norwood, Pfefferbaum, et al., 2004). Therapy may also improve the management of other chronic conditions such as diabetes (Katon, Von Korff, Lin, Simon, Ludman, Bush, et al., 2003). Finding the right diagnosis and treatment, however, requires understanding the story, designing an acceptable therapy, and optimizing that therapy while controlling for adverse reactions.

The second challenge of interpreting in psychiatric encounters is reaching a diagnosis through interpretation when the patient is actively resistant to linking a mental health discussion to past events and current somatic complaints. Foreign-born individuals who have seen enough of American medicine to be able to anticipate psychiatric diagnoses, yet not enough to be convinced that these are treatable conditions prevalent among dispersed traumatized peoples (and not merely an American cultural preoccupation), may unintentionally or even willfully block the psychiatric diagnostic process. Interfering with the work of the clinician is clearly inappropriate, yet it happens and must be considered. Many immigrants link the prevalence of psychiatric diagnoses not with an enhanced clinical system adept at identifying such conditions, but with a pathology in the American social fabric that predisposes American medicine to find mental illness everywhere. Immigrants often perceive dissolution of families, loss of parental authority, decline of religious practice, and breakdown of community as the most obvious social features of the new country. The attenuated role of family and community can thus be seen as the underlying cause of the American predisposition to depression, one that results in an inability to manage loneliness, isolation, and social trauma "normally" and thus requires medical intervention. These social and cultural features of the new home, along with the social stigma of mental illness in the old home, interact to lead patients and interpreters to minimize psychological issues and insist on physical origins for a symptom.

Education of interpreters and communities is critical on this point. Many, if not all, displaced people experience grief. A subset have predisposing conditions, persistent reactions, or traumatic histories that interact with the experience of diaspora to take their grief to another level, or transform it into another diagnostic category altogether. Many such individuals are sad; a much smaller number are unable to function or are likely to pose a risk to self and family. On the surface the affects appear similar, but at the neurological level, distinct neurochemical adaptations are at work.

The third challenge in psychiatric interpreting is to explain to providers the symptoms or concepts that might suggest culturally constructed illnesses — symptoms that would likely go unrecognized by Western professionals as manifestations of depression or PTSD. The presence and skills of the interpreter in the medical interview simultaneously enable and constrain the diagnostic process. On the one hand, as we have seen, the chief complaint and accompanying complaints can be made available through the skill of the interpreter, who finds appropriate linguistic equivalents for the physician or psychiatrist. On the other hand, the resulting expressed complaint may reflect the interpreter's bungled attempt to find an equivalent, or indeed a failure in the interpreter's training.

We return to this point in a more detailed discussion of conceptual equivalents for symptoms or diagnostic terms. A related challenge is that after a psychological diagnosis is made and physical symptoms are linked to past experience, such a linkage may lead the patient away from psychiatric treatments of symptoms toward alternative, culturally defined diagnostic possibilities with alternative treatment implications. We return to this additional challenge in our discussion of culture brokering in mental health interpretation.

The fourth challenge in psychiatric interpreting is the issue of the pattern, rate, and content of the patient's speech, as understood against the background of the home culture's norms. Pressured speech, or the drive to speak quickly, is considered symptomatic of certain affective states. What counts as pressured speech for a Navajo, however, may sound like a normal rate of speech to a Greek or Cantonese speaker. Teaching interpreters the observational skills of the clinician enables them to assist in a task for which they are uniquely positioned. To a psychiatrist it is the precise nature of the confusion, and not simply its presence, that leads to the diagnosis. For example, during Sylvie's medical interview, the interpreter often appeared perplexed, and at one point he threw up his hands in exasperation. "She makes no sense," he said. "Her sentences make no sense." At this point, instead of assuming that the patient herself is disorganized and incoherent, the clinician is better advised to redirect the interpreter to describe the form, cadence, affect, and content of the speech.

Pressured speech is common in anxiety and during manic episodes (American Psychiatric Association, 1994). The patient's thinking may be clear, but the mind is racing and the words come streaming out. By contrast, tangential speech or "flight of ideas" is characteristic of a thought disorder, implying a confused and rambling stringing together of ideas, often sounding nonsensical, that may be encountered in bipolar manic or other psychotic states, such as depression with psychotic features. "Word salad," the random meaningless association of words, is typical of the severely disorganized schizophrenic, but other psychotic states may also express themselves at times in this manner. Neologisms (words invented and given special significance) are commonly encountered in schizotypal personalities, delusional schizophrenics, and some developmentally delayed persons. Finally, certain neurological disorders resulting in aphasia can lead to fluent yet incomprehensible speech, as in cases of Wernicke's aphasia that result from stroke. The point behind these varied permutations is that the precise nature of incoherent speech is a key symptom of the underlying illness, yet the interpreter is the only one capable of describing it, and the clinician is the one responsible for training and directing the interpreter's observations.

The diagnosis of affective disorders or thought disorders through an interpreter is most effective after the interpreter has been oriented to the linguistic detail for which the clinician is listening, such as the tone and cadence of the patient's speech as well as its content. If there is no time for such training and orientation, the clinician must do the work by proxy, quizzing the interpreter to characterize the form and content of the patients' expressions. In Sylvie's case, the interpreter was directed to perform a word-for-word translation of her speech, with the following result:

> The Captain said, "Take them to the woods, not the courthouse, not the church for all to see, not the square, the woods, the woods, the woods." Those woods I played in as a girl. I lost my necklace in those woods. A necklace my grandmother gave me. My grandmother was not Albanian. I think she might have really been Romanian, perhaps a Gypsy. We made a trip to Hungary when I was six. They have beautiful rivers there . . . and woods.

Sylvie begins by remembering a dream she had, but then rambles off tangentially, remembering the woods themselves and her associations with those woods — past events, significant connections both personal and cultural, loved ones, better times. The clinician now can hear that her speech is not "word salad." It lacks neologisms, it is mumbled rather than pressured, and it expresses thoughts that are completely formed but linked in an odd stream-of-consciousness manner. In addition to Sylvie's dysphoria, suicidal thoughts, tangential speech, vivid nightmares, and memory loss, the clinician can now diagnose PTSD and depression, providing a very different pharmacological therapy for the two disorders. The form, cadence, volume, and content of Sylvie's speech were available primarily to the interpreter, yet they provided some of the key symptoms for the diagnosis. After the interpreter understood the distinctions that the clinician was trying to make, the interpreter was able to describe the speech more fully and assist in the clinical assessment. The clinician could then help Sylvie sort out which symptoms were urological or diabetic and which symptoms were somatized, and thus likely to improve with treatment of her PTSD.

The Interaction of Cultural Experience and Cultural Expression: A Case of Neck Pain and Tinnitus

One of the most challenging aspects of cross-cultural medical care and transcultural psychiatry is the bewildering variety of ways in which cultures associate symptoms with illness. The interpreter is left trying to package the interplay of expression and cultural experience into a recognizable form that often lacks a precise linguistic equivalent, or at least one recognizable to a layperson. Consider the case of Preap, an elderly Cambodian man whose family was concerned about his profound weight loss during the preceding year.

Preap presented to a clinic complaining of abdominal pain, head and neck ache, insomnia, and weight loss. He had lost 25 pounds during the past year. He had no significant bowel complaints, but he did exhibit profound anorexia. A standard evaluation, including a physical examination, laboratory work, colonoscopy, endoscopy, chest radiograph, and computed tomographic scan, revealed no evidence of malignancy. During the course of his clinical workup and follow-up visits, Preap frequently mentioned his neck aches and ringing ears. His wife, on the other hand, constantly asked about his blood pressure and wondered whether he had had a stroke. It became apparent that Preap was not sleeping well because of horrible nightmares that had become more pronounced after the recent murder of one of his granddaughters. The nightmares were of Cambodia and his imprisonment under the Khmer Rouge. He awakened repeatedly from dreams of a ghost walking slowly toward him, willing him to die. During this dream he was paralyzed and unable to breathe. He described this as *khmaach sangat* or "the ghost pushes you down," a common experience among Khmer.

Devon Hinton and colleagues (2005) have investigated panic symptoms systematically among 100 Cambodian refugees in a psychiatric clinic in Massachusetts. Symptoms such as sore neck (86%), fear (98%), tinnitus (83%), and cold extremities (91%) were experienced by Cambodians who met *DSM-IV* criteria for panic disorder (American Psychiatric Association, 1994). Sleep paralysis was also experienced by 42% of these patients in the past year. Sleep paralysis is characterized by recurrent nightmares of a dark presence or ghost pursuing the subject and inducing suffocation. The subject has the experience of being paralyzed, unable to move, and overwhelmed by this pursuing presence. Frequently the subject awakens, unable to breathe. The existence of the Khmer term *khmaach sangat* acknowledges that this is a common enough experience among Cambodians to have an abbreviated identifier. Only the interpreter, however, can explain the meaning and context of this term to the clinician, who must then link the term to a symptom complex recognized by Western clinical practice.

In this situation, clinicians unfamiliar with the Cambodian cluster of symptoms reported in the literature might miss key components of panic disorder that would assist in making such a diagnosis. Hinton's work on the ethnopsychiatry of PTSD and panic disorder among Cambodian survivors of the Pol Pot regime underscores the lack of familiarity with such disorders among Western practitioners. Hinton notes that literature is only now emerging on the culturally constructed ways in which large numbers of Southeast Asian refugees (Hmong, Mien, Lao, Khmer, and Vietnamese) express panic, anxiety, depression, and PTSD (Hinton, Pham, Tran, Safren, Otto, & Pollack, 2004). He provides ample documentation of the tendency for traumatized refugees to somatize their complaints. As he notes, "[t]raumatized Southeast Asian refugees, in a state of dysphoria, tend to 'speak corporally.' To decipher this language, the clinician must understand the local ethnophysiology and ethnopsychology, the symbolizing body, and the interpersonal meaning of somatic complaint" (Hinton, Um, & Ba, 2001, pp. 298–299). If clinicians fail to recognize the emerging list of complaints, they will head off in fruitless discussions of possible diagnoses and treatments. On the other hand, if they recognize the link to panic disorder or PTSD, discussing the connection between somatic complaints and mental health issues will present a complex challenge to interpreter and patient alike.

Preap was diagnosed with a panic disorder associated with PTSD. He has been treated with prazosin, clonazepam, and Prozac. Preap perseverates on bodily symptoms in clinic, but he acknowledges that these have improved with the current treatment regimen.

Again, the link between a list of bodily symptoms and a psychiatric diagnosis, or conversely, the recognition of a unique sociocultural manifestation of illness that can lead to such a diagnosis, relies on the clarity of interpretation. The interpreter must be aware of the medicolinguistic challenges encountered during the interview and be prepared to revisit and explore the linguistic ambiguities for both patient and clinician. The interpreter may not be able to link the patient's experience to a diagnosis, but may nevertheless understand that a given term refers to a known cultural entity. In such situations, the interpreter must have both the competence and the permission to act as a cultural broker, guiding the clinician to explore a given phenomenon and its meaning, and offering any relevant cultural background. As a broker, the interpreter must provide examples, meanings, and contexts.

The worst error in such a clinical encounter would be to misunderstand a cultural expression referring to the supernatural — such as this one about ghosts — as evidence of hallucination. In such a case, the clinician–interpreter team would not only fail to link the symptom to a culturally defined experience of panic, but would erroneously conclude that the patient is experiencing psychotic symptoms. This misdiagnosis would stigmatize the patient, undermine his or her confidence in biomedicine, and, most important, fail to relieve suffering.

Actions Implied by Word Choice, Culture, and Social Experience: A Case of Hopelessness and Spiritual Renewal

Saha is a 58-year-old Sinhala shopkeeper who was brought to a primary care clinician by his African American wife. About five months ago, in a drunk driving incident, he caused an automobile accident during which his oldest son was killed. Since then he has had difficulty with headaches and sleep. Lately he has been reading more than before, talking about taking a pilgrimage to Sri Lanka and then India, and making plans to sell the family business. He has taken to meditating and fasting daily, and he is considering becoming a Buddhist monk. He says that he is experiencing *kalakirīma*, a Sinhala expression equivalent to "hopelessness." The social context that led to his diagnosis of depression is obvious. Perhaps it is a reactive depression, perhaps a major depressive episode. Both Saha's Sinhalese relatives and the interpreter immediately recognized the Buddhist underpinnings of *kalakirīma* and its cultural and hence behavioral implications.

In a now classic work, "Depression, Buddhism, and the Work of Culture in Sri Lanka," the anthropologist Gananath Obeyesekere (1985) describes the relationship between symptoms, word choice, cultural attitudes, and the social actions implied by those attitudes. He explains why the language of affect cannot necessarily be used in a technical manner to operationalize a diagnosis and a therapy from a presumed complaint. He writes,

> One of the problems of contemporary psychiatric methodology is the assumption that the language that expresses "depressive affects" can also be operationalized. Yet the attempt to give operational specificity to the vocabulary of emotion is to destroy what is integral to that form of speech (*parole*), namely its intrinsic diffusiveness, multiplicity of meanings, and capacity to assimilate and express emotional states that are not easily differentiated and indeed run counter to the very canons of operationalism.... Furthermore, and I specifically refer here to the vocabulary of suffering and despair, that speech is linked to specific traditions,

such as those of Buddhism and Christianity. It is almost impossible for a Sinhalese person to use words expressing sorrow without articulating them to the Buddhist tradition. Even if all the words he uses do not come from the tradition directly, the larger context of usage will eventually embody it in the doctrinal tradition. The situation is that any kind of affect or sorrow or despair can and must be expressed in ordinary language that is itself for the most part derived from Buddhism or can be articulated to Buddhism. (Obeyesekere, 1985, p. 144)

The Sinhalese term *kalakirīma* means hopelessness, but it also captures the idea of a reaction against life that is linked to the end of life, as well as the notion that suffering is inherent in life (the first of the five Buddhist precepts). When the interpreter expressed *kalakirīma* by using the English word *hopelessness*, this equivalent did not convey the notion of spiritual insight or imply a spiritual course of action in response. Saha's desire to sell his business and renounce his possessions could be seen as extreme and as a threat to self from the perspective of a market-driven society, in which a healthy work ethic implies a healthy person. In the context of Sinhalese society, however, his renunciations are culturally linked to the language of sorrow and suffering, and in fact are implied by the cultural context in which these words evolved.

The SSRI and cognitive–behavioral therapy offered by the psychiatrist were appreciated, and proved helpful, but they did not dissuade Saha from exploring a four-year period of renunciation, meditation, and reconnection to his culture's Buddhist roots. After a year's separation, he and his wife reunited, as she began her own Christian/Buddhist exploration.

Operationalized speech is the process that links reference to intended performance. Words have both a referential and a performative value that is based on use and context. An utterance like "Tiger!" has one reference and intended activity when scanning through an encyclopedia of animals, and quite another when walking through the Indian bush. The context of word use is critical. In the medical care of immigrants, the words used in clinic bridge two contexts simultaneously: the cultural paradigm of the patient's place of origin and the biomedical paradigm of the West, with its highly technical and operational speech.

For these reasons, key words can imply quite different contexts and behaviors for the patient and the clinician, as in the case of Saha. This situation becomes particularly tricky if a word has both technical and vernacular definitions. Words like panic, depression, and anxiety have both lay references and behavioral consequences, as well as *DSM-IV* references and therapeutic consequences.

For these reasons, words derived from Latin and Greek are often used to capture technical definitions and diagnoses. As an example, in cardiology, heart pain is *angina*, and the phrase *heart distress* may mean ischemia or failure. However, in the Farsi language, the term translated *heart distress* rarely signifies angina and far more commonly refers to an affective disorder (Good, 1977). Thus, an interpreter for a Farsi-speaking patient would be in the position of finding equivalent words while managing and explaining their respective referential and performative values to two different audiences. This is why translating between languages with shared linguistic origins, cultural histories, and medical systems, such as English to Dutch or German, is so much easier than translating from

English to Farsi. Yet even European languages and Western social contexts are full of unexpected linguistic challenges.

The philosopher J. L. Austin argues convincingly that speech acts or utterances are in themselves social performances. Among the criteria for an utterance constituting such a performance is that the speaker has the authority to change things by the utterance, and all involved are in agreement on this point. The words "I take you as my lawfully wedded wife" constitute a legally, socially, and financially significant action when spoken during a wedding ceremony by a man 21 years of age or older. Similarly, "you are in contempt of court" has substantial legal implications when uttered by a judge during a court proceeding. Utterances such as "you have lung cancer" or "you are bipolar," when spoken by a physician, are socially meaningful actions for the patient, the workplace, and the third-party payer. The significance of this linguistic insight for cross-cultural medicine is that any utterance may simultaneously have two different performative values in the two cultures present in the consulting room.

Linguistic Denotations of Relationships and Measures of Connection: A Case of Anorexia and Grief

Even as we drift away from operationalized technical speech into a discussion of the patient's history or social context, seemingly straightforward referents can pose problems in clinical interpretation. This possibility is illustrated by the case of Tokiko, a Japanese PhD candidate who presented to her primary care physician in the company of her roommate, who described a 15-pound weight loss and anorexia for six months after Tokiko lost a friend to breast cancer. To refer to this friend, Tokiko used the Japanese word *shinyu*. Her physician considered these symptoms to be rather extreme manifestations of grief and was concerned that perhaps Tokiko was suffering from anorexia nervosa or a major depressive episode. What the clinician could not register is what is immediately apparent to the Japanese speaker. In Japan, friends are denoted sociolinguistically according to the following taxonomy. *Doryo* refers to "work colleagues of the same rank," *nakama* refers to "one's crowd," *nominakama* refers to "one's drinking crowd," *shigotonakama* to "work acquaintances," and *asobinakama* to playmates. Two additional words are used exclusively for close friends: *tomodachi* or "true friend" and *shinyu* or "intimate friend and confidant, best friend." One may have many *tomodachi*, but usually only one *shinyu*. Children do not have *shinyu*, because they are not considered mature enough to understand true intimacy, and one's *shinyu* is typically of the same gender as oneself. Tokiko had lost her *shinyu*, her unique and irreplaceable lifelong girlfriend, to cancer. This was a devastating loss, immediately apparent to a Japanese speaker in Tokiko's word choice, but lost in translation through the equivalent "friend," which is used by English speakers in a much less defined manner and therefore requires significant qualification (Wierzbicka, 1997). Americans tend to view friends, even confidants, as replaceable components. This view varies from person to person, but the idea of a once-in-a-lifetime unique friendship is not the American norm, and we have no single term to reflect that special status.

To make sense of the sociolinguistic implications of the word *shinyu*, the Japanese interpreter must give examples and comparisons and then explain which word was used. This word gives the outsider an insight into the relative importance and valence placed on certain relationships and concepts within a linguistic group. As Anna Wierzbicka argues,

> For a number of disciplines, such as sociology, psychology, anthropology, philosophy, etc., it is important to understand how people categorize and conceptualize relationships with other people. In the abundant literature on the subject, however, human relationships are often interpreted through the lens of one particular ethno-taxonomy, especially that embodied in the (modern) English language. . . . The problem lies largely in the reification of English words such as friend and friendship and their unreflective use as descriptive tools and theoretical constructs in talking about people and human relations in general. (Wierzbicka, 1997, p. 118)

This is the role of the interpreter as culture broker: to interpret, but then try to make sense of the social and conceptual field in which the words and the patient function. Unless clinicians think critically about terms and their social contexts, ethnocentric assumptions and inaccurate glosses can result, blurring important distinctions or eclipsing meanings that would assist in the patient's medical history and diagnosis. Moreover, clinicians must know how to give the interpreter permission to provide conceptual equivalents. After this was done in Tokiko's case, the clinician recognized her condition as a prolonged and profound grief reaction.

For these reasons, what amounts to a few words in one language can become several paragraphs in another. On the other hand, languages that have evolved in close contact with each other, such as French, Italian, and Spanish, have shared histories, literature, religious systems, and geography. Consequently, it is easier to transfer conceptual fields from French to Italian than from Navajo to Russian, where there is little history of contact or coevolution.

Key Words and Operational Paradigms: A Case of Semen Loss

Mr. Lau, a 35-year-old Chinese immigrant, reported being very dizzy. He was aware of nocturnal emissions and felt that he was losing strength. He had been told by his physician that he was iron deficient and anemic, and he was concerned that his health was progressively deteriorating to the point where he would become incapacitated. He was fixating on obtaining rare animal parts from China to replenish his blood, and he seemed obsessed with his regular ejaculations. He began to see an herbalist who detailed exotic concoctions that Mr. Lau should drink to improve his health. His primary care physician referred him to a psychiatrist who, upon hearing this history, was alarmed that Mr. Lau was either delusional or obsessive–compulsive. It was not until Mr. Lau was seen by a physician along with an interpreter who had a background in acupuncture that the social and conceptual field of "blood" and "semen" could be appreciated.

Mr. Lau's apparent obsessions began to appear more reasonable within a Chinese cultural framework. Specifically, the link between his loss of semen and his fix-ation on avoiding phlebotomy and spending money on herbs to "boost" his blood assumed a certain logic.

Obeyesekere (1985) observes that if Americans shared the concept of semen loss, a chief complaint of this sort would be immediately recognizable to a phy-sician. Because they don't, it appears delusional.

> [L]et me practice a piece of reverse ethnocentrism. Take the case of the South Asian male (or female) who has the following symptoms: drastic weight loss, sexual fan-tasies, and night emissions and urine discoloration. In South Asia the patient may be diagnosed as suffering from a disease, "semen loss." But on the operational level I can find this constellation of symptoms in every society, from China to Peru. If I were to say, however, that I know plenty of Americans suffering from the disease "semen loss," I would be laughed out of court even though I could "prove" that this disease is universal. The trouble with my formulation is that while the symptoms exist at random everywhere, they have not been "fused into a conception'" (as se-men loss) in American society. (Obeyesekere, 1985, p. 136)

Kathleen Erwin (2006) notes that the concept of blood as a body part that can be sold as a commodity into the "blood bank" or "blood pool" is still unfamiliar in industrialized Shanghai. Even in the commodity-associated economy of modern China, blood is still invested with a significance derived from traditional Chinese medicine (TCM). Specifically, from a TCM perspective, blood is essential to health, circulating through the body following *chi* (*qi*). Blood is assigned femi-nine gender and seen as a yin presence, whereas *chi* is yang. Blood can be reple-nished, unlike semen (*jing*). The loss of blood through childbirth or menstruation requires replenishment through diet, behavioral restrictions, and nurturing med-ications. Women are thought to tolerate blood loss better than men, because it is part of their physiology and they can replenish blood faster. As Erwin (2006, p. 146) surmises, "The importance of blood and blood health may at least partially explain why many Chinese are reluctant to part with their blood." Blood donation and transfusion in modern Shanghai or among Chinese immigrants to U.S. cities may carry gendered health associations that are unknown to non-Chinese. In Mr. Lau's case, these associations explain why he is noncompliant with the med-ical workup and diverts his resources to expensive preparations from China.

The conceptualization of "blood" in Chinese medicine is an instance of a cultural paradigm that gives meaning to key words and related concepts. Like any paradigm, its clustered meanings imply specific actions and can prompt distinct behaviors. In practice, the paradigmatic gulfs that separate languages and cul-tures demand some of the most troubling and time-intensive work that a clinical interpreter is called to do.

Be it *friend, semen,* or *blood,* the apparently straightforward lexical equivalent in English vacates the conceptual and cultural sense from the original utterance and simultaneously denies its historical significance, thereby impoverishing the patient's medical history. Not only are monolingual, English-speaking physicians ignorant of the cultural field that their patients' languages demarcate; they lack awareness of the complementary manner in which a social system and a culture coalesce around the key words in a given lexicon. Nor can they anticipate the reciprocal shifts in meaning undergone by their biomedical speech when this is transposed into a nonmedical cultural milieu. The point is that key words in patient histories may participate concurrently in several different cultural paradigms, including the culture of origin, the lay culture of the United States, and Western biomedical culture in general.

Therapeutic Paradigms in Conflict: A Case of PTSD and Hot/Cold Idioms of Distress

So far we have focused on history and diagnosis, but let us also offer an example from the perspective of treatment strategies. We turn to a situation in which the diagnosis is not in dispute, yet divergent conceptual paradigms linked to that diagnosis create confusion and interfere with compliance.

Arturo is a 39-year-old first-generation Mexican American male who was hit by a car while riding his bicycle to work, suffering multiple fractures and a head injury. During the weeks after the injury, Arturo experienced insomnia and PTSD intrusive and avoidant symptoms, and he reported difficulties returning to his job as a groundskeeper. He also experienced a number of other stressful and traumatic life events, including a residential fire and an attempted assault. At three months after the injury, he was diagnosed with PTSD. The team physician began low doses of a sedating antidepressant with instructions that the medication be taken in the evening. The team's treatment goal was to titrate the medication up to guideline-level doses. Arturo began the antidepressant, but he proceeded to take it in the morning on an as-needed basis. An in-depth exploration of these issues with his provider revealed that Arturo had adapted the medication regimen to his own culturally configured belief system, which includes a paradigm of hot/cold illness (Foster, 1985). He experienced the medication as giving him a cool feeling deep in his bones, in contrast to his PTSD symptoms, which he experienced as hot. In particular, when Arturo became angry, he felt as if he were going to boil over. He therefore took the medication at the beginning of the day, when he was most likely to encounter situations that would enrage him.

Arturo and his provider continued to discuss these issues during the course of medication treatment. It was imperative for them to explore the paradigms at work together to make sense of Arturo's healing strategies and apparent noncompliance.

The Language-Specific Metaphors Inherent in Words and Their Connection to Cultural Paradigms: Happy Is Up, Sad Is Down

Cultural paradigms, whether in biomedical or lay culture, are constructed by means of metaphor. We have shown how words are part of conceptual systems in which culture, history, and social patterns assign valences and meanings to words as part of that lived culture and shared history. The conceptual systems that shape meaning and link it to action are constructed metaphorically. These are not simply arcane observations about language; they explain how concepts operate and paradigms are formed. As George Lakoff and Mark Johnson (1980) write,

> We have found . . . that metaphor is pervasive in everyday life. Our ordinary conceptual system, in terms of which we both think and act, is fundamentally metaphorical in nature. The concepts that govern our thought are not just matters of the intellect. They also govern our everyday functioning. Down to the mundane details. Our concepts structure what we perceive, how we get around in the world, and how we relate to other people. (p. 3)

They proceed to give English examples of the ways in which spoken metaphor shapes thinking and thereby implies appropriate action. Their examples demonstrate the many levels of metaphor that are at play in language, invisible and unexamined, highlighting as well as hiding conceptual links that suggest operational actions. Speaking most directly to mental health work are the orientational metaphors, in which directions are assigned to concepts as if these associations were both natural and universal. Here their example is "happy is up, sad is down":

Happy Is Up, Sad Is Down

I'm feeling up.
That boosted my spirits.
My spirits rose.
You're in high spirits.
Thinking about her always gives me a lift.
I'm feeling down.
I'm depressed.
He is really low these days.
I fell into a depression.
My spirits sank.
(Lakoff & Johnson, 1980, p. 15)

These are related to other orientational metaphors, such as "conscious is up, unconscious is down" or "having control or force is up, being subject to control or force is down." For example, statements such as "I'm on top of the situation, he's in the upper echelon, his power is on the decline" show how this orientational metaphor constrains our thinking about power. From here it is easy to see how a parallel linkage connects depression and power. The result is that English speakers tend to think about strength, mood, power, and quantities in terms of spatial orientation. Coherence across orientational metaphors of space, medication dosage, and corrective action are unconsciously shaped by culturally based English metaphors. Because metaphorical coherence may or may not also exist in the target language, the translation of metaphorical speech, while often difficult to avoid, nevertheless poses conceptual challenges for an interpreter.

Consider this example: "You're feeling down because your neurotransmitter levels are down. If we can boost these, you'll feel better, and less overwhelmed." Here the English-speaking physician has three parallel orientational metaphors in play:

1. "Feeling down" means either not having energy or displaying symptoms of depression.
2. "Neurotransmitters are down" means that the amount of serotonin per deciliter is more dilute in the patient's synaptic spaces than the physician thinks they should be.
3. "Overwhelmed" means that the events of the patient's life appear to be causing a cessation of efficient functioning.

In English, these three metaphorical notions appear to converge in orientation and thus display a kind of logic and symmetry. However, this orientational congruence may not be so neat in a non-Western language.

When interpreters are translating English sentences into the patient's language more or less word for word, orientational metaphors can become confusing. In a parallel manner, the metaphors that organize concepts in the patient's language require transformation into English speech. Even if idioms are avoided, metaphorical speech is at work in unexamined ways as we think about situations, solutions, and logical consequences. For this reason, shifts in cultural or scientific paradigms are reflected in concomitant changes in language.

Recognizing that thought and language are metaphorical systems is critical in cross-cultural work, because our current biomedical paradigms of physiology, neurochemistry, and neurohormonal regulation are organized just as metaphorically as ordinary vernacular speech. When we attempt to explain the paradigms of diagnosis and treatment that we feel interpreters need or patients require, we are simultaneously teaching our metaphorical systems. Metaphors in speech are typically inherited from past paradigms that are in transition. Because the languages and communities of science share metaphors across national boundaries, such metaphors work well internationally within scientific circles, but not in vernacular speech. For example, in Cold War America we often spoke about "fighting" disease, and we discussed cellular immunity in terms of "attack" and "conquest." Now, in postmodern corporate America, many diseases are no longer "fought" but "managed."

In Summary

We started with histories from patients whose life experiences and origins require interpretation within a framework that makes sense to an English-speaking clinician. For sense to be made, an interpreter is required, a skilled intermediary who must find equivalence between the languages and worlds represented in the examining room. Many aspects of speech itself require trained observation. The rate and content of speech, the expressions used for symptoms, the words referring to social changes, and the cultural systems that contextualize the patient's thoughts are all critical in making a psychiatric diagnosis. Patients may not understand Western biomedical diagnosis and treatment; on the contrary, they may have assigned their symptoms to culturally constructed syndromes that an interpreter must somehow convey to the Western clinician. The interpreter's challenge then becomes culture brokering or navigating between conceptual fields and the links to reasoned actions that are implied in the use of key, culturally defined words. Unwittingly, the words we speak carry relationships to cultural concepts that are known to us but are rendered invisible when our words are interpreted between languages that lack a shared context. Key words will be linked to related words and concepts in the same language that are organized metaphorically into conceptual fields. Such constructs hang together within a given culture and create categories of thought and meaning for members of that culture. These conceptual fields and semantic networks are called into play as people hear words and devise behavioral or therapeutic responses. Yet the same fields and networks that constitute meaning and enable communication are also the sources of misunderstanding and cultural gaps.

Indeed, the complexity of the interpreter's task can lead us to a kind of cross-cultural nihilism, in which we conclude that meaningful conversation through interpretation is impossible. Yet such a conclusion would be false. Many clinicians around the country successfully traverse cross-cultural landscapes of language and meaning and provide effective medical and psychiatric care. Bearing in mind that such a process is complex and nuanced, certain questions inevitably arise: How is it that we are doing it? How do we do it well? How do we do it badly?

TRAINING FOR THE TASK OF MENTAL HEALTH INTERPRETING

With all these challenges, how do we proceed? What is quality interpretation? Several recent articles speak to medicine's growing concern about the impact of interpreters on health care. These articles raise the issue of "quality interpretation" in health care, without a clear definition of what this involves in performance or even in concept. Notably, Flores and colleagues (2003) found that, during pediatric clinical encounters, interpreters averaged 31 errors per encounter at baseline. By far the most common error that they observed was omission (52%), with lower but still substantial rates of "false fluency" (16%), word substitution (13%), editorializing (10%), and addition (8%) (Flores et al., 2003). Alarmingly, they concluded that 63% of all interpretation errors had potential clinical consequences, which in their definition included errors that "altered or potentially altered . . . the history of present illness, the past medical history, diagnostic or therapeutic interventions, parental understanding of the child's medical condition, or plans for any future medical visits" (Flores et al., 2003, p. 9). Ad hoc interpreters (family members or untrained volunteers) were significantly more likely than professional interpreters to make errors of clinical significance (77% vs. 53%). Given what we know about metaphor and conceptual equivalence, on the one hand we are not surprised that interpreters are changing messages, whereas on the other hand we are appropriately concerned about the clinical impact of these changes. Moreover, we are not convinced that such changes result from expert linguistic analysis or professional competence.

A recent article by Aranguri and colleagues (2006) found that, during medical encounters in which conversation focused on lipid management, interpreters made significant revisions of clinician speech. The pattern was similar to the analysis by Flores and associates (2003) with regard to omissions, revisions, and content reduction. However, Aranguri and colleagues (2006) cited numerous additional issues, such as the "loss of small talk" that builds relationships between provider and patient, as well as the reduction in spontaneous utterances by patients. Notably, the number of questions asked of the provider by patients was reduced, because the interpreter often answered questions directly without transmitting them to the provider. One methodological issue affects the observations made by Aranguri and colleagues (2006)—namely, the fact that many of the interpreters in his study were ad hoc, often family members, rather than professionally trained interpreters.

During clinical interpretation at least two dynamics interact: first, the complexities of moving between sociolinguistic contexts and referents, as discussed earlier; and second, the professional demands of the job, notably the difficult and time-consuming necessity of remembering, tracking, and transmitting utterances and side conversations on both sides of the clinical encounter. The first dynamic expresses the sociolinguistic challenge of "can't do it," because no clear lexical equivalent might exist for a given word in one language or the other. The second dynamic expresses the human capacity challenge of "can't do it," because the interpreter might lack the necessary skill or experience.

The linguistic precision and professional skills required in interpretation explain why the use of ad hoc interpreters is inappropriate. An ad hoc interpreter is usually a family member or friend who is presumed to be bilingual. Sometimes it is another clinic or medical center employee conscripted from their usual job to do the task, and occasionally it might even be a stranger kind enough to step in. Repeated studies have shown that ad hoc interpretation is fraught with error. David and Rhee (1998) showed that non-English-speaking patients with ad hoc interpreters were significantly less likely than their English-proficient counterparts to receive information about side effects of treatment. Flores and colleagues (2003) showed that errors made by ad hoc interpreters were significantly more likely to have clinical implications than those made by professional interpreters (77% vs. 53%). The reasons are varied, but the skills required to track and transfer information, and the complexity of the respective contexts and conceptual referents, require practice if interpretation is to be effectively executed. It is ludicrous to expect an ad hoc bilingual person to perform this task with the accuracy and efficiency of a trained professional. These issues are independent of the even more complicated sociolinguistic concerns that are unique to transcultural psychiatry.

Marcos (1979) investigated the use of interpretation in psychiatric encounters and expressed concerns about accuracy, especially in areas of heightened importance. These included overidentification with patients by interpreters, leading to distortion of their responses; issues of confidentiality; and the tendency of interpreters to mask thought disorders through the normalization of patient responses, often by neglecting to transmit evidence of loose associations, delusions, and tangential or circumstantial thinking. When Marcos (1979) examined transcripts involving family members as ad hoc interpreters, he noted instances in which family members simply responded for patients instead of interpreting, and in some instances thereby denied suicidal ideation.

Although these performance errors are not directly related to sociocultural issues, they are indirectly linked by the stigma associated with certain topics, by the need to "save face," or by the ad hoc interpreter's lack of comfort confronting personal topics within the family. Cultural norms and the profound stigma of mental illness in many cultures can influence interpreters' capacity to be objective, meticulous, and discreet if they are not well trained. And this is the critical point: Training, practice in observation, care in transmitting even nonsensical information, and attention to accuracy in affect, rate, and content are all potentially crucial and must be registered against the patient's cultural norms. As we have labored to show, explaining context and conceptual fields (including metaphorical systems and the behaviors implied by key words) is subtle and complex in mental health interpreting. Agility and practice are required to manage the communication and the cultural brokering needed to make sense of the content. Such management can be done well only in situations where these tasks are performed with some frequency, and where interpreters have the training and the time to consider their work outside of a performance setting.

Choosing an Interpreter: Attention to English vs. Target Language Competence

Before considering the essential and optimum topics to cover when training someone in mental health interpretation, it is wise to consider some of the factors to attend to in selecting an appropriate individual to train. Fluency in language and culture seem like obvious criteria, but it is difficult to find interpreters equally fluent in two languages and cultures. In our medical center, for the most demanding work, we have an internal policy of selecting only people who were raised to adulthood in the target language country. In this way, interpreters are sufficiently fluent both in language and in culture to address the sociolinguistic demands outlined earlier. Young people fluent in the target language but raised in the United States lack the sophistication and experience to navigate the two conceptual fields unless they have made substantial efforts to study their mother culture. Part of our reasoning is that if one person in the triadic encounter must bear the onus of additional work in communication and explanation—of divining, so to speak, the other side of the cultural divide—it should be the professional who is paid and trained to do so, and not the patient. As a result, the interpreters' accent and lack of fluency in English may be an issue that will require them to attend classes or consider self-study to strengthen their skills.

What Is Quality Interpretation?

Training to meet the highest standard of mental health interpreting will require designated sessions offered collaboratively by providers, administrators, and interpreters to identify and practice the skills needed for the varied settings and special situations encountered in mental health care.

Standards of Practice

The National Council on Interpreting in Health Care (NCIHC) recently released a document, *National Standards of Practice for Interpreters in Health Care*, which was developed to provide guidelines for training and monitoring the performance of interpreters (National Council on Interpreting in Health Care, 2005). This document offers basic professional standards upon which specialty interpreting and cultural brokering should be based. It is a consensus document developed from a survey of national practices and expert opinion. It details 32 standards, which are organized around the topics of accuracy, confidentiality, impartiality, respect, cultural awareness, role boundaries, professionalism, professional development, and advocacy. When put into practice, these guidelines can ensure accurate and professional interpretation. To meet these standards consistently and accurately will require considerable training and experience in remembering complex messages, transmitting such messages carefully, and tracking the content and details of a conversation. Attention to complete interpretation requires attention to detail and a fairly robust memory. It also requires the presence of mind and professionalism to interrupt clinical conversations to clarify confusion on either side, while simultaneously informing both speakers that confusion exists. Moreover, it requires the ability to participate in the conversation while monitoring it for direction and content to deal with cultural issues and act as an advocate.

These standards of practice acknowledge advocacy as an appropriate role of the mental health interpreter. Interpreters can also be employed as navigators, chronic disease managers, court-appointed interpreters, and clinical interpreters. Each role, although related to the others, implies a distinct skill set and attitude. Therefore, interpretation requires self-awareness and self-tracking on the part of the interpreter to keep in check any potential conflicts between roles that may arise when moving between tasks and practice settings. In some situations the interpreter must act only as an interpreter; even if an advocacy role might seem desirable, to advocate would mean to abandon the role of interpreter. In other situations, interpreters must make it clear they are advocating and have assumed that role instead of simply interpreting. Empathetic providers who might be annoyed by zealous advocacy during clinical interviews, or by chronic disease information added into their conversations, may appropriately take offense at such interventions. A gentle reminder to interpreters of their role in a given setting, and some patience with the complexity of their task, will reinforce the team bond and enhance the professionalism of both interpreter and clinician.

Patterns of Speech and Affect

Mental health interpretation is a special instance of health interpretation in which some standards of practice may prove difficult to fulfill, but none fail to apply. Specialized training is needed to help the interpreter meet the standards of practice that are appropriate to the mental health setting.

The second standard of practice from the NCIHC document is: "The interpreter replicates the register, style, and tone of the speaker" (National Council on

Interpreting in Health Care, 2005, p. 5). This standard is often minimized in actual practice, but if applied it would substantially improve the interpreter's, and thereby the clinician's, attention to affect, rate, register, and pattern of speech.

As we have seen, training in recognizing the aspects of speech that are typical of mood and thought disorders can help interpreters comprehend what they are hearing. Paucity of speech, pressured speech, tangential speech, flight of ideas, word salad, neologisms, fluent aphasia, and Broca's aphasia are some of the more common syndromes. Affect in speech, whether sad, aggressive, terrified, or discordant (e.g., inappropriately happy when content is sad), may appear obvious to any observer but will be most apparent to the interpreter. Affect needs to be communicated to the clinician to provide detail, along with attempts to "replicate the register, style, and tone of the speaker" (National Council on Interpreting in Health Care, 2005, p. 5).

This process of inserting oneself into patients' situations and taking on their emotional state and register is the "hazardous duty" of the medical interpreter. Bear in mind that many interpreters are two steps away from the situation of the patient. If they are members of the same immigrant or refugee community, it is likely that their family members also struggle with the historical, financial, social, ethnic, and educational barriers facing the patient. They, too, may have suffered and they, too, may struggle with the emotional burden of dislocation and social upheaval. This likeness means that identification, projection, transference, and countertransference are all potential complications in the interpreter–patient relationship. The cumulative experience of patient after patient from these communities can create a secondary trauma for interpreters through repeated exposure and close identification with familiar stories of loss, death, grief, and injury. Interpreters may develop generalized anxiety and PTSD through constant exposure to traumatic histories as part of their daily work. Supervision, support systems, and debriefing become important routines to alleviate secondary trauma within interpreter services in mental health settings.

Confidentiality

The professional role of the interpreter may be unclear or distrusted by patients and family. Many patients assume that their physician is a professional who, like a priest or confidant, will keep sensitive information private. However, they may not trust clinic staff or interpreters to adhere to the same professional standards, and justifiably so if they or their friends have ever been injured by careless disclosure or unprofessional gossip. Small communities in which everyone knows the interpreter and the interpreter plays a prominent role confer a central position on that individual. Patients may therefore prefer phone interpretation, using interpreters outside the community. Regardless, reassurance from interpreter and staff that every aspect of the clinical encounter is private and confidential will help establish an environment of trust.

The demands of establishing professional boundaries and rules of confidentiality have to be balanced against the equally important demands of full disclosure and accuracy in interpretation. This is a difficult balance, because a patient who asks the interpreter not to disclose certain information may feel betrayed if such information is subsequently disclosed for medical reasons. Interpreters need to make special attempts to clarify these competing demands for accuracy and full disclosure on the one hand, and confidentiality on the other. The special obligations of the Terasoff law provide an excellent example of the potential for conflict. This statute requires a mental health professional or interpreter to violate a patient's confidence if the patient is deemed a risk to self or others. Awareness and understanding of the Terasoff law is essential for all professionals working in a mental health setting, not least the interpreter.

DIAGNOSES AND SYMPTOMS

As we discussed earlier, the symptoms of psychiatric illness from a Western perspective are formally outlined in the *DSM-IV*. Although Hinton (2001, 2005) and others (Good & Kleinman, 1985) have shown that the *DSM-IV* does not capture the culturally specific criteria for certain disorders, it is nevertheless the best starting place for interpreters who need to familiarize themselves with common diagnoses and symptoms. With this background, interpreters can anticipate the subtleties of affect, speech, and thought that they should convey to assist the provider in characterizing a patient's thinking and mood. Although interpreters are not responsible for drawing distinctions between delirium, delusion, and dementia, and although they should be careful not to project their opinions into an evaluation, it is nevertheless true that knowing these distinctions will help them assist the clinician in sorting through the potentially confusing content and expression of a patient's speech to make a psychiatric diagnosis.

The converse is more difficult. There may be culturally bound syndromes, patterns of speech or content, or symptom complexes that reflect non-Western diagnoses. Interpreters should be trained in broaching this topic with providers so that they can outline for them other diagnostic possibilities in addition to those contained in the *DSM-IV*. If considered or discussed, such alternative diagnoses can enhance the provider's and the health system's credibility with the patient and open a more frank discussion.

The Mental Health System

The history of the mental health system in Europe and the United States is long, and it constitutes a central feature of the evolution of American culture. Three generations ago, troubled individuals were considered crazy, drunk, drug addicts, or just plain melancholy. Within many demographic groups, American culture has evolved beyond this "cuckoo's nest" to a lay appreciation that depression and addiction are illnesses and not failures of character or morality. Most laypeople in the United States understand that psychosis is often chronic and manageable, that various types of therapy can be helpful, and that the serotonin reuptake inhibitors and other antidepressants they see advertised on TV have helped many of their friends and family members manage compulsions, anxiety, or depression. This change has happened in a relatively short time, but it has been reflected and assisted by the popular press and media, not to mention by such formal structures of society as science, law, organized religion, and public education. As a consequence, most Americans are familiar with numerous aspects of psychiatry and the mental health system, whereas many immigrants are not. That said, many of the contradictions and complexities of the system frustrate and confuse even the professionals within it who are laboring to change it.

Practitioners, Agendas, and Practice Settings

Interpreters require a brief introduction to the types of mental health professionals and settings with whom they will work. There are many examples of settings and functions that might seem similar to outsiders, but that in funding, policies, and therapeutic goals are quite different. An example is the role of detoxification centers for drug and alcohol treatment compared with large group homes for the chronically mentally ill. Interpreters need to review the roles of psychiatrists, psychiatric nurses, social workers, and psychologists, as well as the goals of common medications, cognitive–behavioral therapy, dialectical therapy, group therapy, and individual therapy. The timeline and goals of outpatient psychiatry will be unfamiliar to most immigrants from Africa and Asia.

Similarly, the organization of the mental health system, the financial obligations of third-party payers, or the possibility of state or county support within the mental health system is still more opaque to immigrants than to the average American citizen. If interpreters are to act as adequate culture brokers on behalf of a psychiatric team, they need adequate explanation, adequate time, and adequate practice. Their elusive goal is to find linguistic equivalents and to create metaphorical referents that will bridge mutually unintelligible languages. Time is necessary to anticipate and practice the task.

Interpreters need to know how and where the mental health system works—how it varies by agenda and focus according to the setting in which it is practiced. Such settings range from the emergency department, to the involuntary inpatient setting, to the voluntary ward, to the courtroom where patients are committed to a 72-hour hold, to outpatient mental health treatment facilities, to the psychiatrist's office. This is biomedical culture in practice, and interpreters are responsible for finding equivalent phrases to explain this culture so that it makes sense to foreigners.

The goals of medication assessments and symptoms checks, of cognitive–behavioral therapy or of group and individual sessions, must be explained, and their underlying assumptions articulated, if the interpreter is to act as an adequate broker on behalf of Western psychiatry. The difference between chronic psychiatric diagnoses and acute episodes of mental illness must be set forth. The varieties of mood disorders, personality disorders, and affective disorders, as well as their time frame and treatment, must at least be outlined, so that interpreters can avoid their own confusion and personal frustration while helping patients and their families understand the clinician's therapeutic plan. The time and teaching needed for this education must be planned and coordinated; it cannot be done quickly, piecemeal, or in the hallway.

Crisis and Commitment

Interpreters within the mental health system also need to be able to explain how the system approaches threats of suicide and homicide. They need to understand the responsibility of the courts to support the decisions of mental health professionals. These professionals have the legal authority to restrain or confine people who are a threat to themselves or others, just as patients have the legal right to frequent reevaluation. Interpreters need to understand all these legal issues, just as they need to understand why a mental health provider cannot necessarily restrain someone who clearly appears unwell.

Suicidal patients, or those who are a threat to their own safety or the safety of family members, often find themselves engaged with the police and other crisis services. Once these services are set in motion, they operate according to whatever local laws are in effect, such as RCW 71.05 in Washington State, better known as the ITA or Involuntary Treatment Act. This law sets forth the conditions and criteria whereby a patient can be involuntarily detained and treated, as well as the rights of the patient and authority of the state to ensure the patient's safety. Often families and individuals activate the system only to regret it, and then attempt to deactivate detainment that is deemed legally necessary. Or they may see a symptomatic patient released and wonder why the system does not insist on treatment. The confluence of law, intention, behavior, medicine, and treatment settings can be both frightening and confusing. The better an interpreter understands the system, the better he or she is prepared to explain it, to anticipate fears and questions from patient and family, and to facilitate mutual understanding (if not agreement) at an emotionally charged time.

Once past the crisis, patients often want to assume that the illness is over, the medications are no longer needed, and the event was an anomaly in the course of their lives. Yet too often these events are part of a long history of chronic affective illness or even psychosis. The interpreter needs not only to understand these issues, which are often rooted in stigma and denial, but also to anticipate them with the provider and have the means of directing the provider to address them.

Provider Training

Karliner and colleagues (2004) recently surveyed 158 attending physicians, residents, and nurse practitioners from the five general medical practices affiliated with UC-San Francisco. The survey asked about clinicians' satisfaction with their ability to provide care through an interpreter. Although 85% felt they could adequately diagnose, 70% admitted they had trouble eliciting exact symptoms, 69% admitted lack of knowledge of the patient's disease, and 61% admitted lack of knowledge of the patient's culture. Only 45% of the physicians felt they were able to empower their patients with knowledge of diagnosis, treatment, and drug therapy, whereas two thirds said they were unable to empower their patients with knowledge of lifestyle modification. The authors concluded that training in the use of interpreters may help clinicians accomplish these critical tasks for the delivery of care. If such a conclusion is obtained in a general medical setting, it is likely to be still more relevant in a psychiatric setting.

Despite the sophisticated and extensive education necessary to become a health professional, most providers are quite naive about the dynamics and interdependence of language and culture. The process of establishing linguistic equivalence is invisible and unconsidered by most clinicians, who imagine it as a fairly straightforward process. Even a cursory overview of the issues will orient them to the subtleties and complexities of interpreting. After they are able to see beyond the linguistic curtain to the cultural, social, and semantic concepts in flux, they will be able to assist the interpreter.

Providers will be well advised to adopt the following helpful guidelines:

- Speak in clear, short sentences.
- Avoid complex sentence structure.
- Keep to one major idea in each sentence.
- Check with the interpreter and the patient for comprehension.
- Anticipate complex and confusing biomedical concepts and simplify their expression.
- Find useful analogies and metaphors by working with the interpreter.
- Avoid slang, idioms, humor, and examples that might be confusing or offensive.

In this way, providers can manage their speech and work in a manner that facilitates interpretation rather than complicates it.

GUIDELINES FOR TRAINING AND PRACTICE

In conclusion, we review common strategies that will help to manage confusion during the interpreted psychiatric interview. Most of the concerns discussed earlier can be addressed by training both clinicians and interpreters in the general categories of confusion that often emerge in such encounters. Forewarned is forearmed. A look back through our examples suggests the following summary:

Interpretation Challenges for Physician and Interpreter in a Psychiatric Interview

1. *Somatization, or expressing distress through the body, requires interpreters and clinicians to sort through symptoms patiently.*

   Interpreters need training to realize that all grieving and distress are not the same. Some of it crosses into areas of chronic illness and psychosis, where bodily symptoms develop. Therapy must be presented to interpreters and patients alike as a treatment for these symptoms that does not necessarily produce immediate results.

2. *Interpreters and patients resist locating symptoms in psychological and neurochemical processes.*

This is a related interpreter training issue, one that should emphasize the criteria for depression, for example, over and against sadness and grief reactions. It should also stress case reports of effective treatment. Seasoned interpreters are more convincing than clinicians on these points.

3. *The rate, pattern, and content of speech require careful observation against cultural norms for diagnostic purposes.*
   Examples and reminders that interpreters can reveal or obscure these findings through their summary interpretation will help interpreters see their own central role in clarifying symptoms.

4. *Symptoms may suggest culturally constructed illnesses unknown to the clinician.*
   Recognizing such illnesses requires a sophisticated knowledge of the target culture and may not be accomplished at the same level by all providers. Continuing cultural education is needed in the same way that continuing medical education is needed for biomedical concepts.

5. *Unfamiliar symptoms may be uniquely associated with biomedical diagnoses, yet the provider is unaware of the association, or unfamiliar with the culturally specific terminology that links symptom to syndrome.*
   Exposure to relevant literature and examples will prompt clinicians and interpreters alike to investigate whether a given symptom has diagnostic specificity unique to a specific sociolinguistic group.

6. *The patient's words are linked to conceptual paradigms with social and behavioral implications.*
   Permission to broker, training in culture brokering for interpreters, and an efficient means of encouraging brokering for clinicians will address this and related points. It requires teamwork and shorthand communication, and these must be practiced.

7. *The metaphors inherent in English speech are not equally inherent in the target language and can therefore become confusing or contradictory.*
   Here, insight is the first step. Reflection on the language and key metaphors of mental health will help interpreters identify problem areas that require rephrasing.

Interpreter Mental Health Competencies

1. Sensitivity to omissions, deletions, and message change
2. Adherence to professional standards, as detailed in the recently released *National Standards of Practice for Interpreters in Health Care* by the NCIHC (2005)
3. Cultural competence in target and biomedical mental health paradigms
   - *DSM-IV* diagnoses
   - Basic professional job descriptions and institutional functions of the mental health system
   - Key legal features of the mental health system
   - Common symptoms associated with common diagnoses and phrases that express those symptoms in their own culture—a special challenge for younger interpreters not raised in the home country
4. Competence in culture brokering to conduct the elaborate contextual discussions and explanations necessary to bridge the clinical world and the world of the immigrant patient

Many of these gaps and confusions can be managed with patience, training, and practice. In the end, there will be fundamental conceptual and linguistic inequivalences that are insurmountable, but these will be minimized when clinicians and interpreters operate as a trained team with a heightened awareness of the linguistic and cultural landscape that they are traversing together.

REFERENCES

American Psychiatric Association. (1994). *Diagnostic and statistical manual of mental disorders (DSM-IV)* (4th ed.). Washington, DC: American Psychiatric Association Press.

Aranguri, C., Davidson, B., & Ramirez, R. (2006). Patterns of communication through interpreters: A detailed sociolinguistic analysis. *Journal of General Internal Medicine, 21*(6), 623–629.

David, R. A., & Rhee, M. (1998). The impact of language as a barrier to effective health care in an underserved urban Hispanic community. *Mt Sinai Journal of Medicine, 65*(5–6), 393–397.

Erwin, K. (2006). The circulatory system: Blood procurement, AIDS, and the social body in China. *Medical Anthropology Quarterly, 20*(2), 139–159.

Flores, G., Laws, M. B., Mayo, S. J., Zuckerman, B., Abreu, M., Medina, L., et al. (2003). Errors in medical interpretation and their potential clinical consequences in pediatric encounters. *Pediatrics, 111*(1), 6–14.

Foster, G. M. (1985). How to get well in Tzintzuntzan. *Social Science and Medicine, 21*(7), 807–818.

Good, B. & Kleinman, A.K. (1985). Epilogue: Culture and depression. In A. Kleinman & B. Good (Eds.), *Culture and depression* (pp. 134–152). Berkeley, CA: University of California Press.

Good, B. J. (1977). The heart of what's the matter. The semantics of illness in Iran. *Culture, Medicine and Psychiatry, 1*(1), 25–58.

Hinton, D., Um, K., & Ba, P. (2001). A unique panic-disorder presentation among Khmer refugees: The sore-neck syndrome. *Culture, Medicine and Psychiatry, 25*(3), 297–316.

Hinton, D. E., Pham, T., Tran, M., Safren, S. A., Otto, M. W., & Pollack, M. H. (2004). CBT for Vietnamese refugees with treatment-resistant PTSD and panic attacks: A pilot study. *Journal of Traumatic Stress, 17*(5), 429–433.

Hinton, D. E., Pich, V., Chhean, D., & Pollack, M. H. (2005). 'The ghost pushes you down': Sleep paralysis-type panic attacks in a Khmer refugee population. *Transcultural Psychiatry, 42*(1), 46–77.

Karliner, L. S., Perez–Stable, E. J., & Gildengorin, G. (2004). The language divide: The importance of training in the use of interpreters for outpatient practice. *Journal of General Internal Medicine, 19*(2), 175–183.

Katon, W., Von Korff, M., Lin, E., Simon, G., Ludman, E., Bush, T., et al. (2003). Improving primary care treatment of depression among patients with diabetes mellitus: The design of the pathways study. *General Hospital Psychiatry, 25*(3), 158–168.

Kleinman, A. K. (1988). *Rethinking psychiatry: From cultural category to personal experience.* New York: Free Press.

Lakoff, G., & Johnson, M. (1980). *Metaphors we live by.* Chicago: University of Chicago Press.

Marcos, L. R. (1979). Effects of interpreters on the evaluation of psychopathology in non-English-speaking patients. *American Journal of Psychiatry, 136*(2), 171–174.

National Council on Interpreting in Health Care. (2005). *National standards of practice for interpreters in health care* [Online]. Available: www.ncihc.org

Obeyesekere, G. (1985). Depression, Buddhism, and the work of culture in Sri Lanka. In A. Kleinman & B. Good (Eds.), *Culture and depression* (pp. 134–152). Berkeley, CA: University of California Press.

Santos, M., Russo, J., & Zatzick, D. F. (November 2003). *Ethnocultural variations in immediate posttraumatic distress.* Paper presented at the 19th annual meeting of the International Society for Traumatic Stress Studies, Chicago, IL.

Tocher, T. M., & Larson, E. B. (1999). Do physicians spend more time with non-English-speaking patients? *Journal of General Internal Medicine, 14*(5), 303–309.

Ursano, R. J., Bell, C., Eth, S., Friedman, M., Norwood, A., Pfefferbaum, B., et al. (2004). Practice guideline for the treatment of patients with acute stress disorder and post-traumatic stress disorder. *American Journal of Psychiatry, 161*(11 Suppl.), 3–31.

U.S. Census Bureau. (2000). *Population by race for the Unites States: 1990 to 2000.* Washington, DC: U.S. Department of Commerce.

U.S. Department of Health and Human Services. (2001). *Mental health: Culture, race, and ethnicity—A supplement to mental health: A report of the Surgeon General.* Rockville, MD: Public Health Service, Office of the Surgeon General.

Van Ommeren, M., Sharma, B., Sharma, G. K., Komproe, I., Cardena, E., & de Jong, J. T. (2002). The relationship between somatic and PTSD symptoms among Bhutanese refugee torture survivors: Examination of comorbidity with anxiety and depression. *Journal of Traumatic Stress, 15*(5), 415–421.

Waitzkin, H., & Magana, H. (1997). The black box in somatization: Unexplained physical symptoms, culture, and narratives of trauma. *Social Science and Medicine, 45*(6), 811–825.

Wierzbicka, A. (1997). *Understanding cultures through their key words.* New York: Oxford University Press.

Zatzick, D., Jurkovich, G., Russo, J., Roy–Byrne, P., Katon, W., Wagner, A., et al. (2004). Posttraumatic distress, alcohol disorders, and recurrent trauma across level 1 trauma centers. *Journal of Trauma, 57*(2), 360–366.

9

The Role of Family Diversity in the Diagnosis and Treatment of Mood Disorders

AMY E. WEST & GERI DONENBERG

The definition of family has evolved substantially during the past three decades. Because the traditional definition—a biological mother and father and two children—failed to reflect the growing diversity and complexity of families today, the NIMH launched an initiative to redefine the meaning of family. Specifically, the NIMH brought together a consortium of scholars who developed a new and innovative definition of who and what constitutes a family. In this new characterization, family is viewed as a network of mutual commitments, recognizing the role of biological and nonbiological ties among individuals (Pequegnat & Szapocnik, 2000).

A key contribution to the changing view of families has been the recognition that culture plays a significant role in how families function and define themselves. Culture influences all aspects of family life, including health and wellness, sickness and disease, and prevention and treatment. For many groups, mental health and mental illness, as well as decisions concerning treatment for mental health conditions, are viewed through a lens defined by culture. Cultural traditions may encourage treatment or interfere with health-seeking behavior. Moreover, cultural beliefs may at times conflict with best practice. Thus, the diagnosis and treatment of mental health conditions require careful attention to cultural values, attitudes, and beliefs. Unfortunately, psychological diagnostic, assessment, and therapeutic models typically assume universal applicability. Only recently has the role of culture been considered by mental health practitioners. Recent adjustments have been made to add "cultural competence" to graduate curricula, but there has been little effort to ensure true cultural competence in training models or service provision.

Culture is influenced by a variety of factors that extend well beyond race and ethnicity, such as social class, religion, racial and ethnic discrimination, degree of assimilation, and gender politics (McGoldrick, Giordano, & Garcia–Preto, 2006a). Because each of these influences has implications for the diagnosis, assessment, and treatment of mental health problems, a comprehensive understanding of diagnosis and treatment involves attending to these influences as they drive behavior and constitute culture. For example, the degree to which a family has assimilated to the dominant culture can profoundly affect its values, beliefs, status, and access to privileges, thereby shaping its response to mental illness and/ or psychiatric treatment. With assimilation comes stresses of adaptation that may render previously adequate coping strategies no longer effective. As another example, the privilege granted to European Americans is generally unacknowledged in American culture, yet racism continues to exert a profound effect on ethnic minorities, with concomitant effects on their values and cultural experiences. Racial and ethnic prejudice may, even inadvertently, establish boundaries that cannot be crossed or may limit available opportunities, including access to and the quality of mental health services. Thus, working effectively within a cultural context requires a multicultural understanding and an appreciation of the diverse issues that influence the assessment, diagnosis, and treatment of psychopathology.

This chapter addresses some of the key cultural constructs that influence clinical work with families with mood disorders. These include the definition of family, religion and spirituality, level of responsibility for behavior (e.g., collective vs. the individual), the utility of talk therapy, and problem definition. These constructs are explored with a broad focus on four cultural groups—African Americans, Native Americans, Latinos, and Asians—noting similarities and differences in their approach to mental health and treatment. Although we acknowledge the limitations of generalizing across cultural groups with similar backgrounds (e.g., all Latinos), we hope this review provides a meaningful overview and introduction to the ways culture may influence the clinical process, particularly in relation to mood disorders.

Among the many differences across cultural groups is the definition of family, or who constitutes family. For example, European Americans generally consider family to be the traditional nuclear unit, whereas African Americans may cast a broader net that includes a wider network of kin and community. Asian families generally include all ancestors since the beginning of time (McGoldrick et al., 2006a). These differences underscore the need to consider carefully who participates in the therapeutic process, whose opinions are valued, who is the spokesperson for family members, and who must be consulted and included in the treatment. In other words, increased inclusiveness of extended relatives may be appropriate for both African American and Asian families.

Widely varying religious beliefs across cultural groups may also affect use of services, receipt of best practices, and reliance on modern medicine to treat mental health problems. Cultural traditions and values often stem from religious beliefs, and faith can be fundamental to healing. Indeed, "Spirituality ... like culture and ethnicity, involves streams of experience that flow through all aspects of life, from family heritage to personal belief systems, rituals and practices, and shared faith communities. Spiritual beliefs influence ways of dealing with adversity, the experience of pain and suffering, and the meaning of symptoms" (Walsh & Pryce, 2002, p. 337). Religion is frequently used to cope with adversity, garner emotional support, and provide comfort. The African American community, for example, relies heavily on the church for guidance in behavior and decisions. Native American families often turn to shamans or healers to rid family members of disease and illness. Determining best practices for each family will depend on careful attention to these cultural differences.

Cultural groups also vary in their approach to assigning responsibility for individual behavior. Eastern cultures typically emphasize collective responsibility, whereas Western cultures emphasize individual accountability. More specifically, African Americans tend to define identity based on the collective, whereas European Americans characterize identity through individualism. Psychology and psychiatry, too, have tended to emphasize the individual with regard to mental health and mental illness, and both disciplines have failed to recognize the critical role that a community or environment or culture may play in determining behavior. The 1980s witnessed a surge of attention to ethnicity in the mental health field, but this has since dissipated and the focus has shifted away from family and context.

Cultural groups also vary in their attitudes toward "talk" therapy, a staple of Western clinical psychology. Western psychology assumes that talk leads to healing. High levels of verbal interaction, however, may be more appropriate and acceptable for some groups than others. For instance, African Americans and Native Americans may be less willing to disclose to a member of the traditional "white" institution because of mistrust and wariness (Hines & Boyd–Franklin, 2006). For different reasons, some Asian cultures may also discourage verbal exchange because it tends to rely on more symbolic methods of communication. Thus, talk therapy may not be the treatment of choice for some cultural groups.

Finally, definitions of what constitutes a "mental health problem" differ across culture (McGoldrick et al., 2006a). Feelings or behaviors that are considered "problem behaviors" for families in one cultural group may reflect strengths in other cultural groups. For example, although mainstream European American culture may consider dependency and emotionality problematic, other cultures may interpret independence as disrespectful. Understanding what is adaptive in one situation versus another requires an appreciation of the broader context in which the behavior occurs. Differences in perceptions of problem behaviors might also affect help-seeking behavior. Comfort and ease in help seeking is not universal, because some cultural groups are less likely to turn to "outsiders" for assistance.

Incorporation of a culturally sensitive perspective when diagnosing and treating mental health disorders is a complex and multidimensional process. Treatment may involve changing negative cultural attitudes that have been internalized, or managing cultural conflicts in the family or the broader context in which the family exists (McGoldrick, Giordano, & Pearce, 1996b). There are many advantages to using a strengths-based approach, in which the clinician builds on the family's skills and encourages cultural values and behaviors that assist in coping. Similarly, the clinician can help families distinguish deeply held convictions that are barriers to good health, appropriate treatment, and well-being. Indeed, recognizing cultural differences does not mean all cultural attitudes and values should be retained. Some values may be unethical (mistreatment of certain members, oppression of women, racism) or out of sync with current life functions. The task for clinicians operating from a culturally sensitive perspective is to tolerate ambiguities, question values, and carefully evaluate which method of intervention will lead to improved healthy outcomes for family members.

DEFINITION OF FAMILY

Mainstream American culture has traditionally defined the primary family system as the immediate nuclear family. As mentioned earlier, this concept has been changing during the past several decades with the growing recognition of different family structures and the integration of culturally diverse conceptualizations of family. Within the field of psychological research on family process and mood disorders, it has been found that depression in a family member is related to various aspects of family process, including communication, problem solving, family roles, affective experience, and behavioral interaction (Keitner, Miller, Epstein, & Bishop, 1990). In addition, bipolar illness has been found to be associated with family dysfunction, marital conflict, expressed emotion, and poor sibling relationships (Geller, Craney, Bolhofner, Nickelsburg, Williams, & Zimerman, 2002). In general, the literature on family process and mood disorders to date would suggest that considering familial context and involving family members in treatment is important for patient response and recovery. Therefore, cultural differences in the definition of family provide necessary insight into who should be involved in therapy and how.

For example, in many cultural groups, including African American and Native American families, the incorporation of extended kinship networks may be an important aspect of treatment. In African American families, relatives often live in close proximity and rely on each other in times of need. Nearby relatives frequently interchange functions and share responsibilities for childrearing; indeed, it is fairly common for children to be adopted and raised by extended family members who are better off than the child's parents (Hines & Boyd–Franklin, 1996; McAdoo, 1981; Wilson, 1984). Strong family is an essential resource for African American families, particularly in the context of an oppressive society (Boyd–Franklin, 2003; White, 2004). Unfortunately, the strength of the multigenerational family might also introduce blurred boundaries and role confusion (e.g., Who is the mother?) that make family therapy a challenge.

Likewise, in Native American families, the extended family is the basic unit and is frequently misunderstood by those in majority culture who operate under the concept of the nuclear family (Sue & Sue, 1999). Relatives such as aunts, uncles, and grandparents often raise children, and it is not unusual to have children stay in a variety of different households (Hildebrand, Phenice, Gray, & Hines, 1996; Sue & Sue, 1999) with many relatives sharing the responsibilities of childrearing. Again, extended family networks that share familial responsibilities may be confusing to therapists used to operating within a traditional mainstream framework in which the parents are supposed to have sole or primary responsibility for childrearing, and there are often more rigid boundaries between nuclear and extended family members. What is known is that the experience of mood disorder symptoms appears to exist in dynamic interaction with aspects of family process, and therefore it would be important for a treating therapist to explore each family system, determine what roles are played by different members, and involve influential members in the treatment process.

Another important aspect of family definition that may impact the diagnosis and treatment of mood disorders involves gender roles within the family system. How a person understands the roles and responsibilities ascribed to his or her gender may affect how he or she conceptualizes or reports mood symptoms. For example, hallmark symptoms of major depression are feelings of worthlessness, hopelessness, and inadequacy. These kinds of feelings may conflict with family systems that encompass more traditional gender roles, in which a female is submissive and a male is the source of power and decision making for the family. In some Latino cultures, this concept is called *machismo*, and it describes the strong sense of masculine pride and power in the family system that may influence a male's identity (Falicov, 1996). It may be particularly difficult for a male who identifies with the *machismo* principles to accept or admit openly feelings of worthlessness or inadequacy because of the perceived inconsistency of these feelings with his roles and responsibilities within the traditional family system. In contrast, the traditional female role in Latino families is to be submissive, self-sacrificing, and restrained (Avila & Avila, 1995; Sue & Sue, 1999). Because of these traditional roles, and gender-role conflicts that may occur with acculturation or clashes with mainstream views, Latino men and women may present to therapy with unique issues. Men may have difficulty interacting with agencies and individuals outside the family, and may feel that they are not fulfilling their expected roles. They may feel isolated and depressed because of the need to be strong, have difficulty talking about feelings because of perceived weakness, evidence conflicts over the need to be consistent in the male role, and experience anxiety over questions of sexual potency (Sue & Sue, 1999). Latino women may present with conflicts over expectations to meet the requirements of their roles, anxiety when unable to live up to these standards, depression over not being able to live up to these standards, and the inability to act out anger (Sue & Sue, 1999). These culturally bound gender-specific conflicts may be particularly relevant to the understanding and treatment of mood disorders because of how embedded depressive and related symptoms are in this unique social structure. Treatment approaches need to be sensitive to gender roles and gender-role conflicts. For example, a therapist treating a depressed Latino male who appears to adhere to traditional ideas about gender-role fulfillment might work toward helping this patient feel strong and powerful in certain aspects of his life, rather than encouraging him to embrace his vulnerability or be more emotionally expressive, which he may perceive as being weak and which might further contribute to his depressed affect.

In traditional Asian American families, the husband assumes leadership and authority, and the wife is the homemaker and child bearer. The husband plays the role of disciplinarian and the wife is the nurturer. Typically, a wife is dominated by her husband's authority and there is little emotional expression between wife and husband (Lee, 1996a). Like in some Latino cultures, it is apparent how the emphasis on male power and authority may make it difficult for some men to admit they are struggling with feelings of inadequacy or ineffectiveness commonly associated with a mood disorder. In addition, however, it also may be difficult for a woman, who sees her role as primarily caring for others and deferring to her husband, to admit to feeling depressed or unsatisfied without the fear of offending her partner or appearing too self-indulgent. In addition to making the expression of these feelings difficult, it is also important to consider that the feelings of inadequacy, hopelessness, or depression that suggest a mood disorder may have a different etiology, quality, and expression in diverse family systems. For example, it may be difficult for a therapist working within a framework of marital partnership that emphasizes openness, assertiveness, and equality to understand that an Asian woman's sense of inadequacy and hopelessness may not stem from feeling oppressed by her husband, but rather from a fear of not fulfilling her role as an obedient or self-effacing wife. In this case, it would be important for the therapist to explore the genesis of these feelings in a nonjudgmental way to connect with this patient and help her resolve her difficulties.

RELIGION AND SPIRITUALITY

In general, the mainstream conceptualization of mental health and illness is considered scientific and separate from spiritual beliefs or experience. However, this separation is not a universal one. Many cultural groups see spirituality as fully integrated with all aspects of life, and certainly with a sense of psychological well-being. In some cultural groups, spirituality is seen as an imperative aspect of any "recovery" from psychological difficulties. For example, in African American communities, the church often plays a central role in resiliency, health, and wellness. This may stem in part from days of slavery, when religious services served as an important force in dealing with oppression (Hines & Boyd–Franklin, 1996). In present-day African American families, the church often plays a central role in family life, providing a primary social support system, religious education, health promotion, economic assistance, counseling, support groups, and children's socialization (Hines & Boyd–Franklin, 1996). Themes that therapists consider important to address in treatment, such as sensitivity, fulfillment and satisfaction, a sense of purpose, and self-discipline, may be similarly relevant to these families (Hines & Boyd–Franklin, 1996), but perhaps need to be addressed with an understanding of their potential basis in spiritual beliefs, and in a way that acknowledges the church as a powerful source of strength and support in overcoming mood illness.

For some Latino American cultures, the Catholic church often has a powerful influence on family life and interaction between family members. In particular, the religious beliefs of Catholicism espouse the view that personal sacrifice will bring salvation, being charitable is a virtue, and individuals should endure wrongs done against them (Sue & Sue, 1999; Yamamoto & Acosta, 1982). As a result, some Latino patients may have difficulty with being "assertive" or may have a fatalistic attitude that may be frustrating to therapists who do not understand its context. Because cognitive–behavioral, psychoeducational, and other approaches to treating mood disorders tend to rely on empowering the individual toward personal change, these techniques may have to be adapted in this case to be sensitive to the reliance of Catholics on their religious doctrine and its impact on social behavior. In some cases, it may be more effective to build on the strengths of the support of the church community, the power of prayer, or the idea of redemption through personal sacrifice and charity as a means to relieve depressive affect, rather than using more traditional evidence-based techniques.

Asian Americans comprise a diverse cultural group that reflects many religious beliefs and spiritual practices, including Christianity, Buddhism, Hinduism, Taoism, and ancestor worship (Lee, 1996a). In working with Chinese Americans who practice Buddhism, for example, concepts of karma, reincarnation, and compassion may be important to understand and address in therapy. Particularly in treating mood illness, Buddhist and Taoist teachings, which emphasize balance and acceptance, may be helpful in coping with depressive symptoms. In addition, the focus in Chinese culture on interpersonal harmony and familial social support could be utilized (Lee, 1996b). Mindfulness techniques, which have proved useful in treating mood disorders (Segal, Williams, & Teasdale, 2002), actually have their foundation in Eastern ways of thinking that focus on harmony and peaceful acceptance, rather than assertiveness and gaining control over self and circumstances. The recent focus on mindfulness provides an excellent example of the beginning of Western science to adapt and incorporate strengths from other cultural beliefs systems into models of clinical treatment.

The traditional focus of Western science on what is "scientific" often leads many people from other communities to seek out traditional healers who are more sensitive to a holistic and spiritual approach to wellness. In most Native American cultures, a person's spiritual interdependence with the natural environment is a central cultural belief, and many physical and mental illnesses are believed to flow from an imbalance between a person's spirit and the natural world. Therefore, people may prefer to seek the help of a medicine man, who has a traditional and cultural holistic approach to healing and lifestyle, rather than a focus on illness and disease (Sutton & Broken Nose, 1996). Likewise, in Haitian American communities, a belief in voodoo's curative capabilities shapes views about emotional distress and mental illness, and therefore may affect help-seeking behavior, causing Haitians to seek the services of a voodoo rather than a mental health clinician (Bibb & Casimir, 1996). It may be beneficial for a therapist treating a patient with a mood disorder in a more mainstream clinical setting at least to inquire about the use of traditional methods of healing, and be empathic and open to the ways that traditional healing might aid the treatment process. The power to heal may be in the integration of a diversity of techniques for some families, and the willingness of a clinician to embrace these unfamiliar concepts may indeed facilitate rapport and patient response to treatment.

RESPONSIBILITY FOR BEHAVIOR: INDIVIDUALISM VERSUS COLLECTIVISM

Although the fields of psychology and psychiatry have tried to incorporate the importance of culture and context at least theoretically, the models of psychopathology and mental health treatment are still embedded primarily in the concept of individual responsibility for behavior. The assessment, diagnosis, and treatment of mood disorders are no exception. The diagnosis of a mood disorder is made primarily according to the patient's response to diagnostic interview questions, self-report symptom measures, and ideally at least some corroboration of the patient's mood and behavior from a family member. The best practice in terms of psychotherapeutic intervention for a mood disorder is thought to be cognitive–behavioral therapy, which focuses on the patient's control over his or her thoughts and corresponding emotions and behaviors. This patient-centric treatment model is founded on the theoretical assumption that empowering the patient to change his or her patterns of individual thoughts, feelings, and behaviors will affect the symptoms of mood dysregulation. Even alternative treatments, such as interpersonal psychotherapy, psychodynamic psychotherapy, and family systems therapy, all view contextual variables as important only in their interaction with the individual patient, and thus are still inherently individualistic in their approach. Although many of these treatment approaches for mood disorders have received empirical support and are widely used, it is not known how their undeniable foundation in a Westernized view of individual importance may make them less relevant and potentially ineffective for patients with diverse cultural beliefs that do not emphasize individual significance.

Numerous world cultures emphasize the collective good over the individual. In fact, European American culture is more unusual in its emphasis on individualism when compared with cultural beliefs across all societies. For example, in traditional Mexican families, the concept of *familismo*, or family interdependence, emphasizes the sharing between family members, immediate and extended, the responsibilities of nurturing and raising children, financial concerns, companionship between family members, and problem solving (Falicov, 1996). Although most therapists working with patients with mood difficulties likely recognize to some degree the role of external variables and context in the patient's symptoms, within the current framework they are likely to view context as just that—external influences that interact with the individual and can be manipulated through perceptual changes made within the individual. It may be difficult for therapists working within this framework to understand the true extent to which some patients see themselves as connected and fluidly interdependent with family members, so that the concept of "individual" thoughts, feelings, and behaviors may not be a familiar or useful concept. Thus, the tendency to view a mood disorder as a private, internal struggle may not be useful in working with someone from a more collectivistic worldview.

Traditional Japanese family culture also values cohesion and harmony above individual achievement, reflecting a more collectivist worldview (Matsui, 1996). Cohesion is maintained by adherence to a strict hierarchy in which elders and those with more authority are revered and given deference. *Enryo* is a communication style frequently observed in traditional Japanese social interaction in which people emphasize restraint and holding back (Matsui, 1996). The maintenance of social cohesion is of utmost importance within traditional family systems and may have implications for the expression of and communication about mood disorder symptoms, depending on how the person sees the impact on the social flow of the family. The emphasis on personal restraint to maintain social harmony may conflict directly with what is considered "good" treatment for mood disorders—a focus on processing feelings, identifying maladaptive thoughts that contribute to depressive feelings and perpetuating behaviors, and discussing interpersonal struggles and environmental triggers for mood dysregulation. It is possible that a therapist who pushes a patient with these cultural beliefs to share his or her innermost feelings in this way may actually create further turmoil and hardship in his or her attempts to help relieve the patient's mood symptoms. Again, the focus on the individual as a distinct entity, a being that interacts with others but in essence is separate from all others, is a concept that is not shared by all cultures, yet is the foundation for most therapeutic techniques used to treat what we recognize as psychopathological symptoms. Indeed, the concept of individual psychopathology may itself be flawed when considered in a diverse cultural framework. As therapists are faced with ways of thinking from different cultures, which create more fluid boundaries and foster a sense of interdependence between people, Westernized treatment approaches that emphasize empowering the individual towards creating change, personal assertiveness, individualistic thoughts and feelings, may become somewhat uninformed and ineffective.

For many cultural groups, it is not only important to consider the patient in interdependence with his/her family and community, but also within a larger framework of naturalistic and spiritualistic understanding. This understanding might be extremely important in working with Native Americans who adhere strongly to their cultural values. For Native Americans, "mental health" may be much more holistic and spiritual in nature than conventional psychological definitions would suggest (Atkinson, Morten, & Sue, 1999; Trimble, Manson, Dinges, & Medicine, 1984). Often, when problems arise in Native American communities, they cease being problems of the individual and become a problem for the community. Family, kin, and friends coalesce into an interlocking network to observe the individual, draw that person out of isolation, and integrate the individual back into the social life of the group (Atkinson, Morten, & Sue, 1999; LaFromboise, 1988). Whatever distress the individual is experiencing is often seen as arising from inherent weakness as a human, and detachment from spiritually based cultural values and respect for community adherence. Therefore, the traditional healing process, unlike conventional therapies, usually involves more than the client and therapist, but may incorporate traditional healers, significant others, and community members, and often may involve nonconventional techniques, such as acts of atonement, restoration into the good graces of the family and tribe, and intercession with the spirit world (Atkinson, Morten, & Sue, 1999). The goal of therapy, in this sense, is not to focus on empowering the individual and providing the personal insight and strength to change the individual experience, but rather to reintegrate and reestablish interdependence and respect for communal values. In essence, this is a conflict that may arise for many therapists working from an individualistic framework with clients from a collectivist mentality. The differences in emphasis may result in diverse and perhaps conflicting understandings of a mood "disorder's" origin, as well as the most appropriate and effective way to work with the patient toward resolution.

UTILITY OF TALK THERAPY

In addition to a relative emphasis on individualism versus collectivism, another cultural variable that may affect the utility of certain types of therapy in treating mood disorders in diverse populations of families is the use of talking as the primary mode of communication and expression in treatment. As mentioned previously, treatments for mood disorders often stress the verbal processing of feelings, verbal identification of thoughts and beliefs, and discussion of the role of interpersonal interaction and environmental influences in perpetuating negative mood states. In addition, an important part of treatment is often the verbal psychoeducation of patients about mood disorders and their treatment. All these treatment modalities rely on the verbal exchange between patient and therapist, and perhaps others in his or her environment deemed important in the treatment process. For many families with diverse cultural beliefs, this mode of communication and interaction may cause conflict and actually impede the therapeutic process.

As mentioned earlier, Japanese Americans tend to engage in a communication style called *enryo*, which is characterized by a hesitancy to speak out or ask questions (Matsui, 1996). In general, traditional Japanese Americans stress nonverbal over verbal forms of communication, and may consider talking freely excessive and inappropriate. This may cause misunderstanding between therapist and patient in therapy. For example, Root (1998) states that two nonverbal behaviors may be readily misinterpreted between Asian American patients and their therapists: silence and head nodding. A therapist may misinterpret silence as passivity or negativity, versus a communication style that reflects restraint out of respect for authority. Likewise, head nodding, and saying "yes" or "I see" may not necessarily reflect agreement on the part of the patient, but instead may reflect a need to respect authority and wish to avoid conflict. These subtle yet powerful differences in communication styles may have significant implications for therapy, including rapport building, trust, mutual agreement on therapeutic goals, and progress of treatment.

Evidence also exists that communication style might affect the success of counseling for Native American patients. Dauphinias and colleagues (1981) found that Native American students rated both Native American and non-Native American counselors as more credible when they used a culturally relevant counseling style that included nondirective communication. In fact, a heavily verbal approach to the establishment of rapport through repetitive question-and-answer sessions was found to be counterproductive to Native American patients (Atkinson, Morten, & Sue, 1989). Native American culture traditionally values listening and indirect forms of communication. The non-Native American therapist may interpret this silence as resistance or disinterest, when actually it is a useful form of communication for the Native American client (Sutton & Broken Nose, 1996). In this case, joining and rapport building may occur through an increased understanding of nondirective and nonverbal communication patterns, as well as the therapist's openness about differences.

DEFINITION OF PROBLEM

The diagnosis of a mood disorder is made based on a person's (and sometimes family members') report of symptom experience. It follows logically that the diagnosis of a mood disorder is largely contingent on patient and family understanding and interpretation of their struggles or difficulties. The conceptualization of the problem, in turn, may affect whether they seek help at all. If they do present to a mental health provider, the family's cultural context for understanding the "symptoms" may affect their response to what are deemed to be mood disorder symptoms by the provider, and their overall acceptance of the label of mood disorder. Some evidence suggests that the concept of "depression" or "mood symptoms" may be understood and expressed differently among diverse cultural groups. For example, in people from Latin American cultures, it is common for depression to present in somatic terms, rather than in sadness or guilt (Castillo, 1997; Cuellar & Paniegua, 2000). Asian people may show similar experiences in terms of weakness, tiredness, or "imbalance," whereas Native Americans may complain of difficulties with the "heart" (Cuellar & Paniegua, 2000).

In particular, several research findings have reported a prevalence of somatization symptoms among Chinese Americans (Kleinman, 1982; Lee, 1996b; Marsella, Kinzie, & Gordon, 1973; Tseng, 1975), particularly in those with depression (Lee, 1996b; Marsella et al., 1973). Depression appears to be quite common in Chinese Americans, particularly immigrants and refugees, and is thought in part to relate to isolation, lowered social status, grief over loss, war trauma, acculturation stress, financial problems, and other social stressors (Lee, 1996b; Lin, 1986). It is common for Chinese people to present to treatment with complaints of body aches, such as headaches, backaches, and chest pain, as well as exhaustion, weakness, dizziness, difficulty with sleep and appetite, and a sense of hopelessness (Lee, 1996b). Hypotheses differ regarding why Chinese patients tend to manifest depression in somatic symptoms. One hypothesis is that it may be a reflection of cultural values that emphasize the avoidance of shame and protecting one's family from the embarrassment of mental illness. In addition, it may also reflect the traditional Chinese view of holistic health and illness, in which the body and mind are unified (Lee, 1996b).

Circumstances unique to the history of different cultural groups may also affect the patient's understanding and conceptualization of his or her distress. One example in Native American culture is the concept of *intergenerational trauma*, thought to have developed out of the genocide faced by Native Americans upon European contact. European contact was devastating for Native Americans; millions died through genocidal warfare and disease, and entire tribes and communities were completely destroyed (Sutton & Broke Nose, 1996). Many tribes were forced from their native lands, and thousands of Native American children were removed from their families and put into boarding schools, where they were punished severely for speaking their language and practicing customs, and were not allowed any contact with their families (Sutton & Broken Nose, 1996). These practices led to profound cultural trauma, because Native American cultures are rooted in their physical space, family ties, and distinct spirituality (La Due, 1994; Sutton & Broken Nose, 1996). This trauma is often thought to be experienced by Native Americans living today because of their intense connection to their ancestors and the spirit world, and is thought to relate to the incredibly high rates of suicide, violence, homicide, school dropout, teen pregnancy, and substance abuse as part of the legacy of trauma (La Due, 1994; Sutton & Broken Nose, 1996).

In general, it is important to understand how historical, social, and economic factors may influence what are thought of as mood symptoms for some cultural/ethnic groups. For example, chronic depressed mood for at least two years, which might be considered *DSM-IV* dysthymic disorder (American Psychiatric Association, 1994), might also be the result of specific cultural variables, such as racial discrimination or poverty (Castillo, 1997; Cuellar & Paniegua, 2000; Weiss, 1995). Although the relationship of socioeconomic circumstances associated with racial group membership in this country to mood disorder symptoms is not a direct focus of this chapter, it is an imperative part of the contextual framework for understanding differences in mood disorder diagnosis and treatment across culturally diverse families. In addition, the racial discrimination and oppression that is still pervasive in this country has an undeniable impact on all the themes discussed in this chapter, as well as access issues, service utilization, and perceptions about mental health care held by racial and ethnic minority members of society.

Much work remains to be done in psychology and psychiatry to recognize true cultural differences and their impact on mood disorders, and certainly to develop effective models of treatment delivery for culturally diverse families. Yet, progress is being made. If nothing else, the acknowledgment and acceptance of the flaws inherent in the current system of care for diverse families presenting with mood disorders and a commitment of moving toward a more integrated and informed model of interacting with these patients is an important first step.

REFERENCES

American Psychiatric Association. (1994). *Diagnostic and statistical manual of mental disorders* (4th ed.). Washington, DC: American Psychiatric Association.

Atkinson, D. R., Morten, G., & Sue, D. W. (1989). *Counseling American minorities* (3rd ed.). Dubuque, IA: William C. Brown.

Atkinson, D. R., Morten, G., & Sue, D. W. (Eds.). (1999). *Counseling American minorities* (5th ed.). Boston, MA: McGraw Hill.

Avila, D. L., & Avila, A. L. (1995). Mexican Americans. In N. A. Vacc, S. B. DeVaney, & J. Wittmer (Eds.), *Experiencing and counseling multicultural and diverse populations* (3rd ed., pp. 119–146). Bristol, PA: Accelerated Development.

Bibb, A., & Casimir, G. J. (1996). Haitian families. In M. McGoldrick, J. Giordano, & J. K. Pearce (Eds.), *Ethnicity and family therapy* (pp. 86–111). New York: Guilford Press.

Boyd–Franklin, N. (2003). Black families in therapy: Understanding the African American experience (2nd ed.). New York: Guilford Press.

Castillo, R. J. (1997). *Culture and mental illness.* Pacific Grove, CA: Brooks/Cole.

Cuellar, I., & Paniegua, F. A. (Eds.). (2000). *Handbook of multicultural mental health.* San Diego, CA: Academic Press.

Dauphinias, P., Dauphinias, I., & Rowe, W. (1981). Effects of race and communication style of Indian perceptions of counselor effectiveness. *Counselor Education and Supervision, 21,* 31–46.

Falicov, C. J. (1996). Mexican families. In M. McGoldrick, J. Giordano, & J. K. Pearce (Eds.), *Ethnicity and family therapy* (pp. 169–182). New York: Guilford Press.

Geller, B., Craney, J. L, Bolhofner, K., Nickelsburg, M. J., Williams, M., & Zimerman, B. (2002). Two-year prospective follow-up of children with a prepubertal and early-adolescent bipolar disorder phenotype. *American Journal of Psychiatry, 158,* 303–305.

Hildebrand, V., Phenice, L. A., Gray, M. M., & Hines R. P. (1996). *Knowing and serving diverse families.* Englewood Cliffs, NJ: Prentice-Hall.

Hines, P. M., & Boyd–Franklin, N. (1996). African American families. In M. McGoldrick, J. Giordano, & J. K. Pearce (Eds.), *Ethnicity and family therapy* (pp. 66–84). New York: Guilford Press.

Hines, P. M., & Boyd–Franklin, N. (2006). African American families. In M. McGoldrick, J. Giordano, & J. K. Pearce (Eds.), *Ethnicity and family therapy* (pp. 87–100). New York: Guilford Press.

Keitner, G. I., Miller, I. W., Epstein, N. B., & Bishop, D. S. (1990). Family process and the course of depressive illness. In G. I. Keitner (Ed.), *Depression and families: Impact and treatment.* Washington, DC: American Psychiatric Press.

Kleinman, A. M. (1982). Neurasthenia and depression: A study of somatization and culture in China. *Culture, Medicine and Psychiatry, 6,* 117–189.

La Due, R. (1994). Coyote returns: Twenty sweats does not an Indian expert make, bringing ethics alive. *Feminist Ethics in Psychotherapy Practice, 15*(1), 93–111.

LaFromboise, T. (1988). American Indian mental health policy. *American Psychologist, 43,* 388–397.

Lee, E. (1996a). Asian American families: An overview. In M. McGoldrick, J. Giordano, & J. K. Pearce (Eds.), *Ethnicity and family therapy* (pp. 227–248). New York: Guilford Press.

Lee, E. (1996b). Chinese families. In M. McGoldrick, J. Giordano, & J. K. Pearce (Eds.), *Ethnicity and family therapy* (pp. 249–267). New York: Guilford Press.

Lin, K. M. (1986). Psychopathology and social disruption in refugees. In C. Williams & J. Westermeyer (Eds.), *Refugee mental health in resettlement countries* (pp. 61–73). Washington, DC: Hemisphere.

Marsella, A., Kinzie, D., & Gordon, P. (1973). Ethnic variations in the expression of depression. *Journal of Cross-Cultural Psychiatry, 4,* 435–458.

Matsui, W. T. (1996). Japanese families. In M. McGoldrick, J. Giordano, & J. K. Pearce (Eds.), *Ethnicity and family therapy* (pp. 268–280). New York: Guilford Press.

McAdoo, H. P. (Ed.). (1981). *Black families.* Beverly Hills, CA: Sage.

McGoldrick, M., Giordano, J., Garcia–Preto, N. (2006a). Overview: Ethnicity and family therapy. In M. McGoldrick, J. Giordano, & J. K. Pearce (Eds.), *Ethnicity and family therapy* (pp. 1–38). New York: Guilford Press.

McGoldrick, M., Giordano, J. & Pearce, J. K. (2006b). *Ethnicity and family therapy* (2nd ed.). New York: Guilford Press.

Pequegnat, W., & Szapocznik, J. (2000). The role of families in preventing and adapting to HIV/AIDS: Issues and answers. In W. Pequegnat & J. Szapocznik (Eds.), *Working with families in the era of HIV/AIDS* (pp. 3–26) Thousand Oaks, CA: Sage Publications.

Root, M. P. P. (1998). Facilitating psychotherapy with Asian American clients. In D. R. Atkinson, G. Morten, & D. W. Sue (Eds.), *Counseling American minorities* (5th ed., pp. 214–234). Boston, MA: McGraw Hill.

Segal, Z. V., Williams, M. G., & Teasdale, T. D. (2002). *Mindfulness-based cognitive therapy for depression: A new approach to preventing relapse.* New York: Guilford Press.

Sue, D. W., & Sue, D. (1999). *Counseling the culturally different: Theory and practice* (3rd ed.). New York: John Wiley and Sons.

Sutton, C. T., & Broken Nose, M. A. (1996). In M. McGoldrick, J. Giordano, & J. K. Pearce (Eds.), *Ethnicity and family therapy* (pp. 31–44). New York: Guilford Press.

Trimble, J. E., Manson, S. M., Dinges, N. G., & Medicine, B. (1984). American Indian conceptions of mental health: Reflections and directions. In P. Pederson, N. Sartorius, & A. Marsella (Eds.), *Mental health services: The cross cultural context* (pp. 199–220). Beverly Hills, CA: Sage.

Tseng, W. S. (1975). The nature of somatic complaints among psychiatric patients: The Chinese case. *Comparative Psychiatry, 16,* 237–245.

Walsh, F., & Pryce, J. (2002). The spiritual dimension of family life. In F. Walsh (Ed.), *Normal family processes: Growing diversity and complexity* (3rd ed., p. 337). New York: Guilford Press.

Weiss, M. G. (1995). Eating disorders and disordered eating in different culture. *Psychiatric Clinics of North America, 18,* 537–553.

White, J. (2004). Towards a black psychology. In R. Jones (Ed.), *Black psychology* (4th ed.). Hampton, VA: Cobb & Henry Press.

Wilson, M. (1984). Mothers' and grandmothers' perceptions of parental behavior in three-generation black families. *Child Development, 55*(4), 1333–1339.

Yamamoto, J., & Acosta, F. X. (1982). Treatment of Asian-Americans and Hispanic-Americans: Similarities and differences. *Journal of the Academy of Psychoanalysis, 10,* 585–607.

10

Models for the Delivery of Care

AMY M. KILBOURNE

This chapter discusses effective treatment models for managing mood disorders across diverse populations and settings. In addition, the multilevel barriers in translating effective treatment models for mood disorders into real-world settings for vulnerable populations are discussed. A framework to implement treatment models for mood disorders across diverse populations is proposed based on chronic care management principles, as well as innovative strategies that target the multilevel barriers in translating treatment models across different health care settings based on community involvement.

GAPS IN QUALITY OF CARE FOR MOOD DISORDERS ACROSS VULNERABLE POPULATIONS

Quality of care for individuals with mood disorders is suboptimal in general and especially for vulnerable populations, including minority and low-income patients (U.S. Department of Health and Human services, 2001). Vulnerable groups are populations that are disadvantaged based on underlying differences in social status, including racial/ethnic minorities, low-income individuals, rural populations, and individuals with disabilities (Kilbourne, Switzer, Hyman, Matoka, & Fine, 2006b). In the treatment of individuals with mood disorders, particular focus has been paid to disparities in care among racial/ethnic minorities. A recent Surgeon General's report concluded that minorities, and in particular African Americans, compared with whites are less likely to receive adequate care for mental disorders (e.g., fewer outpatient visits, older psychopharmacological medications). Specifically, African Americans were less likely to receive guideline-concordant care for major depression (Surgeon General, 2002). For bipolar disorder, African Americans were more likely codiagnosed with schizophrenia than whites (Kilbourne, Haas, Han, Elder, Conigliaro, & Good, 2005), which can lead to an unstable and inappropriate treatment course. Even when appropriately diagnosed, African Americans compared with whites were less likely to receive adequate posthospitalization outpatient care for bipolar disorder (Kilbourne et al., 2005). Overall, African Americans compared with whites are less likely to remain engaged in mental health treatment for mood disorders (Arean, Alvidrez, Nery, Estes, & Linkins, 2003; Opolka, Rascati, Brown, & Gibson, 2003).

The chief reason for inadequate mental heath care for minorities is that they usually receive their care in community-based health centers or from health care settings that rely on public funding (e.g., Medicaid, Medicare). In addition, most individuals with mood disorders, especially depression, receive mental health care from their primary care providers (Alvidrez, 1999; Charney, Reynolds, Lewis, Lebowitz, Sunderland, & Alexopoulos, 2003; Lebowitz, Pearson, Schneider, Reynolds, Alexopoulos, & Bruce, 1997). These individuals are also reluctant to accept referral to mental health specialists because of stigma regarding mental illness, as well as transportation and financial barriers to specialty care (Cooper, Gonzales, Gallo, Rost, Meredith, & Rubenstein, 2003; Cooper–Patrick, Powe, Jenckes, Gonzales, Levine, & Ford, 1997; Diala, Muntaner, Walrath, Nickerson, LaVeist, & Leaf, 2000, 2001; Glied, 1997; Hirschfeld, Keller, Panico, Arons, Barlow, & Davidoff, 1997; Miranda, Duan, Sherbourne, Schoenbaum, Lagomasino, & Jackson–Triche, 2003; Sirey, Meyers, Bruce, Alexopoulos, Perlick, & Raue, 1999; Snowden, 2001). Mood disorders are less likely diagnosed or treated appropriately in the primary care setting than in mental health specialty settings (Olfson, Marcus, Druss, Elinson, Tanielian, & Pincus, 2002; Sclar, Robison, Skaer, & Galin, 1999; Sirey et al., 1999; Snowden, 2001; Wells, Katon, Rogers, & Camp, 1994).

BARRIERS TO EFFECTIVE MOOD DISORDERS CARE

Many publicly financed primary care practices experience a number of formidable organizational and financial barriers in delivering effective care for mood disorders. The "6 P" framework (Pincus, 2003; Pincus, Hough, Houtsinger, Rollman, & Frank, 2003) describes these barriers as existing at multiple levels: patient, provider, practice, health plan, purchaser, and population (Table 10.1). Patient-level barriers include stigma regarding mood disorders, difficulty in navigating multiple providers, lack of culturally specific mood disorder treatment options, and lack of socioeconomic support mechanisms to continue treatment for mood disorders. Provider barriers include lack of time and training to implement mood disorder treatment in the primary care setting. Health care practices (e.g., physician organizations, clinics, facilities, and so forth) are in general not organized to deliver care for mood disorders because of their acute care focus, because mood disorders require long-term follow-up (i.e., chronic care). At the health plan level, the organizational and financial separation of mental and physical health care has impeded efforts to integrate mood disorder care in primary care settings. Health care purchasers (e.g., Medicaid) lack the incentives or knowledge in choosing health plans and arrangements that promote integrated care. Finally, at the population level, many community-based organizations are not aware of the potential benefits of promoting treatment models for mood disorders in primary care settings.

Patient, provider, and practice barriers need to be considered first when designing mood disorder treatment models for vulnerable groups. Notably, patients are often reluctant to seek mental health care because of lack of knowledge regarding appropriate treatments. Individual cultural beliefs play a major role in attitudes toward mental health treatments as well. Historically, most mental health treatment models sought to change patient behavior without considering these cultural factors. There is a growing realization for the need to differentiate between patient preferences that are grounded in ethnicity or culture from those based on modifiable perceptions or even misleading information, such as urban legends or popular myths arising from unequal access to health care information. For example, minority patients may be reluctant to take antidepressants because of the fear that these drugs act as sedatives and because of provider mistrust. At

Table 10.1 Solutions to Multilevel Barriers to Mood Disorders Treatment Models

Level	Barriers	Solutions
Patient/client	Stigma, lack of culturally specific treatments, navigating multiple providers	Promote culturally specific self-management programs; seamless care management link with community resources
Provider	Lack of time, information; tools to manage mood disorders	Provide outlines of mood disorder treatment guidelines and related tools suitable for primary care; access to specialty expertise
Practice	Lack of resources, organizational strategies to address chronic care	Establish chronic care model to reorganize practice from acute to chronic care focus; link with improved information systems; adapt to community-based settings
Health plan	Misaligned financial incentives, mental health carve-outs, fragmentation of services	Develop provider/system incentives, payment mechanisms; improve information systems to collect longitudinal information on patient mood disorders management and across providers; promote quality improvement in mood disorders
Purchaser	Lack of awareness, "business case" for mood disorders	Educate regarding importance of mood disorders treatment; promote incentives to implement CCM for mood disorders across health plans
Population	Lack of engagement with researchers, mistrust	Engage community stakeholders; adapt models to local needs; increase demand for quality care for mood disorders

CCM, chronic care model.

the same time, some minority groups might be receptive to psychotherapy or faith-based interventions (Brown, Schulberg, & Prigerson, 2000; Cooper, 2001).

Providers, especially those in primary care, lack the time, tools, and training to provide effective mood disorder treatment within their setting. During the clinic visit, chronic illnesses such as mood disorders are often "sidelined" when the patient has other medical problems (Redelmeier, Tan, & Booth, 1998). Research findings also suggest that there is less patient participation in medical decision making when the patient and clinician differ in cultural backgrounds and providers make little attempt to encourage communication (Cooper–Patrick, Gallo, Gonzales, Vu, Powe, & Nelson, 1999). Provider communication barriers may impede joint decision making and treatment (Burgess, Fu, & van Ryn, 2004; King & Brunetta, 1999). For example, in a study that analyzed taped conversations between patients and providers, providers were more likely to communicate in a "verbally dominant" manner with their African American patients compared with their white patients (Johnson, Roter, Powe, & Cooper, 2004). Poor communication can lead to patient mistrust of the provider, and subsequent refusal of treatment. Moreover, providers may often fail to consider the patient's culture within the clinical encounter and subsequently fail to tailor messages about health promotion or disease prevention (e.g., "cultural competence") (Freimuth & Quinn, 2004). Providers who are willing to communicate more with patients are more likely to have patients who are satisfied with their care (Cruz & Pincus, 2002).

Until recently, practice-level barriers have received little attention. Practices (e.g., clinics, offices, outpatient settings) represent important intervention points because they represent the entire clinical encounter that the patient experiences, from check-in with the clerks, to the vital signs check by the nurse or medical assistant, to the physician encounter. In general, primary care practices as they are currently organized do not enhance patient–provider interactions and do not promote successful outcomes for chronic illnesses in general and for mental illness in particular (Bodenheimer, Wagner, & Grumbach, 2002). There is often limited (if any) communication and teamwork between providers from primary care and mental health practices. There are also few treatment models to guide primary care providers in reorganizing their practice to provide chronic, integrated care for mood disorders, especially over a long period of time. Hence, a greater understanding in how these providers do or do not act as a team to provide adequate care for mood disorders is needed. Recently, evidence suggests that practice organizational features such as the availability of physician extenders (e.g., nurses) and more sophisticated clinical information systems are associated with greater continuity of care for chronic illnesses (Casalino, Gillies, Shortell, Schmittdiel, Bodenheimer, & Robinson, 2003; Jackson, Yano, & Edelman, 2005; Kilbourne et al., 2006a). These resources are often out of reach for safety net providers who serve a disproportionate number of vulnerable populations, and who are sensitive to changes in public funding. Still, other organizational attributes, such as a culture committed to quality improvement, are strongly related to improved quality of care and outcomes for chronic conditions independent of funding variations (Jackson et al., 2005; Wagner et al., 1996). Practices with a more entrepreneurial as opposed to a bureaucratic culture were more likely to have patients reporting high levels of patient satisfaction (Meterko, Mohr, & Young, 2004).

Furthermore, some primary care and mental health specialty practices, especially those that serve vulnerable groups, are reluctant to collaborate with researchers to improve coordinated care and implement evidence-based treatment models. First of all, many of these practices face limited funding and existing bureaucratic norms that preclude many interventions established in academic settings from being adopted without an a priori implementation strategy (Kilbourne, Schulberg, Post, Rollman, Herbeck–Belnap, & Pincus, 2004). Providers in these practices may also feel that treatment models are being imposed on them without their input (Sullivan, Duana, Kirchnera, & Henderson, 2005). Researchers can be accused of "using" sites to gain access to patients and conduct studies without any effort to follow up with them to disseminate results or invest in long-term practice changes (Rotheram–Borus, Rebchook, Keyy, Adams, & Neumann, 2000).

The Chronic Care Model Can Reduce Practice-Level Barriers

There has been increasing recognition that primary care practices need to be reorganized to provide better chronic care services. Mood disorders treatment in primary care is impeded as a result of a predominance of an acute care focus in primary care settings and the lack of focus or mechanisms to manage chronic conditions (Kilbourne, Schulberg, Post, Rollman, Herbeck–Belnap, & Pincus, 2004). The Chronic Care Model (CCM) (Bodenheimer et al., 2002; Wagner, Austin, & Von Korff, 1996) has been one of the most widely adopted frameworks designed to reorganize primary care from an acute care to a chronic care focus. The CCM adapted for mood disorders (Figure 10.1) involves an amalgam of provider guideline implementation with patient self-management education and care management delivered by a physician extender who provides longitudinal follow-up care. For example, CCM-based models have been developed and have proved effective for depression in primary care settings (Table 10.2) and, most recently, for bipolar disorder in mental health settings (Bauer, McBride, Williford, Glick, Kinosian, Altshuler, et al., 2006). Most of these studies were randomized, controlled trials in which the CCM-based model reduced affective symptoms and improved quality of life in patients with mood disorders (e.g., Bruce, TenHave, Reynolds, Katz, Schulberg, & Mulsant, 2004; Hunkeler, Meresman, Hargreaves, Fireman, Berman, & Kirsch, 2000; Katon, Von Korff, Lin, Walker, Simon, & Bush, 1995; Simon & Von Korff, 1995; Unutzer, Katon, & Callahan, 2002; Wells, Miranda, Bruce, Alegria, & Wallerstein, 2004). Many of these studies also showed that the CCM was cost neutral (Bauer et al., 2006). The CCM has also been implemented across different treatment settings, including community-based safety net practices and HMOs that serve a disproportionate number of African Americans and Latinos (Berwick & Kilo, 1999; Dietrich, Oxman, & Williams, 2004; Pincus, Pechura, Elinson, & Pettit, 2001; Rubenstein, Parker, Meredith, Altschuler, dePillis, & Hernandez, 2002; Wagner et al., 2001).

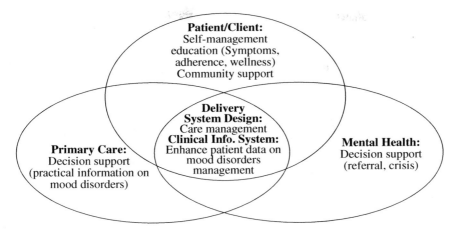

Figure 10.1 Chronic Care Model for mood disorders treatment.

In a recently completed evaluation for a CCM implementation program in low-income clinics, the CCM improved processes and outcomes of care for asthma (Mangione–Smith, Schonlau, Chan, Keesey, Rosen, Louis, et al., 2005).

The CCM includes the following core components: decision support, delivery system design, clinical information systems, self-management, and community support. For depression, decision support includes the use of clinical practice guidelines focused on mood disorders treatment in primary care, often in the form of flow sheets that are palatable to primary care providers. The CCM element of delivery system design promotes a coordinated and integrated approach to managing patients with depression. In doing so, a care manager (i.e., physician extender such as a nurse) collaborates with primary care and mental health providers to ensure that the patient receives adequate treatment and follow-up care in the primary care setting. The care manager also provides ongoing in-person or telephone contact services for patients to ensure that treatment is followed through, and can exchange information between the general medical and mental health providers so that both are aware of the patients' condition. The care manager often will establish a registry to collect ongoing data on patients to track their progress (the CCM clinical information system component). The CCM also emphasizes a patient-centered approach to treatment that incorporates self-management strategies to promote adherence and overall wellness. The goals of patient self-management approaches are to activate, educate, and support patients and families in the management of depression, and to connect patients to culturally specific community organizations or resources whenever appropriate. Self-management education includes discussion on the triggers of affective episodes, improving medication and clinic visit adherence, and navigating across different health care providers. The community component involves the care manager assisting patients in connecting with community organizations for additional support, such as faith-based organizations or mood disorder advocacy groups.

Table 10.2 Examples of Chronic Care-Based Models for Depression

Intervention trials	Collaborative care (Katon et al., 1995)
	Partners in care (Wells et al., 2004)
	Depression in late life—PROSPECT and IMPACT studies (Bruce et al., 2004; Unutzer et al., 2002)
	Telephone care management (Hunkeler et al., 2000; Simon & Von Korff, 1995)
Implementation programs	Institute for Healthcare Improvement Breakthrough Series (Berwick & Kilo, 1999; Wagner et al., 2001)
	RESPECT (Dietrich et al., 2004)
	Quality Improvement for Depression (Rubenstein et al., 2002)
	RWJ Depression in Primary Care (Pincus et al., 2001)

The advantage of the CCM is that it is "manual based" and involves reorganizing existing providers rather than hiring additional teams of providers, as with assertive community treatment or intensive case management programs. Manual-based interventions are ideal for community-based settings with limited funding streams. However, the CCM has not been fully implemented for mood disorders in community-based settings that serve vulnerable groups.

Barriers in Implementing the CCM

Still, evidence suggests that the CCM has not been fully effective in reducing disparities in health care for minority individuals. Foremost is because many of the self-management and care coordination services provided in the CCM were not specifically tailored to address barriers experienced by minority patients, such as language barriers or lack of culturally appropriate materials. Community resources, one of the key components of the CCM, may also be limited in minority communities. For example, effective self-management through a healthy diet is key to weight loss and prevention of diabetes and other chronic illnesses. However, this is difficult to maintain in poor communities with few supermarkets that sell fresh fruits, vegetables, and other healthy foods (Baker, Schootman, Barnidge, & Kelly, 2006). In addition, high crime rates and lack of social capital preclude those living in low-income environments to maintain adequate exercise to prevent chronic illness or to make medical or mental health appointments (Eckert & Galazka, 1986). Nonetheless, a recently completed CCM study focused on improving depression care was found to be equally effective among whites and minorities alike, in part because the intervention encouraged patient choice between antidepressants and counseling, and offered culturally specific services that enhanced community resources (e.g., provided cultural competency training, interpreters) (Miranda et al., 2003).

Additional barriers exist in implementing the CCM for mood disorders beyond the research trial phase, especially at the health plan and purchaser levels (Table 10.1) (Kilbourne et al., 2004). At the health plan level (e.g., Medicaid health plans), the organizational and financial separation of physical and mental health care impedes efforts to coordinate care and increases confusion over which provider is accountable for what condition (e.g., depression presented in the primary care setting). These barriers have been exacerbated with the advent of mental health "carve-outs," disease management programs, and pharmacy benefits management programs that exist separately from health plans. Care for mood disorders is further impeded if some of these providers fail to accept Medicaid patients. Currently, many health plans "carve out" mental health services to separate entities to negotiate lower costs, and many also reduce costs by carving out pharmacy services. This shift has disrupted relationships between primary and mental health providers compared with traditional fee-for-service mechanisms. Primary care providers are therefore less confident in referring patients to specialty services, are less inclined to make informal consultations with mental health specialists even for uncomplicated depression, and are less likely to communicate with the patient's mental health provider in the long run. This shift has also led to a lack of incentives to integrate care for mood disorders in the primary care setting. There are few mechanisms to pay for depression treatment in primary care settings because primary care providers are not reimbursed for mood disorder care, and there is no financial incentive to coordinate services across general medical and mental health specialty providers, leading to fragmentation.

At the health care purchaser level (e.g., Medicare, Medicaid), there is a lack of awareness of the problem with fragmented mental and physical health care. There are also few studies from the health care purchaser's perspective showing the return on investment of treatment models such as the CCM (e.g., improved outcomes, reduced costs). As a result, purchasers do not select plans based on their ability to coordinate care for mood disorders or chronic conditions. Finally, at the population level, many community organizations are not aware of the potential benefits of promoting treatment models for mood disorders in primary care settings.

Strategies to Implement and Sustain the CCM for Mood Disorders

Despite these barriers, there are emerging initiatives to implement the CCM for mood disorders in real-world, primary care settings. These initiatives (Table 10.2) involved organizational changes to tailor the CCM to diverse populations and safety net providers (Berwick & Kilo, 1999), financial incentives to implement the CCM in routine care (Pincus et al., 2001), and community participation in the CCM's operationalization in routine care (Wagner et al., 2001).

Tailoring Treatment Models to Address the Needs of Vulnerable Populations

Chronic Care Model-based mood disorders treatment models that have been successfully implemented within diverse vulnerable populations have shared common features (Miranda et al., 2003; Surgeon General, 2002). These features included customizing CCM elements (e.g., self-management, delivery system design) a priori to address cultural issues among the target population (e.g., incorporating community-based organizations that served specific populations, offering culturally appropriate psychotherapy in conjunction with medications). They also utilized methods for implementing the CCM that maximized participation, such as engaging and working at community-based practices and/or offering self-management sessions at convenient times or holding sessions at convenient locations (e.g., within neighborhoods).

Financial Incentives

There have also been recent efforts to establish financial incentives to encourage primary care providers to adopt CCM components in their settings. Traditionally, providers have been subject to incentives to reduce costly inpatient visits or limited expensive outpatient procedures (e.g., capitation), or productivity bonuses, which discourage the delivery of chronic illness care. Other nonfinancial incentives traditionally used included utilization review or preauthorization (gatekeeping), which also have limited efforts to integrate mental health services.

Emerging incentives that promote chronic illness care are being tested—notably, "pay for performance," which involves paying physicians if they achieve a minimal score on key performance measures linked to quality of care for chronic conditions. National organizations such as the National Committee on Quality Assurance regularly monitor the quality of care for chronic conditions using established, although not necessarily validated, measures of health care processes or clinical outcomes across health plans and provider organizations. (See Table 10.3 for examples of chronic care performance measures for depression and other conditions [National Committee on Quality Assurance, 2006]). Pay-for-performance demonstration programs have been initiated for some of these measures (preventive services, diabetes) (National Committee on Quality Assurance, 2006). Nonetheless, some fear that pay for performance will ensue a backlash among providers, especially those who provide care for vulnerable populations. For example, if a provider has a number of low-income patients who are unable to make regular appointments because of transportation barriers or competing demands, the provider will not be "counted" as delivering adequate quality of care even though the provider made an effort to provide such care. There is also concern that performance monitoring based on intermediate outcomes measures (e.g., glycosylated hemoglobin, cholesterol levels, or depressive symptoms) will result in patient "cherry-picking" (i.e., providers may choose to manage less complex patients). Other nonfinancial incentives such as profiling providers (i.e., comparing them with their peers on quality measures) have been used to some extent, but there is no evidence suggesting their effectiveness in maintaining chronic care management programs for mood disorders.

Other financial incentives that show promise include the establishment of billing codes for mood disorders treatment in primary care or for care management. Allowing primary care providers to bill for extra time for depression management would provide incentives for them to devote extra time to managing

Table 10.3 Examples of Quality Indicators for Mood Disorders and Other Chronic Illnesses

Condition	Measures
Bipolar disorder	Percent of patients prescribed lithium receiving blood, urea, nitrogen/creatinine + thyroid stimulating hormone tests every 6 months
Depression	Percent of patients with a new diagnosis of depression receiving antidepressants for at least 6 months
Mental health, general	Percent of patients with an inpatient psychiatric hospital stay that should receive an outpatient follow-up visit ≤ 30 days from discharge
Diabetes mellitus	Percent of patients with diabetes mellitus type 1 or 2 with the following HbA1C testing: HbA1c poorly controlled (>9), eye exam performed, LDL screening performed, LDL < 130 mg/dL, LDL < 100 mg/dL, kidney disease monitored
Tobacco use	Percent of patients who smoke who received advice to quit smoking, who were recommended smoking cessation medications, or who discussed smoking cessation strategies

HbA1c, glycosylated hemoglobin; LDL, low-density lipoprotein.

mood disorders without having to refer the patient to different mental health providers. Such reimbursement mechanisms may also encourage providers to invest in information technology, care management, or other quality improvement strategies. Still, many primary care providers do not have authorization to bill for depression treatment in primary care, especially in settings in which mental health care has been carved out to a different plan.

In addition, there has been increased demand from health plans to "outsource" or carve out care for patients with multiple chronic conditions to disease management companies to consolidate and reduce treatment costs for these patients. Typically, health plans will subcontract out the care for chronic illnesses (e.g., congestive heart failure, diabetes) to these companies, which in turn provide self-management tools and care management via nurse specialists for these patients. By carving out the care for these conditions, disease management companies promise health plans they will be able to save money in the long run by reducing hospitalization rates. However, many disease management companies do not follow the CCM framework by not involving the patients' providers (Casalino, 2005. This can lead to further fragmentation of health care.

Despite the many challenges, there have been some system- and policy-level solutions proposed to promote the CCM for mood disorders in routine care settings, especially by addressing barriers on the health plan/purchaser side. For example, the Medicare Modernization Act included demonstration programs for chronic care-based models that address patients with multiple comorbidities and across specialties. In fact, the programs that applied for the demonstration support had to cover depression care as part of their services (Centers for Medicare and Medicaid Services, 2004). The RWJ Depression in Primary Care

Program (Pincus, Pechura, Elinson, & Pettit, 2001) was one of the few demonstration programs that funded partnerships between primary care and mental health purchasers, providers, and health plans to align clinical and economic strategies to promote and sustain the CCM for depression care. Some innovative examples that fostered the CCM included a clinician credentialing program that allowed primary care providers to bill for extra time to spend managing depression care or the use of a plan-level care manager to manage conditions across different specialties (Kilbourne et al., 2004).

Still, strategies to implement the CCM have not fully considered diverse patient populations, many of whom suffer from other chronic conditions in additional to mood disorders. Smaller, publicly funded practices may not be able to support customized CCMs for different chronic illnesses. Chronic Care Model strategies that do address multiple illnesses may end up underemphasizing certain conditions (e.g., depression might be "crowded out" in light of other chronic illnesses) (Redelmeier et al., 1998). Even if CCM programs are implemented, patients with multiple chronic illnesses may still be underserved because of client cherry-picking. Recently, Great Britain proposed treatment models that take a "stepped-care" approach and provide different levels of intensive case management depending on the patient's functional status rather than diagnosis. Patients with multiple chronic illnesses, for example, would receive more intensive case management than those with a single chronic illness. However, the extent to which this framework is effective and leads to cost-efficient care has not been explored.

Community Collaborations

Finally, the successful adaptation of the CCM across diverse populations needs to include community-based collaborations. Community members know their clients well and are usually very familiar with the communities they serve, and can initiate innovative strategies to adapt treatment models to local settings (Horowitz, Davis, Palermo, & Vladeck, 2000). Funding agencies (e.g., NIH) have increasingly called on researchers to engage in community-based participatory research programs as a means to understand the origins of disparities and to implement and sustain interventions in the long run (Agency for Healthcare Research and Quality, 2003). Individuals from both research and community settings enjoyed problem solving many of the logistical issues when they worked together (Rotheram–Borus et al., 2000). Although this more hands-on role through community engagement is not always familiar to researchers, building a strong relationship between researchers, communities, and policymakers throughout the research process is critical to the goal of implementing CCM-based treatment models for mood disorders.

Researcher–community collaborations thrive most when researchers bring community members to the table early on, prior to the implementation of the treatment model, to garner their input on its implementation. State-of-the-art frameworks that promote researcher–community (consumer) collaborations have been developed in business and management fields. Foremost among these models have been participatory management (PM) theory, which combines principles of community-based participatory research with shared decision-making techniques used in management research (Din–Dzietham, Porterfield, Cohen, Reaves, Burrus, & Lamb, 2004; Leana & Florkowski, 1992; Miller & Monge, 1986; Valentine, 1996). Participatory management places an emphasis on involving health care consumers and front-line providers (defined as those who are directly providing care for patients) in the process of adapting and implementing a quality improvement initiative such as the CCM as a means to maximize its chances for sustainability in routine care. The core elements of PM include (a) an understanding of usual care and identifying options for adapting a treatment model based on community input, (b) motivation of front-line providers by garnering their input on customizing the model and creative problem solving (e.g., developing menu options for adaptation), and (c) refinement of the treatment model based on input from community members. These elements are implemented using three processes that ensure that input from community providers is incorporated into the development of the treatment model: customization (i.e., through focus groups of community members), evaluation/refinement (i.e., through cross-functional teams), and implementation (Table 10.4). The PM model is designed to involve community-based providers who have not traditionally been involved in research, many of whom care for a disproportionate number of minority individuals. Some of the core elements of PM, notably garnering community input and motivating providers, have increased acceptability, knowledge, and participation of minority individuals in mental health research (Bluthenthal, Jones, Fackler–Lowrie, Ellison, Booker, Jones, et al., 2006; Mulvaney–Day, Rappaport, Alegria, & Codianne, 2006). This growing body of

Table 10.4 Participatory Management Process Outline

PM Process	Procedures	Expected Products/Outcomes
Customization	1. Identification of problem in community, selection of treatment strategy	1. Initial information on usual care in community
	2. Assessment of usual care and barriers via needs assessment	2. Focus groups of providers and consumers to generate ideas to customize treatment model
	3. Options for adapting CCM	3. Provider, consumer buy-in
Evaluation and refinement	Further model refinement for pilot test using an XFT	1. Input from stakeholders to refine model, buy-in using an XFT
		2. Revised treatment model
Implementation	Full scale implementation	Model implementation and formative evaluation, and community feedback

CCM, Chronic Care Model; PM, participatory management; XFT, cross-functional team.

research, encouraged by a positive response to community-based participation, is now focused on the further implementation of effective and sustainable mental health treatment models within these groups.

One of the key components of the PM framework is the cross-functional team. The goals of the cross-functional team are to review input from front-line providers and community members (i.e., from focus groups) and, based on this information, decide on the best approaches to operationalize each CCM core element given the organizational, management, and financial settings of the participating health plans, practices, and community. Cross-functional teams are defined as a small number of people with complementary skills who are committed to a common purpose, performance goals, and approach for which they hold themselves mutually accountable. (McKenzie, 1994). Such teams are typically constituted when a problem or process is sufficiently complicated that information sharing among various specialists is deemed beneficial and/or because various stakeholders must buy into the process in order for it to be successful (Leana & Florkowski, 1992). Cross-functional teams usually involve a committee of key stakeholders (health plan leaders/managers, key providers, consumer groups, study investigators who can resolve issues and develop strategies that involve reorganization of practices) and financial incentives (e.g., identifying care managers, information system upgrades, reimbursement mechanisms for the CCM). The use of cross-functional teams has been found to be associated with a greater likelihood of adapting new products. Cross-functional teams can also lead to greater commitment by stakeholders as well as a richer understanding of potential obstacles and opportunities for researchers (Leana & Florkowski, 1992). Cross-functional teams have been shown to be associated with more innovative approaches to problem solving (McKenzie, 1994), as well as improved patient outcomes in mental health settings (Alexander, Lichtenstein, Jinnett, Wells, Zazzali, & Liu, 2005).

Implementing cross-functional teams may be especially beneficial to health care settings that serve minority clients because as a group the team can leverage resources across different entities (e.g., foundations, charitable organizations, health plans). It can also serve to bring together front-line providers and community advocates through problem-solving barriers to implementation, thus building trust between groups that traditionally have not worked together (Rotheram–Borus et al., 2000).

CONCLUSIONS

For mood disorder treatment models to be successfully implemented across diverse patient populations, researchers need to work with community-based providers to realign organizational and financial incentives that reduce the multilevel barriers to mood disorders treatment. These changes involve reorganizing primary care to provide chronic illness management through integrated, seamless mental health treatment for patients and culturally specific self-management programs. Financial incentives are needed to encourage primary care practices to adapt chronic care treatment strategies. At the same time, PM techniques can be used to engage community providers and get them motivated to change practice above and beyond financial incentives. Overall, researchers ought to involve community-based providers and consumers upfront, when designing and implementing treatment models for mood disorders.

REFERENCES

Agency for Healthcare Research and Quality. (2003, June). *The role of community-based participatory research: Creating partnerships, improving health.* AHRQ publication no. 03-0037. Rockville, MD: Agency for Healthcare Research and Quality.

Alexander, J. A., Lichtenstein, R., Jinnett, K., Wells, R., Zazzali, J., & Liu, D. (2005). Cross-functional team processes and patient functional improvement. *Health Services Research, 40,* 1335–1355.

Alvidrez, J. (1999). Ethnic variations in mental health attitudes and service use among low-income African American, Latina, and European American young women. *Community Mental Health Journal, 35,* 515–530.

Arean, P. A., Alvidrez, J., Nery, R., Estes, C., & Linkins, K. (2003). Recruitment and retention of older minorities in mental health services research. *Gerontologist, 43,* 36–44.

Baker, E. A., Schootman, M., Barnidge, E., & Kelly, C. (2006). The role of race and poverty in access to foods that enable individuals to adhere to dietary guidelines. *Prevention and Chronic Disease, 3,* 76.

Bauer, M. S., McBride, L., Williford, W. O., Glick, H., Kinosian, B., Altshuler, L., et al. (2006). Collaborative chronic care for bipolar disorder, II: Clinical and functional outcome in a 3-year, 11-site randomized controlled trial. *Psychiatric Services, 57,* 937–945.

Berwick, D., & Kilo, C. (1999). Idealized design of clinical office practice: An interview with Donald Berwick and Charles Kilo of the Institute for Healthcare Improvement. *Managed Care Quarterly, 7,* 62–69.

Bluthenthal, R. N., Jones, L., Fackler–Lowrie, N., Ellison, M., Booker, T., Jones, F., et al. (2006). Witness for wellness: Preliminary findings from a community–academic participatory research mental health initiative. *Ethnicity and Disease, 16,* S18–S34.

Bodenheimer, T., Wagner, E. H., & Grumbach, K. (2002). Improving primary care for patients with chronic illness. *Journal of the American Medical Association, 288,* 1775–1779.

Brown, C., Schulberg, H. C., & Prigerson, H. G. (2000). Factors associated with symptomatic improvement and recovery from major depression in primary care patients. *General Hospital Psychiatry, 22,* 242–250.

Brown, C., Schulberg, H., Sacco, D., Perel, J., & Houck, P. (1999) Effectiveness of treatments for major depression in primary medical care practice: A post hoc analysis of outcomes for African American and white patients. *Journal of Affective Disorders, 53,* 185–19.

Bruce, M., TenHave, T., Reynolds, C. F., Katz, I., Schulberg, H. C., & Mulsant, B. H. (2004). A randomized trial to reduce suicidal ideation and depressive symptoms in older primary care patients: The PROSPECT Study. *Journal of the American Medical Association, 291,* 1081–1091.

Burgess, D. J., Fu, S. S., & van Ryn, M. (2004). Why do providers contribute to disparities and what can be done about it? *Journal of General Internal Medicine, 19,* 1154–1159.

Casalino, L. P. (2005). Disease management and the organization of physician practice. *Journal of the American Medical Association, 293,* 485–488.

Casalino, L., Gillies, R. R., Shortell, S. M., Schmittdiel, J. A., Bodenheimer, T., & Robinson, J. C. (2003). External incentives, information technology, and organized processes to improve health care quality for patients with chronic diseases. *Journal of the American Medical Association, 289,* 434–441.

Centers for Medicare and Medicaid Services. 2004. *The Chronic Care Improvement Program* [Online]. Available: http://www.cms.hhs.gov/medicarereform/ccip/

Charney, D. S., Reynolds, C. F., Lewis, L., Lebowitz, B. D., Sunderland, T., & Alexopoulos, G. S. (2003). Depression and bipolar support alliance consensus statement on the unmet needs in diagnosis and treatment of mood disorders in late life. *Archives of General Psychiatry, 60,* 664–672.

Cooper, L. A., Brown, C., Vu, H. T., Ford, D. E., & Powe, N. R. (2001). How important is intrinsic spirituality in depression care? A comparison of the views of white and African-American primary care patients. *Journal of General Internal Medicine, 16,* 634–638.

Cooper, L. A., Gonzales, J. J., Gallo, J. J., Rost, K. M., Meredith, L. S., & Rubenstein, L. V. (2003).The acceptability of treatment for depression among African-American, Hispanic, and white primary care patients. *Medical Care, 41,* 479–489.

Cooper–Patrick, L., Gallo, J. J., Gonzales, J. J., Vu, H. T., Powe, N. R., & Nelson, C. (1999). Race, gender, and partnership in the patient–physician relationship. *Journal of the American Medical Association, 282,* 583–589.

Cooper–Patrick, L., Powe, N. R., Jenckes, M. W., Gonzales, J. J., Levine, D. M., & Ford, D. E. (1997). Identification of patient attitudes and preferences regarding treatment of depression. *Journal of General Internal Medicine, 12,* 431–438.

Cruz, M., & Pincus, H. A. (2002). Research on the influence that communication in psychiatric encounters has on treatment. *Psychiatric Services, 53,* 1253–1265.

Diala, C., Muntaner, C., Walrath, C., Nickerson, K. J., LaVeist, T. A., & Leaf, P. J. (2000). Racial differences in attitudes toward professional mental health care and in the use of services. *American Journal of Orthopsychiatry, 70,* 455–464.

Diala, C., Muntaner, C., Walrath, C., Nickerson, K. J., LaVeist, T. A., & Leaf, P. J. (2001). Racial/ethnic differences in attitudes toward seeking professional mental health services. *American Journal of Public Health, 91,* 805–807.

Dietrich, A. J., Oxman, T. E., & Williams, J. A. (2004). Re-engineering systems for the primary care treatment of depression: A randomized, controlled trial. *British Medical Journal, 329,* 602.

Din–Dzietham, R., Porterfield, D. S., Cohen, S. J., Reaves, J., Burrus, B., & Lamb, B. M. (2004). Quality care improvement program in a community-based participatory research project: Example of Project DIRECT. *Journal of the National Medical Association, 96,* 1310–1321.

Eckert, J. K., & Galazka, S. S. (1986). An anthropological approach to community diagnosis in family practice. *Family Medicine, 18,* 274–277.

Freimuth, V. S., & Quinn, S. C. (2004). The contributions of health communication to eliminating health disparities. *American Journal of Public Health, 94,* 2053–2055.

Glied, S. (1997). The treatment of women with mental health disorders under HMO and fee-for-service insurance. *Women and Health, 26,* 1–16.

Hirschfeld, R., Keller, M., Panico, S., Arons, B., Barlow, D., & Davidoff, F. (1997). The National Depressive and Manic-Depressive Association consensus statement on the undertreatment of depression. *Journal of the American Medical Association, 277,* 333–340.

Horowitz, C. R., Davis, M. H., Palermo, A. G., & Vladeck, B. C. (2000). Approaches to eliminating sociocultural disparities in health. *Health Care Financial Review, 21*, 57–74.

Hunkeler, E. M., Meresman, J. F., Hargreaves, W. A., Fireman, B., Berman, W. H., & Kirsch, A. J. (2000). Efficacy of nurse telehealth care and peer support in augmenting treatment of depression in primary care. *Archives of Family Medicine, 9*, 700–708.

Jackson, G. L., Yano, E. M., & Edelman, D. (2005). Veterans Affairs primary care organizational characteristics associated with better diabetes control. *American Journal of Managed Care, 11*, 225–227.

Johnson, R. L., Roter, D., Powe, N. R., & Cooper, L. A. (2004). Patient race/ethnicity and quality of patient–physician communication during medical visits. *American Journal of Public Health, 94*, 2084–2090.

Katon, W., Von Korff, M., Lin, E., Walker, E. L., Simon, G. E., & Bush, T. (1995).Collaborative management to achieve treatment guidelines. *Journal of the American Medical Association, 273*, 1026–1031.

Kilbourne, A. M., Haas, G. L., Han, X., Elder, P., Conigliaro, J., & Good, C. B. (2005). Racial differences in the treatment of veterans with bipolar disorder. *Psychiatric Services, 56*, 1549–1555.

Kilbourne, A. M., Pincus, H. A., Kirchner, J., Schutte, K., Haas, G. L., & Yano, E. M. (2006a). Management of mental disorders in VA primary care practices. *Mental Health Services Research, 33*, 208–214.

Kilbourne, A. M., Schulberg, H. C., Post, E. P., Rollman, B. L., Herbeck–Belnap, B., & Pincus, H. A. (2004). Translating evidence-based depression-management services to community-based primary care practices. *Milbank Quarterly, 82*(4), 631–659.

Kilbourne, A. M., Switzer, G., Hyman, K., Matoka, M., & Fine, M. J. (2006b). Advancing health disparities research: A conceptual framework for detecting, understanding, and reducing disparities in vulnerable populations. *American Journal of Public Health, 96*, 2113–2121.

King, T. E., Jr., & Brunetta, P. (1999). Racial disparity in rates of surgery for lung cancer. *New England Journal of Medicine, 341*, 1231–1233.

Leana, C., & Florkowski, G. (1992). Employee involvement programs: Implementing psychological theory and management practice. *Research in Personnel and Human Resources Management, 10*, 233–270.

Lebowitz, B. D., Pearson, J. L., Schneider, L. S., Reynolds, C. F., III, Alexopoulos, G. S., & Bruce, M. L. (1997). Diagnosis and treatment of depression in late life: Consensus statement update. *Journal of the American Medical Association, 278*, 1186–1190.

Mangione–Smith, R., Schonlau, M., Chan, K. S., Keesey, J., Rosen, M., Louis, T. A., et al. (2005). Measuring the effectiveness of a collaborative for quality improvement in pediatric asthma care: Does implementing the Chronic Care Model improve processes and outcomes of care? *Ambulatory Pediatrics, 5*, 75–82.

McKenzie, L. (1994). Cross-functional teams in health care organizations. *Health Care Supervision, 12*, 1–10.

Meterko, M., Mohr, D. C., & Young, G. J. (2004). Teamwork culture and patient satisfaction in hospitals. *Medical Care, 42*, 492–498.

Miller, K., & Monge, P. (1986). Participation, satisfaction and productivity: A meta-analytic review. *Academy of Management Journal, 29*, 727–753.

Miranda, J., Duan, N., Sherbourne, C., Schoenbaum, M., Lagomasino, I., & Jackson–Triche, M. (2003). Improving care for minorities: Can quality improvement interventions improve care and outcomes for depressed minorities? Results of a randomized, controlled trial. *Health Services Research, 38*, 613–630.

Mulvaney–Day, N. E., Rappaport, N., Alegria, M., & Codianne, L. M. (2006). Developing systems interventions in a school setting: An application of community-based participatory research for mental health. *Ethnicity and Disease, 16,* S107–S117.

National Committee on Quality Assurance. *The health plan and employer data information set 2006 measures* [Online]. Available: http://www.ncqa.org/Programs/HEDIS/Hedis%202004%20 Summary %20Table.pdf

Olfson, M., Marcus, S. C., Druss, B., Elinson, L., Tanielian, T., & Pincus, H. A. (2002). National trends in the outpatient treatment of depression. *Journal of the American Medical Association, 287*(2), 203–209.

Opolka, J. L., Rascati, K. L., Brown, C. M., & Gibson, P. J. (2003). Role of ethnicity in predicting antipsychotic medication adherence. *Annals of Pharmacotherapy, 37*(5), 625–630.

Pincus, H. A. (2003). The future of behavioral health and primary care: Drowning in the mainstream or left on the bank? *Psychosomatics, 44,* 1–11.

Pincus, H. A., Hough, L., Houtsinger, J. K., Rollman, B. L., & Frank, R. G. (2003). Emerging models of depression care: Multi-level ('6 P') strategies. *International Journal Methods Psychiatry Research, 12,* 54–63.

Pincus, H. A., Pechura, C. M., Elinson, L., & Pettit, A. R. (2001). Depression in primary care: Linking clinical and systems strategies. *General Hospital Psychiatry, 23,* 311–318.

Redelmeier, D. A., Tan, S. H., & Booth, G. L. (1998). The treatment of unrelated disorders in patients with chronic medical diseases. *New England Journal of Medicine, 338,* 1516–1520.

Rotheram–Borus, M. J., Rebchook, G. M., Kelly, J. A., Adams, J., & Neumann, M. S. (2000). Bridging research and practice: Community–researcher partnerships for replicating effective interventions. *AIDS Education and Prevention, 12*(5 Suppl.), 49–61.

Rubenstein, L. V., Parker, L. E., Meredith, L. S., Altschuler, A., dePillis, E., & Hernandez, J. (2002). Understanding team-based quality improvement for depression in primary care. *Health Services Research, 37,* 1009–1029.

Sclar, D., Robison, L., Skaer, T., & Galin, R. (1999). Ethnicity and the prescribing of antidepressant pharmacology: 1992–1995. *Harvard Review of Psychiatry, 7,* 29–36.

Simon, G. E., & Von Korff, M. (1995). Recognition, management and outcomes of depression in primary care. *Archives of Family Medicine, 4,* 99–105.

Sirey, J., Meyers, B., Bruce, M., Alexopoulos, G., Perlick, D., & Raue, P. (1999). Predictors of antidepressant prescriptions and early use among depressed outpatients. *American Journal of Psychiatry, 156,* 690–696.

Snowden, L. R. (2001). Barriers to effective mental health services for African Americans. *Mental Health Services Research, 3,* 181–187.

Sullivan, G., Duana N., Kirchnera, J., & Henderson, K. L. (2005). Reinventing evidence-based interventions? *Psychiatric Services, 56,* 1156–1157.

Unutzer, J., Katon, W., & Callahan, C. M. (2002). Improving mood-promoting access to collaborative treatment investigators. Collaborative care management of late-life depression in the primary care setting: A randomized controlled trial. *Journal of the American Medical Association, 288,* 2836–2845.

U.S. Department of Health and Human Services. (2001). *Surgeon General: Mental health: Culture, race, and ethnicity. A supplement to mental health: A report of the Surgeon General.* Rockville, MD: U.S. Department of Health and Human Services.

Valentine, N. M. (1996). A national model for participative management and policy development. *Nursing Administration Quarterly, 21,* 24–34.

Wagner, E. H., Austin, B. T., & Von Korff, M. (1996). Organizing care for patients with chronic illness. *Milbank Quarterly, 74*, 511–544.

Wells, K., Katon, W., Rogers, B., & Camp, P. (1994). Use of minor tranquilizers and antidepressant medications by depressed outpatients: Results from the Medical Outcomes Study. *American Journal of Psychiatry, 151*, 694–700.

Wells, K., Miranda, J., Bruce, M. L., Alegria, M., & Wallerstein, N. (2004). Bridging community intervention and mental health services research. *American Journal of Psychiatry, 161*, 955–963.

11

Factoring Culture Into Outcomes Measurement in Mental Health

MATT MENDENHALL

A comprehensive understanding of outcomes measurement in the mental health field should be based on an analysis of at least four different points of view, including those of consumers,[1] practitioners, researchers, and funding/policy bodies. An initial premise for the current discussion is that stakeholder perspectives emerge from each group's distinct relationship to outcomes measurement as a socially situated process. Additionally, an analysis of differences among stakeholder perspectives on outcomes reveals important implications for mental health service delivery systems and for consumer empowerment. Finally, although outcomes measurement operates broadly in mental health services, this discussion will apply the subject specifically to mood disorders treatment.

Measurement of outcomes in mental health services occurs within conceptual frameworks that are built upon the theories, research, and policies that inform and direct mental health services. In turn, these theories, research knowledge, and policies are based on socially constructed definitions for mental illness. Thus, measuring progress for individuals diagnosed with mental illnesses occurs within the context of beliefs and ideas that are (a) held by practitioners, (b) perpetuated by researchers, and (c) institutionalized through policy and funding agendas. For example, a perspective that views mental illness primarily as a persistently debilitating and chronic condition holds different implications for outcomes work than a perception of mental illness as situational and episodic. This distinction may hold particular salience for people diagnosed with mood disorders because of how disorders (e.g., depression) are diagnosed (discussed further later). Exploring differences in stakeholder perspectives regarding outcomes measurement may contribute to increased collaboration across stakeholder groups, fuller inclusion of consumers in a range of decision making, and increased relevancy of outcomes data.

The work of this chapter contributes to the study of how conceptual dimensions of culture influence our understanding of mental illness and mental health treatment. The concept of culture refers here most basically to a set of values, beliefs, and practices that a group of people hold in common based on their relationship to some environment or challenge. Cultural groups are often defined in ethnic and national terms; however, cultures can also be identified by profession, religion, or other types of association. A broad sense of culture serves as a helpful context in which to consider implications for how the identified stakeholders relate to mental health outcomes measurement. A case is made that outcomes measurement has the potential both to empower and to alienate further consumer populations (Rose, 2005). An empowering outcomes measurement model is one that explicitly places consumer perspectives and contributions at the center of this social process. A central task for this chapter is to identify implications of framing outcomes measurement as a social process with multiple stakeholders.

The conceptual framework needed to complete this task depends first on operationalizing three basic concepts: stakeholder perspective, mental illness, and outcomes. These concepts are briefly defined and applied to the subject of how stakeholders relate to outcomes in mental health treatment. The construction of a working conceptual framework then proceeds through four stages. The first stage involves positing the value of enhanced collaboration in outcomes measurement for the field. The second stage involves describing differences in stakeholder perspectives regarding outcomes measurement. The third stage provides a simple model for outcomes measurement with three dimensions. Finally, the fourth stage recognizes criticisms of tying human services funding to an outcomes measurement paradigm. A brief case example then demonstrates how the framework applies to a specific area in mental health.

CONCEPTUALIZATION

Stakeholder Perspective

Stakeholders within mental health service delivery systems include the individuals, professions, and organizations that play some part in funding, developing, delivering, and receiving services. Stakeholder perspectives in mental health are shaped by their roles and statuses within the mental health field. For example, practitioners need an outcomes model that can account for the complexity of consumers' *real worlds*, as well as for the limited time and resources available for both practice and measurement activities. For researchers, an outcomes model ideally involves processes to include practitioner and consumer input to improve the relevancy of research to the phenomenon being studied. Researchers also need an outcomes model that can account for the rigor and complexity of generating reliable and valid information. For funders and policy makers, an outcomes measurement model needs to produce accurate and compelling information about services for constituencies, and to demonstrate effectiveness in improving broad social problems. For consumers and participants, the outcomes paradigm can manifest as yet another professionalized and abstract construct that professionals use to do something to or label consumers. Unless consumers have an active role in understanding and naming their own outcomes, the process of outcomes measurement becomes another instance in which professionals name a reality for vulnerable people. Consumers' perspectives on an outcomes framework may depend on the level of empowerment (i.e., setting their own outcomes goals) fostered by the provider. An outcomes process that builds in meaningful consumer participation may serve as a mechanism for increased self-determination.

Mental Illness

Mental illness, as a concept, is often referred to as a *social construction*, meaning that the defining elements of mental illness are situated socially. A common example used to explain the social construction of mental illness relates to how the same behaviors that designate the status of healer or shaman in some cultures actually distinguish people in another culture as having mental illnesses. Stephen and Suryani (2000) make an argument to distinguish the " shaman's vocation as emerging from an inner process clearly distinguishable from psychosis or madness" (p. 6). Thus, the meaning of behaviors, the function of behaviors in society, and the consequences of those behaviors vary according to culture and are (to some degree) socially constructed.

Another simple example regarding the social construction of mental illness relates to behaviors associated with grieving the death of a significant other. A study by Bonanno and colleagues (2005) indicated that measures of grief processing and grief avoidance had predictive power for study participants in the United States, but not for participants from the People's Republic of China. Clements and associates (2003) provide a review of cultural perspectives related to grief, and identify multiple dimensions within which cultures define "appropriate" grieving. In some cultures, active grieving is expected for long periods of time, up to a year or longer. In other cultures, the expectation is to "move on" quickly, and if grief is still apparent after two weeks, something must be wrong. Survivors may be judged as having grieved too long or not long enough, too intensely or not intensely enough—that is, according to whether they have adhered to culturally prescribed/accepted ways. If the culturally defined grieving parameters are breached, the person may be considered within a culture to have depression, anxiety, or some other maladaptive response, and could be referred for treatment. The same behavior (e.g., displaying depressive symptoms for a year) could indicate mental health (e.g., respect for the deceased) or mental illness (e.g., clinical depression). Perception and measurement of *successful outcomes* from grief treatment relates to the perception that the survivor's behavior has returned to an accepted expression of grieving within a culture. Outcomes measurement regarding any mental illness should be informed by applicable cultural dimensions.

Taking one more step into this example regarding the socially constructed nature of grief and depression, the treatment and outcomes scenario may become even more complicated for a person with depression who experiences a loss. Does the person's grief become dismissed as simply part of the depression? When treatment for grief within depression faces the outcomes test, what is measured? The issue here relates to how social construction and generalized conceptions of mental illness may confound treatment and outcomes measurement because of the complexity involved in the personal experience of mental illnesses.

The complexity of diagnosing can be demonstrated through a brief discussion regarding the *DSM-IV-TR* (American Psychiatric Association, 2000). A diagnosis of depression or a bipolar condition indicates that a number of symptom criteria have been met. Regarding the diagnoses of major depressive disorder or a bipolar disorder, distinctions that need to be made from the *DSM-IV-TR* include establishing the natures, frequency, and recentness of major depressive episodes and/or manic episodes. Diagnosing a major depressive episode entails (at least initially) determining that, of the nine symptoms listed in the *DSM-IV-TR*, the consumer experienced at least five. The intention here is not to criticize the *DSM-IV-TR* (see, instead, Kutchins & Kirk, 1997), but to acknowledge that mental illness is in part socially defined, not explicitly and empirically determinable, and that there are consequences for reifying mental illness (i.e., treating a conceptual abstraction as if it were self-evident and independent of our conceptual and social processes).

Outcomes

Outcomes measurement has become prominent in human services. In their forward to an National Association of Social Workers Press book, *Outcomes Measurement in the Human Services: Cross-Cutting Issues and Methods*, Feldman and Siskind (1997) consider the prominence of outcomes measurement:

> Many human service professionals know that they are successful in relieving the pain that so many people experience because of poverty, social stress, or mental illness. However, self-perceptions are no longer enough. The development of valid outcomes measures will help attract the resources and community recognition our work so richly deserves. (p. xvi)

Outcomes are often contrasted with a similar term: *outputs*. Although outputs are measures of what the provider or program does (e.g., number of sessions or classes held), *outcomes* are distinguished as the changes that occur for consumers (United Way of America, 1996). Additionally, the changes that occur for consumers are thought to be associated in some way with having received the service or intervention. Outcomes data are supposed to demonstrate the level of impact or effectiveness that a service or intervention has had for a person or within a population. Funders perceive that outcomes measurement is a mechanism for ensuring accountability. Differences in the type of outcomes or outputs valued by each of the stakeholders relate to their interests. For example, payers may be more interested in outputs (i.e., services delivered), whereas consumers would be more naturally focused on improvement in depressive symptoms.

FRAMEWORK CONSTRUCTION I: VALUE OF OUTCOMES COLLABORATION

Feldman and Siskind (1997) go on to provide a starting point for understanding the importance of developing a conceptual framework for outcomes measurement that promotes collaboration:

> As a rule, the current attacks on the human services professions are not supported by empirical data that demonstrate deficiencies or failures, but rather by the absence of reliable data that can either affirm or reject their promises of efficacy. In such a vacuum, public debates are shaped more on *ideology, rhetoric,* and *political muscle* than by systematic empirical data. (p. xv, emphasis added)

Perhaps practitioners consider the outcomes framework used by researchers as ideological because that framework does adequately address the important values, complexity, and methodological concerns related to practice (and vice versa). Perhaps political processes (i.e., "political muscle") are considered as uninformed by practice and research to the degree that timely and meaningfully presented outcomes information are not available. Finally, it is possible to consider that consumers may perceive the outcomes measurement paradigm as a lot of rhetoric when they don't have a voice in selecting their own outcomes and measures. Effective collaboration relies on understanding and integrating the perspectives of those who share concerns, just as much as it relies on a common understanding of the issues to be addressed (Edelman, 1988). If, as alluded to earlier, the current models for outcomes measurement effectively exclude consumer voices (and thus their self-determination), a charge can be issued to practitioners, researchers, and funding/policy bodies to evolve toward an outcomes model that is more inclusive of consumer voice so that consumers (as a stakeholder group) can participate in shaping data that are used in policy and research agendas.

FRAMEWORK CONSTRUCTION II: STAKEHOLDER PERSPECTIVE ON OUTCOMES MEASUREMENT

Outcomes information within any field of practice is generated by and utilized within a definitive set of dimensions and meanings distinct to the culture of that practice. Cultural factors that influence outcomes measurement are considered here for funders, practitioners, and researchers. Although consumer groups are also important stakeholders, consumer perspectives are not discussed here, because professionals have the ultimate responsibility to increase the clarity, relevance, and consistency of the outcomes paradigm to facilitate consumer participation in the outcomes process more meaningfully. The lack of clarity and cohesion among the conceptual frameworks of the three professional cultures potentially contributes to at least three negative consequences: (1) the gap between research and practice, (2) perceived conflicts with funders, and (3) a failure to include client/participant perspectives meaningfully.

As a funding source, the United Way of America (1996) considers that the "bottom line" of outcomes measurement is to identify clearly the benefits for participants that can be associated in some way with the participant's involvement with a program or intervention. A common method of further clarifying this type of perspective is to compare the terms *outcomes* and *outputs*. Outputs are often defined as the products of the program's activities (United Way of America, 1996). Thus, although outcomes measure what happens for the client, outputs measure what the provider does (e.g., the number of sessions or number of classes provided). For funding bodies, the important factors in outcomes measurement include the type, extent, and sustainability of the benefits for consumers or consumer systems. Consumer systems can be specified as individuals, families, or communities.

Funder perspectives are informed by focused missions to solve social problems. The importance of outcome data relates to helping the funder demonstrate their own impact—at an aggregate level—on the social problem of interest. This same perspective could also be attributed to policy-making bodies, with an added consideration that these bodies are accountable to their constituencies to fulfill certain mandates and sanctions. Thus, outcomes data are a medium for policy and funding bodies to be accountable to their constituencies and communities for the use of resources.

A practitioner's perspective on outcomes measurement is complicated by the reality that practitioners must identify and balance multiple variables in making treatment decisions with consumers. Consumers present with complicated, situation-specific challenges that do not always fall clearly into treatment protocols or outcome frames. Consumers bring unique cultural identities with a wide variety of values and beliefs, so that cultural differences related to age, ethnicity, and socioeconomic status may complicate the task of forming a common view between consumer and provider on both the problem and solution. Identifying pertinent characteristics of the challenges brought by consumers requires an ability to identify important information as it emerges, and so the process of measurement (of outcome indicators) is often viewed as distinct from the process of actually working with consumers to create the outcomes. Working with consumers involves therapeutic processes such as forming a trusting relationship, creating a safe space to explore, doing the work of encouraging a consumer to understand new ideas and possibilities for change, and holding a consumer accountable in appropriate ways. Although therapeutic relationships need to be fluid in their development (i.e., allowing for significant changes in problem and solution definition), outcome measures are necessarily concrete (measurement of before-and-after conditions) and not as available to emerging issues.

Even more specifically, the time and labor required to form measurable outcomes or to locate existing measures that apply to the wide variety of challenges becomes a barrier for practitioners. Outcomes measurement may be perceived to take time away from working with consumers that is already limited for practitioners. Throughout this discussion, it should not to be implied that practitioners do not perceive the importance of being accountable for demonstrating effective practices.

A researcher's perspective on outcomes is also complicated, but for different reasons, and a comprehensive presentation would be beyond the reach of this chapter (see McCall & Green, 2004). Briefly, the concerns related to a research perspective of outcomes include factors related to establishing a level of confidence in the knowledge (i.e., outcomes results) about the impact that a program or intervention has on a social problem at both the aggregate and individual levels. For example, researchers are concerned with (a) the level of precision in defining the concepts used to represent the benefits referred to in the United Way definition, (b) the reliability of the tools used to measure those benefits, (c) the validity of both the measures and the conclusions formed regarding the data associated with the measures, and (d) an increased ability to predict occurrence of the outcome, as a dependent variable predicted by an independent variable. The culture of research is defined by the paradigm of scientific inquiry.

FRAMEWORK CONSTRUCTION III: THREE DIMENSIONS OF OUTCOMES MEASUREMENT

This section begins with descriptions for a set of concepts used in developing a basic outcomes measurement model. At this point, it may be helpful to refocus on the stated purpose of the text, which is *to identify cultural factors that influence the diagnosis, treatment, and research on mood disorders.* In this regard, the aim for this chapter remains to explore cultural factors associated with outcomes measurement in mental health (i.e., stakeholder perspective, social construction of the operative terms, and sociopolitical criticisms), not to present a comprehensive outcomes measurement model.[2] The proposed benefits to this type of approach reach beyond the "how-to" level and instead include the fostering of (a) a common language for practitioners, researchers, and funders; (b) increased attention to the complexities of mental illness; (c) increased conceptual precision needed to facilitate drawing valid conclusions from data; and (d) a renewed focus on promoting consumer voice in defining the situation and solutions.

Literature that promotes outcomes work as central to the therapeutic process in mental health services describes outcomes work as parallel and facilitative to therapeutic objectives, not as disruptive and antithetical (Hatry, 1997; Ogles, Lambert, & Fields, 2002; Rossi, 1997; Wiger & Solberg, 2001). Three dimensions of outcomes measurement are key components for bridging practice/research/funding/consumer gaps. These dimensions also facilitate the effective use of outcomes measurement in therapeutic practice. These dimensions include (a) specifying the type of change/outcome expected, (b) identifying explicit strategies for measuring the expected change/outcome, and (c) presenting a three-stage model for illustrating the complexity involved with identifying the

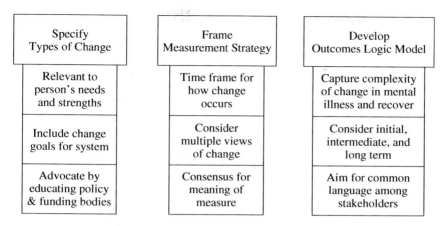

Figure 11.1 Three dimensions for planning for outcomes measurement.

sustained and grounded benefits for people with mental illnesses. Figure 11.1 illustrates the dimensions of this model and the associated tasks. It is essential to clarify how an outcomes paradigm is situated among practitioners and researchers so that the process of outcomes measurement can be more easily utilized by client/participant groups and more meaningfully communicated to funding and policy bodies. Figure 11.1 provides at least some starting ideas on developing a framework to account for and integrate perspectives and interests of the different stakeholders.

Type of Change

First, outcomes can reflect many different types of change for consumer systems. Changes for consumer systems may include, but are not limited to, attitude, knowledge, skill, behavior, status, functioning, circumstances, and quality of life. Davidson (2003) and Davidson and colleagues (2005) describe multiple elements of recovery in mental health that could serve as focal points for helping consumers/participants accept and overcome challenges associated with disability. Outcomes measurement based on Davidson's work might include *redefining self* so that social roles are not defined only in terms of being mentally ill, *overcoming stigma*, and actively *managing symptoms*. Another consideration for providers is that not all outcomes need be focused on measuring traits of and changes at the client/participant level. For example, community-level strategies to reduce the stigma associated with mental illness, and policy-level work can also be defined as important outcomes. A multidimensional approach to improving the quality of life for people diagnosed with mental illness includes understanding the many types of changes that can be fostered for the client/participant, but also for the community and practitioner. Finally, another nuance relates to selecting appropriate outcomes. For example, consumers with severe and persistent mental illnesses may never obtain the typical long-term outcome of placement in independent employment. However, these consumers may benefit in many ways from supported employment settings. If expectations and measures do not include outcomes that are obtainable for more severely disabled consumers, benefits from the program will not be demonstrated, and important support systems may be lost to the client/participant. Funding and policy bodies need to understand that the potential for employment may vary and that positive outcomes should be customized to consumer's situations.

Measurement Strategy

A second dimension for developing valuable and valid outcomes measurements is the overall measurement strategy. Recommendations for developing an overall strategy begin with clearly identifying the type of change you are interested in measuring and reporting on, including how and when measurements will occur. When selecting a measurement tool or process, be specific about (a) what type of change is being fostered within an intervention, (b) how long the change is expected to take, and (c) which indicators of more abstract changes (e.g., attitude) are accepted by key stakeholders. Standardized measures that have been tested for reliability and validity are helpful in ensuring that the results probably relate more to the phenomenon than to some type of error or bias. However, standardized measures that are irrelevant to target changes may be reliable but not be able to demonstrate change that is actually occurring. When therapeutic goals are reflected in the measurement tools, continue to remember that the measurement *tools* are different than the consumer's *experience*, which is much more complicated than any single measure or even a set of measures can fully assess. A measurement tool is not the phenomenon itself and can misrepresent or miss the changes that are actually occurring. Thus, when reporting or interpreting a score from an assessment tool (standardized or not) for any type of consumer system change, the possibility for error, bias, and misuse should be kept in mind.

One strategy that practitioners can use to increase validity when interpreting outcomes data is to attempt to measure progress/change measuring more than one perspective, on more than one type of change, or with multiple measurement methods. This type of measurement strategy is referred to as *triangulating* in the collection of information about a phenomenon. For example, a school-based mental health therapy program can obtain assessments of a child's progress in forming positive relationships from multiple points of view (e.g., the child, parent, and teacher). Indicators of progress could include the frequency of a child's disruptive behavior, a teacher's perspective on the child's academic behaviors (e.g., completing academic work during the scheduled time), and academic performance on standardized tests. In this way, progress demonstrated through one of the measures can be checked or supported with similar progress on the other measures. The triangulating technique is not exclusively related to collecting outcomes data. Therapeutic strategies often rely on multiple perspectives on a consumer's progress. In this way, an explicit outcomes measurement strategy can be understood as complementary with therapeutic strategies.

Three-Stage Logic Model

The third dimension for incorporating an outcomes measurement process into a therapeutic practice is the development of a logic model that will identify how initial, intermediate, and long-term outcomes logically relate. With this type of model, the types of change, acceptable indicators, and measures of those indicators are explicitly identified. Figure 11.2 demonstrates potential steps that support a long-term goal for improving quality of life in consumer populations.

Initial outcomes might include identifying specific aspects of attitude and knowledge that are believed to improve the intermediate outcomes of skills and behavior gains, which in turn are designed to improve functioning and quality of life. Another way to understand this process is as steps to operationalize, from consumer perspectives, the abstract concept of quality of life in terms of attitude, knowledge, skills, and behavior. Each of these steps can be measured as an outcome, generating data that can be used to create meaningful reports on the most relevant benefits of treatment. Clearly, the client/participant should maintain a central role in choosing how the outcome types are defined and then how they can be measured.

At this point, restating an earlier citation of Feldman and Siskind (1997) may help to refocus the discourse: "As a rule, the current attacks on the human services professions are not supported by empirical data that demonstrate deficiencies or failures, but rather by the absence of reliable data that can either affirm or reject their promises of efficacy" (p. xv). Human service professionals have an opportunity, through forming and reporting on client-generated outcome logic models, to communicate critical components of working with various populations. In this way, outcome reporting becomes a vehicle to bridge the gap between researchers and practitioners. More specifically, practitioners can help researchers identify the critical elements of change for consumer populations, because consumers have had a direct role in defining outcomes. In these dialogs regarding the identification of the critical elements of change, researchers can facilitate the movement toward greater conceptual precision. Researchers can

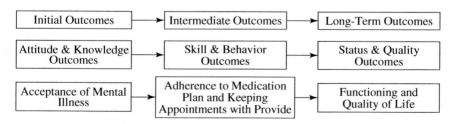

Figure 11.2 Example of a logic model.

then develop and offer measures for the indicators of change as identified by consumers, working also with practitioners to increase the reliability and validity of these measures. Practitioners can give feedback regarding the usability of the measurement tools. Also, researchers and practitioners can work together to map out the complexity of mental illness and treatment to communicate the needs of mentally ill consumers to funding and policy bodies.

The discussion of this simple model does not presuppose that these collaborative activities are not already occurring. However, the gap between practice-based and research-based knowledge continues to be discussed, and both practitioners and researchers continue to seek ways to influence funding policies. Perhaps a methodology for fostering collaboration and influencing policy already exists in a simple framework, such as the one presented, for being explicit and precise about (a) types of change, (b) measurement strategies, and (c) logic models that reflect greater detail regarding the complexity of the challenges faced by mental health consumers. The goal of this chapter has not been to present an innovative and comprehensive framework for outcomes measurement. Instead, the goal has been to consider how a cultural view of outcomes measurement might inform increased collaboration among the stakeholders in mental health services by aligning distinct points of view into a common and comprehensive conceptual framework. A simple outcomes logic model format may provide enough of a conceptual foundation for practitioners, researchers, and funders to work more collaboratively toward holding consumer voice at the center of determining effectiveness in mental health treatment.

A brief application of these guidelines follows regarding the experience and treatment of depression. Selecting the types of change to measure for a person experiencing depression should be based on the understanding that depression is thought to involve both genetic and environmental factors. Thus, pertinent outcomes might include medication compliance, behavioral changes, and residential stability. Also, meaningful outcomes for treatment of depression may differ for unipolar and bipolar experiences (National Alliance on Mental Illness, 2006).

Standardized measures exist to measure depression. For example, the CES-D (Radloff, 1977) has a long history of use, established psychometric properties, and includes 20 items on which consumers self-rate. Alternatively, narrative approaches to therapy may facilitate consumers in describing and reconstructing their understanding of experiences and options. Measures related to this approach may involve consumer-constructed scales, such as those found with solution-focused approaches (DeJong & Berg, 2002). Triangulation of outcomes measurement might assemble multiple methods and gain ratings from not only the consumer, but also the consumer's family or other caregivers.

A logic model framework might then propose an informal theory for how these different outcomes are connected. For example, one might first consider that a consumer's attitude, in the form of acceptance of illness (or lack thereof), may be based on misconceptions about the illness or fear of stigma regarding depression. When misconceptions are cleared and stigma is confronted, the consumer may then attempt to explore increased social venues for which behavioral skills are lacking. Finally, with improved behavioral skills, a supported employment opportunity may arise that could provide a greater sense of self-sufficiency.

FRAMEWORK CONSTRUCTION IV: CRITICISMS OF THE OUTCOMES PARADIGM

Describing a conceptual framework for outcomes measurement should include acknowledgment of the criticisms and accepted limitations regarding the trend of tying human service funding to outcomes reporting (Clegg, 2005; Hudson, 1997; Mullen & Streiner, 2004; Rossi, 1997; Witkin & Harrison, 2001). Hatry (1997), for example, describes a limitation related to the use of outcomes in human services: "I believe that no human service official can with fairness be held fully accountable for outcomes, because in the real world many other factors in addition to the subject program affect outcomes" (p. 4). Criticisms often address the inherent oversimplification involved in reducing human experience and progress to measurable terms (Lather, 2004; Mullen & Streiner, 2004). Additionally, mental health treatment providers articulate that many of the meaningful factors of progress in mental illness and treatment are difficult to measure (Weisz, Sandler, Durlak, & Anton, 2005). Positivist perspectives and linear ways of studying and understanding human and social phenomena do not always capture or account for the complexity of all factors or of how those factors interrelate (Mullen & Streiner, 2004). Furthermore, the demands for producing outcomes data place a heavy burden on providers whose time and resources are already stretched. Measurement and data analysis are labor-intensive endeavors and often require specific conceptual skills to generate meaningful, reliable, and valid data (Gambrill, 1997, 2005). Concerns are also expressed about the potential for the outcomes measurement process to erode the clinical discretion of practitioners and, instead, further empower managers, policy makers, or funders. Empowerment of nonclinical stakeholders may occur through increased power to issue outcomes mandates (i.e., to produce specific outcome results) and required use of manualized evidence-based practices (Lather, 2004).

A comprehensive critique of the outcomes paradigm is beyond the scope of this chapter.[3] Yet, pressure for increased accountability through outcomes measurement and reporting is unlikely to fade because of such criticisms. Therefore, mental health practitioners and researchers have an important stake in ensuring that these types of concerns shape the role that outcomes measurement has in a society. Specifically, advocates should work to promote clarity regarding how outcomes measurement can best represent concerns related to the complexity of human problems, to professional autonomy, and to public policy.

CASE APPLICATION

School-based mental health programs were designed to improve mental health outcomes for children and youth with serious emotional disturbances by increasing access to services and by decreasing the stigma associated with receiving mental health treatment (Taylor & Adelman, 2000). A core document describing the prevalence of and difficulties associated with serious emotional disturbance in children and youth is the *Report of the Surgeon General's Conference on Children's Mental Health* (U.S. Public Health Service, 2000). The Surgeon General's conference report estimates that between 10% and 20% of children and adolescents, nationally, have a need for mental health treatment. The report estimates that only 20% of children known to have mental health needs actually receive treatment. Additionally, the National Alliance for Mental Illness website reports that approximately 20% of youth will have one or more major episodes of depression by adulthood, and that at any one time about 2% of school-age children and about 4% of adolescents have a major depressive episode (National Alliance on Mental Illness, 2006).

Ideally, development of an outcomes measurement framework for a school-based mental health program would be grounded in the research literature that describes important factors associated with positive impacts for the target population. Two factors are distilled from the literature to provide a foundation for an outcomes framework. First, as Craft (1998) articulates, "[t]he range of psychological, educational, family, and neighborhood problems affecting children, especially those with emotional disturbances or those in crisis, is extremely complex" (p. 1). The importance of considering complexity as a factor is also highlighted in a document provided by the Center of Mental Health in Schools (2000): "The findings also underscore that addressing major psychological problems one at a time is unwise because the problems are interrelated and require multifaceted and cohesive solutions" (p. 4). Second, the problems that children have are most appropriately understood as contextually based, not individually based. Weist and Christodulu (2000) state this succinctly: "Too many times children are held accountable for their problems when many emotional and behavioral problems in youth are strongly determined by the environment; we attempt to 'fix' the student, when the real problem lies elsewhere" (p. 196). Other factors certainly exist and would be important to identify; however, these two factors (complexity and context) suffice for describing the outcomes measurement process within the case example. As presented here, a significant number of children and youth who need services are experiencing, either currently or at some time in adolescence, major depressive episodes. Outcomes measurement should distinguish between emotional disturbances that are demonstrated in acting out behaviors (e.g., oppositional defiant disorder and ADHD) and emotional disturbances that are demonstrated through internalized behaviors (e.g., depression and anxiety).

An application of the dimensions to school-based mental health programs includes discussion about the value of outcomes measurement, stakeholder characteristics, and outcomes measurement dimensions. First, Weist and Christodulu (2000) describe the importance of being able to document positive outcomes to develop a wide array of funding streams. Pfeiffer and Reddy (1998) report a comprehensive review of mental health programs for children that includes a program's ability to demonstrate accountability and effectiveness as one of the seven characteristics of effective programs. Second, the stakeholders in this case

include children, parents, teachers, school administrators, mental health therapists, allied treatment staff, physicians, and funding sources. Outcomes logic
models can identify the specific types of changes that relate to both acting out and
internalizing behaviors and conditions. For children, valued outcomes might include being perceived more positively by peers and adults, feeling successful in
the classroom and home, and increased understanding about their emotions and
experiences. Parents might focus more on improved interactions at home, fewer
calls from the teacher regarding problem behaviors (or in the case of depression,
more classroom involvement), and increased understanding about their child's
emotional challenges. Teachers may value school-based programs related to increased knowledge about children's mental health issues, strategies to keep children in the classroom, and minimizing overall classroom interruptions so they can
delivery academic material to all students in the classroom. School administrators consider a school-based program's value in terms of the program's impact on
absenteeism, readiness to learn, and assessment for educational supports. Allied
treatment staff may value increased resources in the school building to meet all
students' needs, and increased communication regarding student's ongoing challenges. For physicians, the continuity of care, progress reports, and facilitation for
keeping appointments might be considered priority outcomes. Finally, funding
sources must have valid and meaningful evidence of the impact to continue to
secure funding and maintain accountability to their constituencies.

Types of Change Related to School-Based Services

An outcomes framework takes into consideration the analysis of identified factors
and stakeholder perspectives just described. Often the types of changes measured
involve academic progress. Academic progress can be measured in terms of
standardized test scores, quarterly grades, or specific positive behaviors that the
teacher observes. A teacher could be asked to rate a referred student's (a) ability to
listen and follow directions, (b) ability to complete work during the scheduled
time, (c) need for monitoring and support to complete work, and (d) quality of
work. Other indicators, or types of targeted change, might include attendance,
tardiness, behavior disruptions, participation in activities, parental involvement,
teacher knowledge of mental health issues, and specific concepts from a theoretically based intervention that deals with social skills, behavior issues, and self-
confidence. Concepts from theoretically based interventions can be operationalized and measured to demonstrate progress in the terms of the intervention.

Measurement Strategy Related to School-Based Services

Although standardized scores are certainly an important indicator, two challenges
arise related to this indicator. First, the test is given only once per year in many
locations. Measuring change and reporting positive results with one data point
per year is difficult. Second, a question can be asked here: Can mental health
therapy fairly take credit for significant changes on standardized tests? In this case,
so many other school interventions are in place and operating that it would be

difficult to determine which part of the improved scores could be attributed to school-based mental health services. On the other hand, behaviors such as following directions, completing work during scheduled time, and need for monitoring are all more specific indicators that could be measured and more fairly attributed to a school-based therapy intervention. Teachers could be asked to rate these types of facilitators to learning before and after mental health treatment or at the beginning and end of the school year. Response options should be specific enough to allow consistency in rating. Another important measurement strategy is to gain input from the child, parent, and teacher regarding progress on some similar measure. In this way, comparisons can be made and progress from one point of view can be supported or challenged by another perspective.

Logic Model Application

A logic model provides a conceptual map that identifies how a school-based therapist expects to reach a long-term impact objective. A primary objective for a school-based mental health program might be to increase the child's exposure to learning opportunities through strategies to limit behavior disruptions, to increase classroom participation and quality of work completion, and to improve peer relationships. The long-term outcome of these types of objectives might be measured as fewer office referrals for disruptive behaviors, increased number of times the students raise their hands, or increased number of positive interactions with peers. An intermediate outcome might be improved ratings by the child, parent, and teacher on a measure of social skills. Finally, the initial outcome could relate to attendance and tardiness or to the child asking for help from the teacher. The logic of this model can be stated succinctly. Children who feel unsuccessful at school may simply not attend or may be late to avoid the challenges, and children who are experiencing depressive symptoms may not actively engage in solving problems. A therapist works with the child toward creating some feelings of success so that a child attends more regularly and seeks out help from school adults. This may take some strategizing with the teacher and helping the teacher understand the "plan." Because of increased attendance, the child works with the therapist and teacher at school, and with the parents at home, to improve skills in social situations. The child uses these skills and is able to stay in the classroom for longer periods of time each day, thus having more opportunities to learn. Of course this is a very simple example and the complexities related to emotional disturbances, poverty, and the range of teacher competence in working with emotionally disturbed students require greater sophistication. The logic as stated, however, provides some clear opportunities for outcomes definition, measurement, and reporting.

CONCLUSION

In summary, this level of conceptual abstraction reveals important policy, research, and practice implications for the mental health service delivery system.

If outcomes data are going to be increasingly used to influence decisions about funding treatments and research in mental health, then outcomes data should become increasingly relevant and inclusive. A model that promotes collaboration among all stakeholders and places the voice of the consumer at the center of the process will not only promote empowerment (i.e., inclusion) of consumer populations, but should also increase the relevancy of the resulting data.

The same concepts that facilitate understanding of how cultural diversity (e.g., in terms of race and ethnicity) impacts treatment decisions can also facilitate a deeper understanding of how diverse perspectives influence outcomes measurement. The position taken here is that deconstructing stakeholder perspectives, related to views on outcome measurement, provides an opportunity to identify common elements of measuring consumer progress. This chapter describes a process for practitioners to use in reconsidering or reconstructing the value and place of outcomes measurement in practice. The proposed process begins by recognizing that outcomes measurement has important social implications, such as its capacity to inform policy and funding agendas. Outcomes measurement is a socially constructed mechanism that can be used by all the stakeholders for different purposes. Practitioners with this view on outcomes might be more inclined to discover ways to empower consumers, through this mechanism, to participate in and influence social policy.

When the value and utility of outcomes measurement in our society are perceived, the next step involves recognizing that each stakeholder group approaches and understands outcomes measurement quite differently. These differences, although expected, create the potential for discordance in the use of outcomes data as information to inform policy and research agendas, which ultimately impact consumers and practitioners. Within the context of differences regarding perceptions on outcomes measurement, three dimensions of outcomes measurement provide a framework for engaging in outcomes measurement: type of change, measurement strategy, and a three-stage logic model framework. These three dimensions are not presented as a comprehensive model, but instead as a common language to use in the discussion regarding stakeholder perspective. Finally, criticisms regarding the outcomes paradigm heighten our awareness regarding interactions between outcomes measurement and the complexity of human problems, the role of social construction in mental health, protecting professional autonomy (while maintaining accountability), and policy implications.

This chapter has approached the subject by describing a contextualized outcomes process that considers the social functions of and differing views regarding outcomes measurement. Within such a context, three dimensions guide practitioners in incorporating an outcomes approach into practice. This approach provides a conceptual framework that is both sensitive to racial and ethnic cultural differences (through individualized change identification and logic models), but is also accountable for differences in how outcomes data may be collected and interpreted by the professional stakeholders in mental health services. Research and policy agendas built on a contextualized outcomes process stand to become increasingly relevant to the needs of diverse populations and increasingly collaborative among researchers, policy makers, and practitioners.

NOTES

1. The term *consumers* is used in this chapter to refer to people who receive mental health services.

2. References used in this chapter are good sources for learning about outcomes logic models (Mullen & Magnabosco, 1997; Ogles, Lambert, & Fields, 2002; United Way of America, 1996; Wiger & Solberg, 2001). It is helpful to read several sources on outcomes models because multiple perspectives provide the opportunity to form a more comprehensive perspective. Outcomes measurement is a process with multiple dimensions, which become clearer when different perspectives are viewed.

3. A thorough understanding of the pertinent aspects of impact measurement, data collection, data analysis, and generating valid conclusions as well as sociopolitical aspects would require a different approach and certainly could not be done in a single chapter (see instead Mullen & Magnabosco, 1997). These topics are often treated in distinct handbook formats because the theory, assumptions, and methods are complex.

REFERENCES

American Psychiatric Association. (2000). *Diagnostic and statistical manual of mental disorders* (4th ed., text rev.). Washington, DC: American Psychiatric Association.

Bonanno, G. A., Papa, A., Lalande, K., Noll, J. G., & Zhang, N. (2005). Grief Processing and Deliberate Grief Avoidance: A Prospective Comparison of Bereaved Spouses and Parents in the United States and the People' s Republic of China. *Journal of Consulting and Clinical Psychology*, 73(1), 86–98.

Center for Mental Health in Schools, (2000). Addressing barriers to student learning and promoting healthy development: A usable research-base. *Addressing Barriers to Learning*, 5(4), 1–4.

Clegg, S. (2005). Evidence-based practice in educational research: A critical realist critique of systematic review. *British Journal of Sociology of Education*, 26(3), 415–428.

Clements, P. T., Virgil, G. J., Manno, M. S., Henry, G. C., et al. (2003). Cultural perspectives of death, grief, and bereavement. *Journal of Psychosocial Nursing & Mental Health*, 41(7), 18–26.

Craft, S. F. (1998). School-based mental health services: Going where the children are. In S. Craft & J. Hutto, (Eds.). *Focus on mental health issues*. South Carolina Department of Mental Health, p. 1-9, Columbia, South Carolina.

DeJong, P., & Berg, I. K. (2002). *Interviewing for solutions* (2nd ed.). Pacific Grove, CA: Brooks/Cole.

Davidson, L., Tondora, J., Staeheli, M., O'Connell, Frey, J., & Chinman, M.J., (2003). In A. Lightburn & P. Sessions (Eds.), *Community Based Clinical Practice*. Recovery guidelines: An emerging body of community-based care for adults with psychiatric disabilities. London: Oxford University Press.

Davidson, L., O'Connell, Tondora, J., Lawless, M., & Evans, A. C., (2005). Recovery in serious mental illness: A new wine or just a new bottle. *Professional Psychology Research and Practice*, 36(5). 480–487.

Edelman, M. (1988). *Constructing the political spectacle*. Chicago: University of Chicago Press.

Feldman, R. A., & Siskind, A. B. (1997). Forward. In E. J. Mullen & J. L. Magnabosco (Eds.), *Outcomes measurement in the human services: Cross cutting issues and methods*. p. xv-xviii. Washington, DC: NASW Press.

Gambrill, E. (1997). *Social work practice: A critical thinker's guide*. New York: Oxford University Press.

Gambrill, E. (2005). Critical thinking, evidence-based practice, and mental health. In S. A. Kirk (Ed.), *Mental disorders in the social environment* (pp. 247–269). New York: Columbia University Press.

Hatry, H. P. (1997). Outcomes measurement and social services: Public and private sector perspectives. In E. J. Mullen & J. L. Magnabosco (Eds.), *Outcomes measurement in the human services: Cross cutting issues and methods*, p. 3–19. Washington, DC: NASW Press.

Hudson, W. W. (1997). Assessment tools as outcomes measures in social work. In E. J. Mullen & J. L. Magnabosco (Eds.), *Outcomes measurement in the human services: Cross cutting issues and methods, p. 68–80.*. Washington, DC: NASW Press.

Kutchins, H., & Kirk, S. A. (1997). *Making us crazy*. New York: Free Press.

Lather, P. (2004). Scientific research in education: A critical perspective. *British Educational Research Journal*, 30(6), 759–772.

McCall, R. B., & Green, B. L. (2004). Beyond the methodological gold standards of behavioral research: Considerations for practice and policy. *Social Policy Report: A Publication of the Society for Research in Child Development*, 18(2), 3–17.

Mullen, E. J., & Magnabosco, J. L. (Eds.). (1997). *Outcomes measurement in the human services: Cross cutting issues and methods*. Washington, DC: NASW Press.

Mullen, E. J., & Streiner, D. L. (2004). The evidence for and against evidence-based practice. *Brief Treatment and Crisis Intervention*, 4(2), 111–121.

National Alliance on Mental Illness. (2006). *Depression in children and adolescents* [Online]. Available: http://nami.org

Ogles, B. M., Lambert, M. J., & Fields, S. A. (Eds.). (2002). *Essentials of outcome assessment*. New York: John Wiley & Sons.

Pfeiffer, S. I., & Reddy, L. A. (1998). School-based mental health programs in the United States: Present status and a blueprint for the future. *School Psychology Review*, 27(1), 84–96.

Radloff, L. S. (1977). The CES-D scale: A self-report depression scale for research in the general population. *Applied Psychological Measurement*, 1, 385–401.

Rose, S. M. (2005). Empowerment: The foundation for social work practice in mental health. In S. A. Kirk (Ed.). *Mental disorders in the social environment* (pp. 247–269). New York: Columbia University Press.

Rossi, P. H. (1997). Program outcomes: Conceptual and measurement issues. In E. J. Mullen & J. L. Magnabosco (Eds.), *Outcomes measurement in the human services: Cross cutting issues and methods, p. 20–34*. Washington, DC: NASW Press.

Stephen, M., & Suryani, L. K. (2000). Shamanism, psychosis, and autonomous imagination. *Culture, Medicine and Psychiatry*, 24, 5–40.

Taylor, L., & Adelman, H. (2000) Toward ending the marginalization and fragmentation of mental health schools. *Journal of School Health*, 70(5), 171–178.

United Way of America. (1996). *Measuring program outcomes: A practical approach.* United Way of America.

U.S. Public Health Service. *Report of the Surgeon General's Conference on Children's Mental Health: A national action agenda.* Washington, DC: Department of Health and Human Services, 2000.

Weist, M. D., & Christodulu, K. V. (2000). Expanded school mental health programs: Advancing reform and closing the gap between research and practice. *Journal of School Health, 70*(5), 195–200.

Weisz, J. R., Sandler, I. N., Durlak, J. A., & Anton, B. S. (2005). Promoting and protecting youth mental health through evidence-based prevention and treatment. *American Psychologist, 60*(6), 628–648.

Wiger, D. E., & Solberg, K. B. (2001). *Tracking mental health outcomes: A therapist's guide to measuring client progress, analyzing data, and improving your practice.* New York: John Wiley & Sons.

Witkin, S. L., & Harrison, W. D. (2001). Whose evidence and for what purpose? *Social Work, 46*(4), 293–296.

12

Psychopharmacology and Culture

MARTHA SAJATOVIC & MATTHEW A. FULLER

Modern psychopharmacology, the science of drug or medication treatment for mental disorders, was ushered in by such groundbreaking developments in the treatment of mood disorders as tricyclic and SSRI antidepressants for depression, and lithium, anticonvulsant compounds, and atypical antipsychotics for the treatment of bipolar disorder. However, although these developments in psychopharmacology have led to substantial improvements in health outcomes for many individuals suffering from mood disorders, in other cases biological or social factors may lead to differing or even suboptimal medication response in some populations. The relationship between psychopharmacology and culture is complex and still not entirely understood.

Response to psychopharmacology may differ or be less than anticipated for a variety of reasons, including the diagnosis of the individual being treated, medical or psychiatric comorbidity, the biological processes that occur in the individual ingesting the medication, treatment nonadherence, other medications or alternative treatments the individuals may be taking concurrently, and culturally based expectations of treatment, such as expected rate of recovery or threshold for medication-related adverse events. Additionally, environmental factors such as alcohol or smoking may affect response to medication treatments among groups of individuals.

With respect to psychiatric diagnosis, commonly accepted and utilized treatment guidelines for both depression and bipolar disorder recommend first-line, "gold-standard" medication treatments (American Psychiatric Association, 2000, 2002). In some cases, variation in symptom reporting and interpretation of symptoms across cultures may lead to imprecise or incorrect psychiatric diagnoses (Dilsaver & Akiskal, 2005). The issues in diagnosis and assessment of mood disorders that form the basis for psychopharmacological decision making are addressed by Marin and Escobar in this volume. In current psychiatric treatment guidelines, culture-specific diagnoses may be addressed in only a very limited way (American Psychiatric Association, 2000, 2002), leaving clinicians considering psychopharmacology for these conditions with few resources or evidence-based suggestions. The meaning of culture-specific diagnoses and relationship to standardized *DSM* diagnoses have been addressed in this volume by Guarnaccia. Additionally, Westermeyer has provided a discussion of treatment modalities and culture that includes cultural issues in the acceptability of various types of treatments, including psychotherapy. This chapter specifically addresses the issue of medication treatments across cultures and the current literature on biological and social factors that appear to affect medication tolerability and effectiveness.

CULTURAL ISSUES IN MEDICATION TREATMENTS

Biological Factors: Pharmacokinetics

Pharmacokinetics involves the way a drug moves through the body, usually via oral ingestion, absorption by the stomach and small intestine, first-pass metabolism through the liver, and entry into the systemic circulation (Jacobson, Pies, & Greenblatt, 2002; Wilkinson, 2005). From the systemic circulation, drugs can then act on target organs such as the brain, or go to peripheral storage sites such as fat or muscle (drug distribution). For drugs that are administered intramuscularly or intravenously, the drug goes from fat (adipose) tissue directly to the systemic circulation. For this reason, psychotropic medications that are available in intramuscular formulations, such as some of the benzodiazepines (lorazepam and others), or antipsychotics (ziprasidone and others) are particularly useful in emergency situations when a rapid response is desired (Fuller & Sajatovic, 2005). Although this can be considered beneficial from an efficacy point of view (e.g., when needed to calm individuals who may be very agitated and potentially harmful to themselves or others), the potential for serious adverse effects such as hypotension (severely low blood pressure) is generally substantially greater for drugs administered intramuscularly or intravenously than for drugs administered orally (Fuller & Sajatovic, 2005).

From the systemic circulation, most psychotropic medications are metabolized by the liver and then cleared/eliminated by the kidneys. Some drugs, such as lithium, are cleared in intact form by the kidneys without going through the hepatic/liver metabolic process. Individuals with impaired liver or kidney functioning are particularly prone to developing adverse effects from psychotropic medication as a result of excessive accumulation of a drug and/or the breakdown product of a drug or drug metabolite. Those who abuse alcohol or other substances that may cause hepatic (liver) damage may be more likely to experience toxic effects of commonly prescribed medication treatments for mood disorders such as all the antipsychotic compounds or some anticonvulsants.

Biological Factors: Genetic Variables

It has been demonstrated that differential effects from medications among groups of diverse ethnicity can be the result, in part, from variations in the genetically controlled activity of enzyme systems responsible for the metabolism/breakdown of psychotropic medications (Fuller & Sajatovic, 2005; Nemeroff, DeVane, & Pollack, 1996; Richelson, 1997). The cytochrome (CYP) P450 enzyme in the liver is critical in the breakdown of medications and toxins that an individual may ingest, and in the case of psychotropic medications, the most important CYP groups are CYP1, CYP2, and CYP3 (Nemeroff et al., 1996). Many psychotropic medications are oxidatively metabolized by CYP enzymes and are broken down into inactive compounds or less active metabolites. Some drugs are noted to be enzyme inducers, whereby the oxidative reaction is facilitated and the parent drug (medication the individual originally ingests) is broken down more quickly. In clinical settings, this could result in lower or even therapeutically suboptimal concentrations of medication in the systemic circulation.

In contrast to enzyme inducers, some drugs are enzyme inhibitors, whereby the oxidative process is slowed and the concentration of parent drug in the systemic circulation remains relatively elevated. In some instances it may be possible that the individual being treated for a mood disorder may be prescribed multiple medications that are CYP inhibitors, potentially putting the individual at risk for toxic effects resulting from accumulation of the parent drug in the systemic circulation. There is an extensive and growing literature on clinically significant CYP drug interactions (Fuller & Sajatovic, 2005; Michalets, 1998; Wilkinson, 2005). It has been documented that genetic differences in the presence or activity of certain CYP enzymes can account for a substantial amount of observed interindividual variability in systemic circulation levels of certain psychotropic compounds. "Slow metabolizers" are individuals who have low or no activity of an enzyme. Because of reduced rates of breaking down a medication, these slow metabolizers may accumulate high levels of active drug, and possibly experience more side effects related to the elevated levels. Extensive metabolizers have higher levels and activity of the CYP enzyme, sometimes resulting in lower systemic circulation levels, and possibly lower therapeutic effects of medication. Several interethnic differences in the P450 enzymes have been identified:

- CYP1A2: The enzyme CYP1A2 is involved in the hepatic metabolism of a variety of psychotropic compounds, including antipsychotics such as clozapine, haloperidol, and olanzapine; some antidepressants, such as fluvoxamine and imipramine; the anticholinesterase inhibitor (dementia treatment) tacrine; and the β-blocker (sometimes used to treat anxiety symptoms or bipolar symptoms) propranolol. A minority of whites, Asians, and African Americans are slow metabolizers with respect to this enzyme (Richelson,1997). Additionally, activity of this enzyme is known to decline with aging (Jacobson et al., 2002).
- CYP2C19: The enzyme CYP2C19 has low activity (slow metabolism) in 18% to 23% of Asians, 3% to 5% of whites, and 2% of African Americans (Richelson, 1997). Drugs that are broken down by the CYP2C19 enzyme (i.e., substrates) include the antidepressants amitriptyline, imipramine, and citalopram. In a clinical

setting, the care provider prescribing these compounds to Asian patients should consider the fact that approximately one in five Asian individuals may be more prone to developing adverse effects/toxicity and may choose to lower/slow medication dosing accordingly.

- CYP2D6: The enzyme CYP2D6 has low activity in 3% to10% of whites, and as many as 2% of African Americans and Asians (Richelson, 1997). CYP2D6 is involved in the metabolism of many psychotropic and nonpsychotropic compounds, including antidepressants, antipsychotics, and mood stabilizers. The antidepressants paroxetine, fluoxetine, sertraline, and fluvoxamine are inhibitors of this enzyme, potentially leading to greater likelihood of drug toxicity in slow metabolizers. Conversely, the mood-stabilizing medication carbamazepine is an inducer of CYP2D6.

Recently, the U.S. Food and Drug Administration approved a commercially available CYP450 test that potentially allows for metabolic profiling (De Leon, 2006). The pharmacogenetic test uses a DNA microarray, the AmpliChip CYP450, that determines the genotype for P450 (CYP) 2D6 and CYPC19 (De Leon, 2006). How useful the CYP testing may become in routine clinical settings remains to be determined.

In addition to interethnic variance with respect to the CYP isoenzymes, it has also been reported that there are ethnic differences in the isoenzymes alcohol dehydrogenase (ADH) and aldehyde dehydrogenase, the enzymes that are important in the breakdown of alcohol. Individuals who have slower rates of alcohol metabolism have elevated blood acetaldehyde with the consumption of ethanol (Wall, 2005). These individuals may exhibit relative insensitivity to the effects of alcohol, such as vomiting or skin flushing, and may have a lower risk of alcoholism (Wall, 2005). Asian and Jewish populations may be particularly prone to alcohol intolerance (Choi, Son, Yuang, Kim, Lee, Chai, et al., 2005; Cook, Luczak, Shea, Ehlers, Carr, & Wall, 2005; Hasin, Aharonovich, Liu, Mamman, Matseonae, Carr, & Li, 2002; Neumark, Friedlander, Durst, Leitersdorf, Janne, Ramchandani, et al., 2004), and their genetic phenotype may be protective against alcohol dependence (Garver, Tu, Cao, Aini, Zhou, & Israel, 2001). Hasin and colleagues (2002) have noted that Sephardic Jews had a higher prevalence of the ADH2*2 allele of the ADH gene compared with Ashkenazis, and that ADH2*2 is associated with lower lifetime DSM-IV alcohol dependence severity.

Alcohol abuse is common among individuals with mood disorders, particularly among individuals with bipolar disorder (Grant, Stinson, Hasin, Dawson, Chou, Ruan, & Huang, 2005), and use of alcohol and the resultant medical and psychiatric sequelae clearly affect prescribed psychotropic medication tolerability and response. However, the literature on genetic polymorphism and alcohol dependence is not entirely consistent, and further research is needed to elucidate clearly the relationship between genetic polymorphisms and risk of alcohol abuse, as well as how this may potentially affect individuals who are also suffering from mood disorders.

The human N-acetylation polymorphism is another genetic trait phenotypically expressed by differences in N-acetyltransferase activity. Similar to CYP, individuals may be rapid or slow metabolizers of therapeutic agents (Anitha &

Banerjee, 2003). Compounds such as the benzodiazepine clonazepam and the monoamine oxidase inhibitor (MAOI) antidepressant phenelzine involve acetylation in the metabolic process. It has been reported that among some ethnic groups, such as Hmong immigrants in the United States and Dravidian ethnic communities of Southern India, slow acetylation individuals may predominate, on the order of 75% (Anitha & Banerjee, 2003; Straka, Hansen, Benson, & Walker, 1996).

Compared with pharmacokinetics, pharmacodynamics—the body's response to drugs—have been less studied with respect to ethnic variability. Pharmacodynamic response has been noted to be a function of neuron receptor number and the affinity of those receptors to various chemical compounds, and the processes of signal transduction (movement of signals from outside the cell to inside the cell), cell responsivity, and homeostatic regulation (Turner, Scarpace, & Lowenthal, 1992). Clinical response to antidepressant medications, a cornerstone of treatment for mood disorders, appears to be affected by differential interactions between dopamine and serotonin (two key neurotransmission substances) systems in the central nervous system, and these interactions appear in some cases to be modified by genetic differences in the enzymes that interact with dopamine (Arias, Serretii, Lorenzi, Gasto, Catalan, & Fananas, 2006). Arias and colleagues (2006) analyzed the catechol-O-methyltransferase enzyme-coding gene (COMT-22qll), which intervenes in the degradative pathways of catecholaminergic neurotransmitters (responsible for breakdown/inactivation of the important neurotransmitter dopamine) in depressed patients of European origin. The group noted that individuals carrying the Met/Met genotype had greater likelihood of treatment nonremission, and concluded that the COMT gene could have a small and indirect effect on clinical response to SSRI antidepressant medication by slowing down the antidepressant action (Arias et al., 2006). Although allelic and genotypic profiles for the polymorphism did not differ significantly between two subgroups in the analysis (Spanish and Italian), the authors noted that both subgroups present a Southern European common genetic origin (Arias et al., 2006). More studies are needed on the interaction between neurotransmitters known to be important in psychotropic drug mechanism of action, polymorphism, and drug response across groups of varying ethnicity.

Environmental Factors

In addition to genetic variation, individuals across ethnic groups and subgroups may differ greatly in socially determined patterns of use of substances that affect tolerability and response to a variety of psychotropic medications. Examples include smoking, the use of recreational drugs, and the ingestion of caffeine. For many psychotropic compounds, these environmental factors have clinically significant effects on drug serum concentration, drug elimination, drug tolerability, and response. For example, it is known that cigarette smoking may lower blood levels of some psychotropic compounds such as clozapine (Derenne & Baldessarini, 2005), and smoking status should be determined prior to determining a dosing regimen for individuals on clozapine.

Another environmental factor that may have strong social determinants and that may differ across cultural settings is the use of complementary and alternative medicine (CAM). CAM use may be particularly important for individuals with mood disorders. Data from a national household telephone survey conducted in 1997–1998 ($n = 9585$) found that 16.5% of respondents self-reported using CAM, with utilization significantly greater in individuals with mental disorders (21.3%) compared with those without mental disorders (12.8%) (Unutzer, Klap, Sturm, Young, Marmon, et al., 2000). Individuals who see their psychiatric care providers less frequently may be particularly likely to use CAM (Alderman & Kiepfer, 2003). A recent survey of 31,044 adults found a similar widespread use of CAM, with higher use rates in women than men (21% vs. 16.7%, $p < .0001$), and in those of multiple races (32.2%), Asians (24.6%), or Native Americans or Alaskan natives (21.9%) compared with whites (19.1%) or blacks (14.3%) (effect of race, $p < .0001$) (Kennedy, 2005).

The report by Kennedy (2005) illustrates the complex relationship between conventional medical care/medication taking and use of CAM. Many individuals use herbal treatments as a complement to conventional prescribed medications. Herb use is relatively common among adults who use prescription medication (20.6%) or over-the-counter medications (20.6%). However, there is also evidence that herbs are often used as an alternative to conventionally prescribed medication treatments. Adults who delay (27.7%) or avoid (27.2%) recommended medical care because of cost are more likely to use herbs than those who do not delay or avoid care ($p < .001$) (Kennedy, 2005). The implications of this are important. Populations that are poor and underserved, as is the case for many minority populations, may be particularly likely to use CAM and may be less likely to use conventional pharmacological interventions.

The issue of CAM use among individuals with psychiatric illness including mood disorders is important from a clinical and psychopharmacological viewpoint because it is known that some alternative compounds may worsen or precipitate psychiatric symptoms (Boerth & Caley, 2003; Fahmi, Huang, & Schweitzer, 2002). Additionally, some commonly utilized CAMs may interact with frequently prescribed psychotropic agents (Edie & Dewan, 2005). As noted in previously in the discussion of pharmacokinetics, ingested drugs undergo a fairly complex process of absorption, distribution, metabolism, and elimination. Herbal compounds and other alternative treatments may interact with prescribed medications at any point during this process. For example, it has been reported that St. John's wort is a potent inducer of CYP3A, another liver isoenzyme. Thus when a patient receiving a drug such as human immunodeficiency virus protease inhibitors also takes St. John's wort, the desired medication response ("therapeutic failure") may not occur (Flexner, 2000; Wilkinson, 2005). Unfortunately, the processes of interaction may be multiple and varying, and are still not well understood for many herbal compounds (Fuller & Sajatovic, 2005). Table 12.1 illustrates selected herbal compounds that may alter gastrointestinal absorption and metabolism of prescribed drugs.

Unfortunately, although herb and natural supplement use is common, particularly in minority populations in the United States, it has been reported that

Table 12.1 Herbal Compounds That May Alter Metabolism and Gastrointestinal Absorption of Drugs

Herbal Medications That May Alter Metabolism	Herbals Medications That May Alter Gastrointestinal Absorption
Virginia snakeroot, Serpenteria (*Aristolochia serpenteria*)	California buckeye (*Aesculus californica*)
Indian root, Raiz del indio (*Aristolochia Watson*)	Ohio buckeye (*Aesculus glabra*)
Sagebrush (*Artemisia tridentata*)	Horse chestnut (*Aesculus hippocastanum*)
Common barberry (*Berberis vulgaris*)	Aloe
Button bush (*Cephalanthus*)	Uva, Ursi, Manzanita, bearberry (*Arctostaphylos*)
Greater celandine (*Chelidonium*)	Cayenne, African bird peppers (*Capsicum*)
Balmony, Turtlehead (*Chelone*)	Sodium copper chlorophyllin, Chlorophyll
Fringtree (*Chionanthus*)	Mormon tea, American ephedra, Canutillo (*Ephedra viridis*)
Wahoo, Burning bush (*Euonymus*)	Rhamnus frangula, Buckthorn
Goldenseal (*Hydrastis*)	Maravilla (*Mirabilis multifulorum*)
Blue flag (*Iris versicolor*)	Wager ash, Hop tree (*Ptelea*)
Verconicastrum, Culver's root (*Leptandra*)	California buckthorn (*Rhamnus californica*)
Oregon grape, Algerita (*Mahonia*)	Buckthorn (*Rhamnus frangula*)
American mandrake (*Podophyllum*)	Cascara sagrada (*Rhamnus purshiana*)
	Senna
	Yucca

Adapted with permission from Fuller and Sajatovic (2005)

only approximately one third of individuals who take CAM share this information with a conventional health care provider (Kennedy, 2005). Wang and colleagues (2001) have reported that the use of CAM has increased among individuals with major depression, and have recommended that general practitioners, mental health specialists, and alternative medicine providers be aware of their patients' use of both conventional medical services and CAM, because there may be interaction between the conventionally prescribed drugs and alternative agents.

TREATMENT OF MOOD DISORDERS

Medications utilized to treat individuals with mood disorders include, primarily, antidepressant agents, traditional mood-stabilizing agents, and antipsychotic agents (American Psychiatric Association, 2000, 2002). Other compounds such as anxiolytics or sedative–hypnotics are also frequently utilized to help manage symptoms such as restlessness or insomnia. However, these compounds are frequently used on a temporary basis or may be part of a medication regimen to assist in the treatment of common comorbidities such as anxiety. There are some identified differences across ethnic groups in use of these agents as well as in apparent tolerability and response.

Antidepressant Therapy

Antidepressant agents are generally considered to be equally effective for the management of major depression. These agents are often classified based on their chemical structure or pharmacological action. Classes include the TCAs and related compounds that inhibit the reuptake of norepinephrine and serotonin (5HT), SSRIs, dopamine reuptake inhibitors, serotonin/norepinephrine reuptake inhibitors, serotonin antagonists, noradrenergic antagonists, and MAOIs.

Anecdotal reports and cultural surveys of prescribing patterns suggest that antidepressant dosage requirements may differ among racial groups (Sramek & Pi, 1996). Pi and colleagues (1993) reviewed studies on Asian/non-Asian TCA psychopharmacology and concluded that although anecdotal reports suggest a difference between Asian and non-Asian populations in the pharmacokinetics of TCAs, controlled studies have not consistently validated these finding. Roy–Byrne and colleagues (2005) recently noted that among ethnic minority patients with mood and anxiety disorders treated with SSRI antidepressants, Hispanic and Asian patients appeared to have a slightly lower response rate, whereas Asians had the highest rates and Hispanics had the lowest rates of "full response." There were no treatment interactions by minority group membership for depressed patients, and overall speed of response and adverse effects were similar across groups (Roy–Byrne et al., 2005). In another report, it was suggested that African American patients may require lower doses of both TCAs and SSRIs than white patients with depression to achieve a similar clinical response (Varner, Ruiz, & Small, 1998).

Data on prescribing patterns with respect to ethnicity are also rather inconsistent. In one study of 407 Hispanic and non-Hispanic whites, investigators examined differences in prescribing SSRIs and non-SSRI antidepressants in the primary care arena (Sleath, Rubin, & Huston, 2001). Hispanic ethnicity did not influence antidepressant prescribing; both groups were equally likely to be prescribed SSRI and non-SSRI antidepressants (Sleath et al., 2001). Another report noted that African Americans are less likely than whites to receive adequate pharmacotherapy for unipolar depression (U.S. Department of Health and Human Services, 2001) and are less likely to receive treatment with SSRI-type compounds (Melfi, Croghan, Hanna, & Robinson, 2000). Recently, Hong and colleagues (2006) completed a prospective six-week study evaluating plasma concentrations, efficacy, and adverse reactions to sertraline in Chinese versus white patients. White depressed patients received significantly higher dosages than Chinese depressed patients ($p = .012$).

It has been speculated that differences in prescribing patterns may relate to varying expectations of treatment that may vary across cultures. Cooper and colleagues (2003) surveyed 829 white, African American, and Hispanic adults who had been diagnosed with depression, and they evaluated the acceptability of antidepressant medication and individual counseling. African American and Hispanic patients had lower odds than whites of finding antidepressant medication acceptable. Furthermore, African Americans had lower odds and Hispanics had higher odds of finding counseling acceptable in comparison with white subjects.

Mood-Stabilizing Medication

Traditional mood-stabilizing medications include lithium and the anticonvulsant medications valproate, carbamazepine, and lamotrigine. Wing and colleagues (1997) studied the pharmacokinetics of lithium in 16 Chinese adults with bipolar disorder who were receiving lithium. The combined plasma and urine data revealed that the pharmacokinetics of lithium in Chinese adults appear similar to white patients receiving lithium. Similar conclusions were made by Lee and colleagues (1998), who studied the pharmacokinetics of lithium in eight Taiwanese/Chinese bipolar patients.

In another study, 58 patients with bipolar I disorder received a longitudinal follow-up after their first psychiatric hospitalization (Fleck, Hendricks, DelBello, & Strakowski, 2002). Comparisons were made between African American and white patients in medication prescribed and compliance. Compared with whites, African Americans received antipsychotics for a significantly greater percentage of follow-up, were more likely to receive antipsychotics when not psychotic, and were more likely to receive first-generation antipsychotics. In addition, they also had poorer treatment adherence (Fleck et al., 2002).

Recent work by Kilbourne and Pincus (2006) evaluated the pattern of psychotropic medication use among a group of veterans with bipolar disorder. They found that compared with whites, African Americans were significantly less likely to receive lithium and SSRIs and more likely to receive first-generation antipsychotics and any antipsychotic. It is not clear whether these findings reflect a perception that African American patients are more likely to exhibit psychotic features and therefore be given a diagnosis of schizophrenia or that clinicians believe that the increased risk of metabolic side effects associated with second-generation antipsychotic agents poses a greater risk for African Americans.

In addition to pharmacokinetic and pharmacodynamic differences that are related to ethnicity, cultural interpretation of adverse effects can have an impact on therapy. In a study conducted in Hong Kong, Lee and colleagues (1992) systematically assessed adverse effects experienced by bipolar patients treated with lithium. They found that Chinese patients experienced side effects similar to those reported by patients treated in the United States. These were primarily weight gain, polydipsia (excessive fluid drinking), polyuria (excessive/frequent urination), metallic taste, and a decrease in creativity. Interestingly, the cultural interpretation of these side effects differed. The Chinese patients viewed the polydipsia and polyuria as signs of lithium's efficacy, whereas whites were more concerned about these symptoms as adverse effects (Lee et al., 1992). Conversely, the Chinese patients were significantly more concerned about the fatigue they experienced compared with their control subjects, even though the prevalence and degree of fatigue was similar between groups.

Antipsychotic Medications

Antipsychotic compounds include the older typical/conventional medications as well as the more recently developed atypical antipsychotic medications risperidone, olanzapine, quetiapine, aripiprazole, ziprasidone, and clozapine. Early work showed that the mean dose of chlorpromazine for mania was lower in Japanese than in Western populations (Okuma, 1981). However, until relatively recently, antipsychotic medications were primarily utilized as episodic/intermittent treatment for situations in which individuals had a mood disorder (either mania or depression) that was accompanied by psychotic symptoms such as hallucinations or paranoia. More recently, the atypical antipsychotic medications have become much more widely utilized as maintenance therapies for bipolar disorder (American Psychiatric Association, 2002). In contrast, the antipsychotic compounds have long been a cornerstone of treatment for chronic psychotic conditions such as schizophrenia. For this reason, the majority of the published literature on antipsychotic therapy among groups of varying ethnicity is derived from populations with schizophrenia. However, useful information may still be derived from these reports, because there is often considerable overlap in symptoms and functional status among individuals with bipolar illness and schizophrenia.

Little information in the literature exists regarding cultural differences in antipsychotic use among mood-disordered populations. However, Fleck and colleagues (2002) evaluated 58 patients with bipolar I disorder who were recruited at the time of their first psychiatric hospitalization and were monitored longitudinally for as long as two years. Compared with whites, African Americans received antipsychotics for a significantly greater percentage of time, were more likely to receive antipsychotics when not psychotic, and were significantly more likely to receive first-generation antipsychotics. Kilbourne and Pincus (2006) noted that African Americans with bipolar disorder were significantly more likely to receive antipsychotic medications compared with non-African Americans with bipolar disorder.

Further work by Fleck and colleagues (2005) evaluated rates of medication nonadherence, self-perceived reasons for nonadherence, and attitudes associated with nonadherence in African American and white patients with bipolar disorder. Nonadherence was present in more than 50% of patients. More than 20% of patients in each group mentioned physical side effects from medications as a reason for nonadherence. Furthermore, African American patients were more likely to state patient-related factors as reasons for nonadherence compared with whites. In particular, African American patients had a greater fear of becoming addicted to medications, and had the feeling that medications were symbols of mental illness.

It appears that there are few pharmacokinetic differences of antipsychotics among African Americans, whites, and Hispanics (Bond, 1991). However, in a study evaluating the prescribing of antipsychotic medication to patients with schizophrenia in cross-cultural clinical programs, dosage requirements for Asian and Hispanic patients were noted to be less than that received by patients in the general sample (Collazo, Tan, Sramek, Sramek, & Herrera, 1996). Ruiz and colleagues (1999) evaluated the response to antipsychotics in whites, African Americans, and Hispanic patients with schizophrenia. They found that Hispanic patients needed lower doses of antipsychotics compared with whites and African Americans to achieve a similar clinical response. When weight was taken into consideration, African Americans required similar dosages as whites to achieve a response. Another study involving 20 Asian and 20 white patients with chronic schizophrenia who were treated with clozapine evaluated dosage, plasma levels, and clinical and side effect profiles to determine whether differences existed (Ng, Chong, Lambert, Fan, Hackett, Mahendran, et al., 2005). Asian patients received significantly lower dosages of clozapine compared with whites, even though plasma concentrations were similar between groups. Compared with whites, Asian patients seem to require a lower dosage to achieve clinical efficacy.

African Americans are less likely than whites to receive adequate pharmacotherapy for schizophrenia (U.S. Department of Health and Human Services, 2001), are less likely to receive second-generation antipsychotics (Herbeck, West, Ruditis, Duffy, Fitek, Bell, et al., 2004; Kuno & Rothbard, 2002; Opolka, Rascati, Brown, & Gibson, 2004), more likely to receive depot (long-acting injectable) antipsychotics (Valenstein, Copeland, Owen, Blow, & Visnic, 2001), and more likely to be prescribed excessive doses of first-generation antipsychotics (Diaz & De Leon, 2002). Copeland and colleagues (2003) reported that the use of second-generation antipsychotics in veterans with schizophrenia was less, and clozapine much less, among African Americans and Hispanics than among whites.

Arnold and colleagues (2004) evaluated the interaction of gender and ethnicity on the use of depot antipsychotics and the dosing of antipsychotics in a group of 167 inpatients with psychotic disorders including psychotic mood disorders. African American men received depot antipsychotics more frequently than African American women and white patients (Arnold et al., 2004). African American men and women with psychotic mood disorders were more likely to be discharged on high doses of antipsychotics compared with whites. No ethnic or gender differences were found in the dosing of antipsychotics in patients with schizophrenia spectrum disorders. Conversely, a study from Great Britain found that dosages of olanzapine and clozapine did not significantly differ between Asians, African Americans, and whites (Taylor, 2004). These data point to a potential for increased risk of extrapyramidal side effects and tardive dyskinesia for African Americans. Furthermore, the greater use of first-generation antipsychotics over the second-generation antipsychotics in this ethnic group may contribute to lower rates of adherence, with eventual psychiatric hospitalization and a worse clinical outcome.

Emsley and colleagues (2002) compared the response to antipsychotic treatment in three ethnic groups of patients with schizophrenia. Fifty African American individuals, 63 individuals of mixed descent, and 79 whites with schizophrenia or schizoaffective disorder were assessed using the Positive and Negative Syndrome Scale (PANSS). Baseline PANSS scores were significantly higher among the African American and mixed-descent patients. Patients of mixed descent showed the greatest mean percent reduction in PANSS total scores, followed by African Americans and whites. The numbers of responders, defined as a reduction of 40% or more in PANSS total scores, showed a similar pattern.

Last, a group of 88 African Americans, 198 Whites, and 65 Latinos with schizophrenia who were part of the initial phase of the San Diego site of the Schizophrenia Care and Assessment Program (a longitudinal naturalistic study of the course of schizophrenia treatment) were studied for differences in symptom expression (Barrio, Yamada, Atuel, Hough, Yee, Berthot, & Russo, 2003). The symptoms were measured using the PANSS. Analyses were conducted to determine whether ethnic differences would be more apparent in positive scale symptoms than in negative and general scale symptoms of the PANSS. Multivariate analysis of covariance revealed no significant ethnic differences on the scale scores.

CONCLUSION

In summary, there appears to be a rather complex relationship between psychopharmacology and culture that is affected by an individual's biological and inherited makeup, environmental factors such as use of substances or alternative treatments, socially determined treatment practices, and individual and societal expectations and interpretations of treatment. Although developments in pharmacological treatments for mood disorders during the past two decades have been impressive, it is clear that medication treatments are not "one size fits all." A supplement to the Surgeon General's report on mental health, which focused on minority mental health, documented an unfortunate dearth of minorities in published NIMH-funded research studies in which less than 7% of patients were identified as minorities and there were no separate analyses of minority subgroups (U.S. Department of Health and Human Services, 2001). Additional research is urgently needed to elucidate more clearly the relationships between medication treatments and treatment response/outcomes among individuals of varying ethnicity.

REFERENCES

Alderman, C. P., & Kiepfer, B. (2003). Complementary medicine use by psychiatry patients of an Australian hospital. *Annals of Pharmacotherapy*, 37(12), 1779–1784.

American Psychiatric Association. (2000). Practice guideline for the treatment of patients with major depressive disorder (revision). *American Journal of Psychiatry*, 157 (4 Suppl.), 1–45.

American Psychiatric Association. (2002). Practice guideline for the treatment of patients with bipolar disorder (revision). *American Journal of Psychiatry*, 159(4) 1–82.Anitha, A., & Banerjee, M. (2003). Arylamine N-acetyltransferase 2 polymorphism in the ethnic populations of South India. *Indian Journal of Molecular Medicine*, 11(1), 125–131.

Arias, B., Serretii, A., Lorenzi, C., Gasto, C., Catalan, R., & Fananas, L. (2006). Analysis of COMT gene (Val 158 Met polymorphism) in the clinical response to SSRIs in depressive patients of European origin. *Journal of Affective Disorders, 90,* 251–256.

Arnold, L. M., Strakowski, S. M., Schwiers, M. L., Amicone, J., Fleck, D. E., Corey, K. B., & Farrow, J. E. (2004). Sex, ethnicity, and antipsychotic medication use in patients with psychosis. *Schizophrenia Research, 66,* 169–175.

Barrio, C., Yamada, A. M., Atuel, H., Hough, R. L., Yee, S., Berthot, B., & Russo, P. A. (2003). A tri-ethnic examination of symptom expression on the Positive and Negative Syndrome Scale in schizophrenia spectrum disorders. *Schizophrenia Research, 60*(2–3), 259–269.

Boerth, J. M., & Caley, C. F. (2003). Possible case of mania associated with ma-huang. *Pharmacotherapy, 23*(3), 380–383.

Bond, W. S. (1991). Ethnicity and psychotropic drugs. *Clinical Pharmacology, 10*(6), 467–470.

Choi, I. G., Son, H. G., Yuang, B. H., Kim, S. H., Lee, J. S., Chai, Y. G., et al. (2005). Scanning of genetic effects of alcohol metabolism gene (ADH1B and ADH1C) polymorphisms on the risk of alcoholism. *Human Mutation, 26*(3), 224–234.

Collazo, Y., Tam, R., Sramek, J., Sramek, J., & Herrera, J. (1996). Neuroleptic dosing in Hispanic and Asian inpatients with schizophrenia. *Mt Sinai Journal of Medicine, 63*(5–6), 310–313.

Cook, T. A., Luczak, S. E., Shea, S. H., Ehlers, C. L., Carr, L. G., & Wall, T. L. (2005). Associations of ALDH2 and ADH1B genotypes with response to alcohol in Asian Americans. *Journal of Studies on Alcohol, 66*(2), 196–204.

Cooper, L. A., Gonzales, J. J., Gallo, J. J., Rost, K. M., Meredith, L. S., Rubenstein, L. V., et al. (2003). The acceptability of treatment for depression among African-American, Hispanic, and white primary care patients. *Medical Care, 41*(4), 479–489.

Copeland, L.A., Zeber J.E., Valenstein M. & Blow, F.C. (2003). Racial disparities in the use of atypical antipsychotic medications among veterans. *American Journal of Psychiatry, 160,* 1817–1822.

De Leon, J. (2006). AmpliChip CYP450 test: Personalized medicine has arrived in psychiatry. *Expert Review of Molecular Diagnostics, 6*(3), 277–286.

Derenne, J. L., & Baldessarini, R. J. (2005). Clozapine toxicity associated with smoking cessation: Case report. *American Journal of Therapy, 12*(5), 469–471.

Diaz, F. J., & De Leon, J. (2002). Excessive antipsychotic dosing in 2 U.S. state hospitals. *Journal of Clinical Psychiatry, 63*(11), 998–1003.

Dilsaver, S. C., & Akiskal, H. S. (2005). High rate of unrecognized bipolar mixed states among destitute Hispanic adolescents referred for 'major depressive disorder.' *Journal of Affective Disorders, 84*(2–3), 179–196.

Edie, C. F., & Dewan, N. (2005). Which psychotropics interact with four common supplements? *Current Psychiatry, 4*(1), 17–30.

Emsley, R. A., Roberts, M. C., Rataemane, S., Pretorius, J., Oosthuizen, P. P., Turner, J., et al. (2002). Ethnicity and treatment response in schizophrenia: A comparison of 3 ethnic groups. *Journal of Clinical Psychiatry, 63,* 9–14.

Fahmi, M., Huang, C., & Schweitzer, I. (2002). A case of mania induced by hypericum. *World Journal of Biological Psychiatry, 3*(1), 58–59.

Fleck, D. E., Hendricks, W. L., DelBello, M. P., & Strakowski, S. M. (2002). Differential prescription of maintenance antipsychotics to African American and white patients with new-onset bipolar disorder. *Journal of Clinical Psychiatry, 63*(8), 658–664.

Fleck, D. E., Keck, P. E., Corey, K. B., & Strakowski, S. M. (2005). Factors associated with medication adherence in African American and white patients with bipolar disorder. *Journal of Clinical Psychiatry, 66*(5), 646–652.

Flexner, C. (2000). Dual protease inhibitor therapy in HIV-infected patients: Pharmacologic rationale and clinical benefits. *Annual Review of Pharmacology and Toxicology*, 40, 649–674.

Fuller, M., & Sajatovic, M. (2005). *Drug information handbook for psychiatry* (5th ed.). Hudson, OH: Lexi-Comp.

Garver, E., Tu, G. C., Cao, Q., Aini, M., Zhou, F., & Israel, Y. (2001). Eliciting the low-activity aldehyde dehydrogenase Asian phenotype by an antisense mechanism results in an aversion to ethanol. *Journal of Experimental Medicine*, 194(5), 571–580.

Grant, B. J., Stinson, F. S., Hasin, D. S., Dawson, D. A., Chou, S. P., Ruan, W. J., & Huang, B. (2005). Prevalence, correlates, and comorbidity of bipolar I disorder and axis I and II disorders: Results from the National Epidemiologic Survey on alcohol and related conditions, *Journal of Clinical Psychiatry*, 66(10), 1205–1215.

Hasin, D., Aharonovich, E., Liu, X., Mamman, Z., Matseoane, K., Carr, L. G., & Li, T. K. (2002). Alcohol dependence symptoms and alcohol dehydrogenase 2 polymorphism: Israeli Ashkenazis, Sephardics, and recent Russian immigrants. *Alcoholism, Clinical and Experimental Research*, 26(9), 1315–1321.

Herbeck, D. M., West, J. C., Ruditis, I., Duffy, F. F., Fitek, D. J., Bell, C. C., et al. (2004). Variations in use of second-generation antipsychotic medication by race among adult psychiatric patients. *Psychiatric Services*, 55, 677–684.

Hong Ng, C., Norman, T. R., Naing, K. O., Schweitzer, I., Kong Wai Ho, B., Fan, A., et al. (2006). A comparative study of sertraline dosages, plasma concentrations, efficacy and adverse reactions in Chinese versus Caucasian patients. *International Clinical Psychopharmacology*, 21(2), 87–92.

Jacobson, S. A., Pies, R. W., & Greenblatt, D. J. (2002). *Handbook of geriatric psychopharmacology* (pp. 1–23). Washington, DC: American Psychiatric Publishing.

Kennedy, J. (2005). Herb and supplement use in the U.S. adult population. *Clinical Therapeutics*, 27(11), 1847–1858.

Kilbourne, A. M., & Pincus, H. A. (2006). Patterns of psychotropic medication use by race among veterans with bipolar disorder. *Psychiatric Services*, 57, 123–126.

Kuno, E., & Rothbard, A. B. (2002). Racial disparities in antipsychotic prescription patterns for patients with schizophrenia. *American Journal of Psychiatry*, 159, 567–572.

Lee, C. F., Yang, Y. Y., & Hu O. Y. (1998). Single dose pharmacokinetic study of lithium in Taiwanese/Chinese bipolar patients. *Australian and New Zealand Journal of Psychiatry*, 32(1), 133–136.

Lee, S., Wing, Y. K., & Wong, K. C. (1992). Knowledge and compliance toward lithium therapy among Chinese psychiatric patients in Hong Kong. *Australian and New Zealand Journal of Psychiatry*, 26, 444–449.

Melfi, C. A., Croghan, T. W., Hanna, M. P., & Robinson, R. L. (2000). Racial variation in antidepressant treatment in a Medicaid population. *Journal of Clinical Psychiatry*, 61, 16–21.

Michalets, E. L. (1998). Update: Clinically significant cytochrome P450 drug interactions. *Pharmacotherapy*, 18(1), 84–112.

Nemeroff, C. B., DeVane, C. L., & Pollack, B. G. (1996). Newer antidepressants and the cytochrome P450 enzyme system. *American Journal of Psychiatry*, 153, 311–320.

Neumark, Y. K., Friedlander, Y., Durst, R., Leitersdorf, E., Janne, D., Ramchandani, V. A., et al. (2004). Alcohol dehydrogenase polymorphisms influence alcohol-elimination rates in a male Jewish population. *Alcoholism, Clinical and Experimental Research,* 28(1), 10–14.

Ng, C. H., Chong, S. A., Lambert, T., Fan, A., Hackett, L. P., Mahendran, R., et al. (2005). An inter-ethnic comparison study of clozapine dosage, clinical response and plasma levels. *International Clinical Psychopharmacology,* 20(3), 163–168.

Okuma, T. (1981) Differential sensitivity to the effects of psychotropic drugs: Psychotics vs normals; Asian vs Western populations. *Folia Psychiatr Neurol Jpn,* 35(1), 79–87.

Opolka, J. L., Rascati, K. L., Brown, C. M., & Gibson, P. J. (2004). Ethnicity and prescription patterns for haloperidol, risperidone, and olanzapine. *Psychiatric Services,* 55, 151–156.

Pi, E. H., & Simpson, G. M. (2005). Cross-cultural psychopharmacology: A current clinical perspective. *Psychiatric Services,* 56, 31–33.

Richelson, E. (1997). Pharmacokinetic drug interactions of new antidepressants: A review of the effects on the metabolism of other drugs. *Mayo Clinic Proceedings,* 72(9), 835–847.

Roy–Byrne, P. P., Perera, P., Pitts, C. D., & Christi, J. A. (2005). Paroxetine response and tolerability among ethnic minority patients with mood or anxiety disorders: A pooled analysis. *Journal of Clinical Psychiatry,* 66(10), 1228–1233.

Ruiz, P., Varner, R. V., Small, D. R., & Johnson, B. A. (1999). Ethnic differences in the neuroleptic treatment of schizophrenia. *Psychiatry Quarterly,* 70(2), 163–172.

Sleath, B. L., Rubin, R. H., & Huston, S. A. (2001). Antidepressant prescribing to Hispanic and non-Hispanic white patients in primary care. *Annals of Pharmacotherapy,* 35(4), 419–423.

Sramek, J. J., & Pi, E. H. (1996). Ethnicity and antidepressant response. *Mt Sinai Journal of Medicine,* 63(5-6), 320–325.

Straka, R. J., Hansen, S. R., Benson, S. R., & Walker, P. F. (1996). Predominance of slow acetylators of N-acetyltransferase in a Hmong population residing in the United States. *Journal of Clinical Pharmacology,* 36(8), 740–747.

Taylor, D. M. (2004). Prescribing of clozapine and olanzapine: Dosage, polypharmacy, and patient ethnicity. *Psychiatric Bulletin,* 28, 241–243.

Turner, N., Scarpace, P. J., & Lowenthal, D. T. (1992). Geriatric pharmacology: Basic and clinical considerations. *Annual Review of Pharmacology and Toxicology,* 32, 271–302.

Unutzer, J., Klap, R., Sturm, R., Young, A. S., Marmon, T., et al. (2000). Mental disorder and the use of alternative medicine: Results from a national survey. *American Journal of Psychiatry,* 157(11), 1851–1857.

U.S. Department of Health and Human Services. (2001). Mental health: Culture, race, and ethnicity: A supplement to mental health: A report of the Surgeon General. Rockville, MD: U.S. Department of Health and Human Services.

Valenstein, M., Copeland, L. A., Owen, R., Blow, F. C., & Visnic, S. (2001). Adherence assessment and the use of depot antipsychotics in patients with schizophrenia. *Journal of Clinical Psychiatry,* 62(7), 545–551.

Varner, R. V., Ruiz, P., & Small, D. R. (1998). Black and white patients' response to antidepressant treatment for major depression. *Psychiatry Quarterly,* 69(2), 117–125.

Wall, T. L. (2005). Genetic associations of alcohol and aldehyde dehydrogenase with alcohol dependence and their mechanisms of action. *Therapeutic Drug Monitoring,* 27(6), 700–703.

Wang, J. L., Patten, S. M., & Russell, M. L. (2001) Alternative medicine use by individuals with major depression. *Canadian Journal of Psychiatry,* 46(6), 528–533.

Wilkinson, G. R. (2005) Drug metabolism and variability among patients in drug response. *New England Journal of Medicine, 352*(21), 2211–2221.

Wing, Y. K., Chan, E., Chan, K., Lee, S., & Shek, C. C. (1997). Lithium pharmacokinetics in Chinese manic-depressive patients. *Journal of Clinical Psychopharmacology, 17*(3), 179–184.

13

Legal and Ethical Issues in Research Relating to Mood Disorders

SANA LOUE

Significant legal and ethical issues exist in the context of research with participants who have been diagnosed with mood disorders. Many of these issues relate to the informed consent process, such as the capacity of the prospective research participant to provide or withhold his or her consent to participation, the ability of the individual to understand the information that is provided to him or her by the research team, the designation of a surrogate for consent to participate and the standard to be used by the surrogate in providing or withholding that consent, and the standard by which to assess and balance the risks and benefits that may result from participation. The resolution of these issues in a specific context may be rendered even more difficult as individuals with mood disorders age and develop additional conditions that may impact their ability to understand and process information, such as stroke, dementia, hearing loss, and vision loss, and/or encounter circumstances, such as placement in a nursing home or an assisted living situation, that reduce their actual or perceived ability to participate in research free of coercion or duress.

Conducting research with individuals suffering from mood disorders is critical if we are to improve our understanding of the epidemiology of mood disorders, our ability to assess individuals' capabilities, and our ability to develop and implement more effective and supportive interventions. Yet past history demonstrates the vulnerability of cognitively impaired, mentally ill, and institutionalized persons to abuse in research (Advisory Committee on Human Radiation Experiments, 1996; Bein, 1991; Garnett, 1996; *Kaimowitz v. Michigan Department of Health*, 1973; Lubasch, 1982; Rothman, 1991; *Scott v. Casey*, 1983; *Valenti v. Prudden*, 1977). An outright prohibition against the participation of mentally ill individuals in research would shield them from the potential for such abuse, but would also result in a loss of their individual autonomy and possibly exacerbate their societal isolation and stigmatization. Such a prohibition would also contravene the ethical principle of distributive justice, which seeks an equitable distribution of the burdens and the benefits of research across groups and populations. In addition, future generations would be deprived of important scientific knowledge critical to the amelioration and/or prevention of the disease and the improvement of care. Consequently, individuals suffering from mental illness, including mood disorders, may face the twin dangers of exploitation and overprotection. Our challenge is to foster such research while simultaneously protecting mentally ill research participants from potential exploitation and abuse.

THE REQUIREMENT OF INFORMED CONSENT

Ethically and legally, researchers are required to obtain the informed consent of an individual to enroll an individual into a study. This ethical requirement derives from several international documents, including the Nuremberg Code and the Helsinki Declarations, and has been integrated into U.S. law by federal regulations. These federal regulations state that "no investigator may involve a human being as a subject in research . . . unless the investigator has obtained the legally effective informed consent of the subject or the subject's legally authorized representative" (Code of Federal Regulations, 2007, § 46.116).

The federal regulations, however, do not provide specific guidance to researchers who wish to conduct studies with cognitively impaired individuals, including those whose decision-making abilities are diminished as a result of mental illness. Regulations applicable to all research participants mandate the presence of four elements in a valid informed consent process:

1. The individual from whom consent is to be obtained must be given the information necessary to make a decision.
2. The individual must understand the information.
3. The prospective participant must have the capacity to consent.
4. The consent of the individual to participate must be voluntary (Faden & Beauchamp, 1986; Meisel, Roth, & Lidz, 1977).

It cannot be emphasized enough that informed consent is a process that continues from the time of recruitment and enrollment throughout the study; it is not and should not be construed as the mere presentation to and signing of a document by the prospective research participant.

Enhanced procedures during this informed consent process may be ethically required to ensure that research participants who have been diagnosed with a mental illness are able to provide valid informed consent. Still other enhancements may be required to protect those who are suffering from cognitive impairment as a result of their mental illness, dementia, or other age-related process, resulting in their heightened vulnerability. Vulnerable participants are those individuals with "insufficient power, prowess, intelligence, resources, strength, or other needed attributes to protect their own interests through negotiations for informed consent" (Levine, 1988, p. 72). However, the mere fact of having been diagnosed with a mental illness, such as bipolar disorder, should not serve as the basis for automatically assuming that the individual lacks capacity (National Bioethics Advisory Commission, 1998). These additional enhancements and protections are discussed later in the context of maximizing understanding, assessing capacity, balancing the risks and benefits of participation, and specifying the mechanisms for indicating consent.

Assessing Capacity to Consent

The terms *capacity* and *competence* are often used synonymously, but they actually represent distinct concepts. The term *capacity* is used here to refer to an individual's decision-making ability. In contrast, the term *competence* reflects a legal judgment that an individual has a minimal level of mental, cognitive, or behavioral functioning to perform or assume a specified legal role (Bisbing, McMenamin, & Granville, 1995; Loue, 2001). It is important to recognize that although being diagnosed with a particular condition is relevant to incapacity for informed consent, it is not determinative of the issue (High, Whitehouse, Post, & Berg, 1994). For instance, the course of bipolar disorder or major depression may fluctuate, so that there may be periods of time during which an individual is able to understand and to give legally valid consent. Additionally, the course of bipolar disorder may change over time, and older individuals may be more impaired than younger persons.

Symptomatology and Capacity

In general, it is presumed at the commencement of research studies that a prospective participant has capacity to consent, unless there is some reason to believe that he or she does not or that the capacity to give consent may be limited in some way. However, if a study focuses on a disorder involving either permanent cognitive impairment (such as mental retardation), progressive impairment (such as Alzheimer's disease), or fluctuating impairment (such as may occur with major depression or bipolar disorder), an assessment of capacity should be conducted at the commencement of participation.

This is particularly important with individuals who have been diagnosed with more severe mood disorders. Research findings suggest that decreased motivation to protect their interests may reduce the ability of depressed patients to make decisions or may impact the nature of these decisions (Elliott, 1997; Lee & Ganzini, 1992). In fact, hospitalized depressed patients have been found to experience decision-making difficulties approximately half as frequently as individuals diagnosed with schizophrenia (Grisso & Appelbaum, 1995). This means that roughly one quarter of hospitalized depressed patients suffer impairment of their decision-making abilities.

Individuals with bipolar disorder may also experience decision-making difficulties. The manic phases are characterized by elevated mood, impulsivity, and reduced attention. These features are associated with poor decision making related to relationships, employment, and financial matters (American Psychiatric Association, 2000). It has been hypothesized that these same symptoms may impair individuals' decision-making ability in the context of research (National Bioethics Advisory Commission, 1998).

Longitudinal studies involving participants with bipolar disorder or major depression or other mood disorder may find two or more forms of impairment even within the same individual. For instance, individuals may experience fluctuating impairment resulting from the progression of their bipolar disorder but, as they age, they may develop Alzheimer's disease or other neurological illness, resulting in additional levels of progressive impairment. Because capacity and decision-making ability may vary during the course of the study, depending upon the length of the study and the progression of the disorder or disease, it is also recommended that assessments of capacity and decision-making ability be conducted periodically during the course of an individual's participation in research, unless that participation is of very short duration.

Factors Affecting Capacity

Although a decreasing proportion of individuals with mental illness are now institutionalized in mental health care facilities or hospitals, the capacity of those individuals who are so confined may be impacted by the fact of institutionalization alone. It has been observed that individuals who are essentially removed from the world are effectively stripped of their concept of "self" (Goffman, 1962), and a perception of self is integral to the ability to provide informed consent (Annas & Glantz, 1997). In some such instances, individuals may lack the capacity to provide informed consent. However, it is also possible that individuals accustomed to the regimentation associated with institutionalization may become confused or frightened with any change in routine. Absent a careful assessment, signs of that confusion may be mistaken for signs of diminished capacity.

Although current federal regulations severely curtail the possibility that research will be conducted in prisons, they do not foreclose this possibility (Code of Federal Regulations, 2006). It has been estimated that 16% of adult inmates in state prisons and local jails are mentally ill (Ditton, 1999). In fact, there are three times as many mentally ill persons housed in prisons and jails than are confined in mental hospitals (Metzner, Cohen, Grossman, & Wettstein, 1998). Individuals suffering from mood disorders and confined in prisons or jails, even if initially possessing capacity, may experience diminished capacity to provide informed consent as a result of inadequate medication, incorrect medication, and actions taken by prison authorities in misguided attempts to control through discipline their apparently psychotic and/or bizarre behaviors. One physician explained the impact of segregation policies on individuals suffering from various mood disorders as follows:

> Prisoners who are prone to depression and have had past depressive episodes will become very depressed in isolated confinement. People who are prone to suicidal

ideation and attempts will become more suicidal in that direction. People who are prone to disorders of mood, either bipolar... or depressive will become that and have a breakdown in that direction.... (Kupers, 2003, as cited in Abramsky & Fellner, 2003, p. 152)

An individual's ability to respond to questions posed or to perform well on a test of cognitive ability may also be impacted by iatrogenic and specific institutional factors (Kennedy, 2000). The individual's ability to concentrate, or his or her level of awareness may be affected by his or her medications. It is likely that older individuals will utilize a greater number of medications resulting from the existence of comorbid medical conditions. Environmentally induced stress, such as sleep deprivation and recent bereavement, resulting in depression and a decline in functional ability, may also adversely impact the individual's decision-making ability (American Psychiatric Association, 2000). Physiological causes, such as fluctuations in the blood sugar of individuals with diabetes, sodium deficiency, and electrolyte imbalances, can also affect cognition. Older individuals are more prone to medical illness and are more likely to experience adverse drug reactions or drug intolerances (Routledge, O'Mahony, & Woodhouse, 2004). Because a determination of (in)capacity is so complex, it has been suggested that a determination of (in)capacity be verified through reliance on second opinions or the services of individuals who are consent specialists (Bonnie, 1997).

Assessing Capacity

It is critical that the conditions under which capacity is to be assessed maximize the likelihood that an accurate finding will be achieved. First, it is important that the individual who is to assess capacity be matched appropriately with the prospective research participant (Kennedy, 2000). For instance, a woman with a history of sexual abuse as a child may continue to be intimidated by males in a position of authority and power and may be less forthcoming when interviewed by a male research team member than she might be with a female. It has been suggested by some commentators that the assessment and monitoring of an individual's capacity to consent and to participate in a study is best done by the research team of a study in collaboration with family members (Keyserlingk, Glass, Kogan, & Gauthier, 1995). Four exceptions to this basic premise have been noted:

1. When project staff does not have the requisite skill to assess or monitor the participants' capacity
2. When there is a strong danger of conflict of interest
3. When the individual had previously executed an advance directive for research while he or she still had capacity, but the document requires interpretation
4. When the protocol does not have the potential to confer a direct benefit on the participant and it involves more than minimal risk

The assessment of capacity may be particularly difficult in situations involving researchers and prospective participants with differing religious or cultural backgrounds. For instance, an individual may report having visions of religious figures, frequently seeing shadows, having the ability to speak with deceased persons, or receiving messages from angels or directly from God or a higher power. Some faiths view these behaviors as gifts and encourage their devotees to develop and share their visions with others (Beit-Hallahami, 1997; Kildahl, 1972; Malony & Lovekin, 1985). In such instances, it may be difficult, without sustained and in-depth contact with an individual, to determine whether these voiced abilities reflect psychotic delusions and hallucinations or are reflective of shared spiritual beliefs—or both.

Receiving Information

Federal regulations now require that the following information be provided to all research participants during the informed consent process: (a) a statement that the study involves research, an explanation of the purposes of the research, the expected duration of the subject's participation, a description of the procedures required for participation, and the identification of any procedures that are experimental; (b) a description of any reasonably foreseeable risks or discomforts to the research participant; (c) a description of any benefits from the research that may be reasonably expected for the research participant or others; (d) a disclosure of appropriate alternative procedures or courses of treatment, if any, that might be advantageous to the research participant; (e) a statement describing the extent to which confidentiality of records identifying the research participant will be maintained; (f) for research involving more than minimal risk, an explanation regarding whether any compensation or any medical treatments are available if injury occurs and, if so, what they consist of or where further information may be obtained; (g) an explanation of whom to contact for answers to pertinent questions about the research and the rights of research participants, and whom to contact in the event of a research-related injury to the research participant; and (h) a statement that participation is voluntary, that a refusal to participate will not involve any penalty or loss of benefits to which the research participant is otherwise entitled, and that the participant may discontinue participation at any time without penalty or loss of benefits to which the subject is otherwise entitled (Code of Federal Regulations, 2007).

In addition to these mandated disclosures, federal regulations indicate that the following information may be provided to research participants when appropriate: (a) a statement that the particular treatment or procedure may involve risks to the research participant (or to the embryo or fetus, if the subject is or may become pregnant) that are currently unforeseeable, (b) anticipated circumstances under which the participation of a research participant may be terminated by the investigator without regard to the subject's consent, (c) any additional costs to the subject that may result from participation in the research, (d) the consequences of a participant's decision to withdraw from the research and procedures for orderly termination of participation by the subject, (e) a statement that significant new findings developed during the course of the research that may relate to the subject's willingness to continue participation will be provided to the subject, and (f) the approximate number of subjects involved in the study (Code of Federal Regulations, 2007).

The provision of information may become even more complex when there exist differences in language and/or culture. For instance, prospective participants, even within the United States, may not be predominantly English speaking or may not speak English at all. In such instances, careful translation of the informed consent documents will be necessary. This process requires more than the literal translation of the words; rather, the sense of what is said must also be conveyed in the translation. The effective transmission of the information requires that the translation be done at a reading level that is commensurate with the abilities of the intended recipient; the translation of a two-syllable word into a three-syllable Spanish word for an individual with limited education will not be effective. And, because the provision of information is a continuing process throughout the duration of the study, mechanisms must be developed and implemented that will facilitate communication with the non-English-speaking participants throughout the course of the investigation.

Ensuring Understanding

It is critical that individuals understand that they are participating in research and that the procedures that they will undergo may not yield any direct benefit to them. A number of studies have found that many research participants may not understand either that they are participating in research rather than receiving clinical care, or the nature of the procedures that they will undergo in conjunction with their participation (Fletcher, 1973; Gray, 1975; Hassar & Weintraub, 1976; Howard, DeMets, & The BHAT Research Group, 1981; McCollum & Schwartz, 1969; Park, Slaughter, Covi, & Kniffin, 1966; Riecken & Ravich, 1982). Research suggests that among severely mentally ill individuals, the ability to understand is related both to the level of psychopathology and the quality of the information that is presented (Benson, Roth, Appelbaum, Lidz, & Winslade, 1988).

The ability of an individual with a mood disorder to process the information provided will vary with the disorder and with the severity of the symptoms at any given time. Symptoms of major depression include depressed mood; feelings of worthlessness; reduced interest and pleasure in many activities; changes in appetite, sleep patterns, and energy level; and difficulty in concentration (American Psychiatric Association, 2000). Individuals suffering from major depression may also experience difficulties in processing information and reasoning (Baker & Channon, 1995; Hartlage, Alloy, Vazquez, & Dykman, 1993). Individuals with bipolar disorder in a depressed state may also experience similar difficulties.

The National Bioethics Advisory Commission (2001) has recommended that the informed consent procedure be tailored to the specific abilities of each individual participant to receive and process information. For instance, in addition to severe depression, some elderly participants may have hearing or vision impairments that further impede their ability to understand the information in the form in which it might be presented; therefore, accommodations must be made for these limitations to ensure that potential research participants understand the substance of the information being presented. A number of suggestions have been made to maximize understanding, including the use of a clear and simple presentation format for the information (Bergler, Pennington, Metcalfe, & Freis, 1980), the provision of sufficient time to enable the individual to process the information given to him or her (Morrow, Gootnick, & Schmale, 1978), and discussion of the information with the physician (Williams, Rieckmann, Trenholme, Frischer, & Carson, 1977). The individual may be asked to restate or summarize in his or her own words the information provided to confirm that he or she understood. Tailored questions, whether in multiple-choice, true/false, or essay format, may be asked of the participant after the presentation of the information to ascertain whether and how much the prospective participant understood of the information presented (Bonnie, 1997; Flanery, Gravdal, Hendrix, et al., 1978; Hassar & Weintraub, 1976; McCollum & Schwartz, 1969; Roth, Lidz, Meisel, Soloff, Kaufman, Spiker, & Foster, 1982; Williams et al., 1977). One commentator has suggested that a family member participate with the cognitively impaired member during the informed consent process to ensure understanding and provide concurrent consent (Bonnie, 1997).

Voluntariness

The life situation of many individuals with major depression and bipolar disorder may affect their ability to consent or to refuse consent to participate in research. One research study found that 21% of adults with serious mental illness live below the poverty threshold, compared with 9% of the general adult population (Barker et al., 1992). Many homeless individuals suffer from mental illness (Isaac & Armat, 1990). A lack of adequate medical care may be associated with the poverty that they experience. Consequently, the possibility of participation in research with its attendant psychiatric and medical care may represent an otherwise unavailable and unattainable resource, leading individuals to disregard the risks that may be inherent in participation and to overemphasize the likelihood that they will obtain a direct benefit from their participation (National Bioethics Advisory Commission, 1998).

Some individuals may be dependent on others for their physical care, for attention to their personal needs, or for their medical care. This is particularly true of those individuals who have been hospitalized in psychiatric units as a result of the severity of their disease. They may fear that if they refuse to participate in a particular research study, they will suffer the withdrawal of such assistance, a diminution in the quality of this assistance, or complete abandonment (Annas & Glantz, 1997). Individuals may also be concerned that they will disappoint their caregiver or care provider if they refuse to participate (Sachs & Cassel, 1989). Some individuals may also believe that they would not have been offered the possibility of participation in a study unless the researcher believed that their participation would yield some clinical benefit to them personally. They may believe this despite all assertions by the research team that they may not receive any personal benefit from their participation and only future patients will derive any benefit from the new-found knowledge gained through the study. This misconception is known as the *therapeutic misconception* (Grisso & Appelbaum, 1998).

Voluntariness is an issue of especial concern in a variety of other circumstances. First, incarcerated individuals suffering from mood disorders may have limited ability to exercise freedom of choice because of the coercive nature of their imprisonment (Abramsky & Fellner, 2003). This potential for coercion provides the basis for the severe restrictions on the conduct of research among prisoners (Code of Federal Regulations, 2006; Council of International Organizations for Medical Sciences, 2002).

Second, the concept of autonomy that is reflected in the requirement of voluntariness, as it is operationalized in U.S. regulations, is based on the idea of individual sovereignty. In many cultures, however, the "self" is defined in relation to those to whom he or she is connected, and the wishes of the individual are subordinated to those of the immediate or extended family (Fox & Swazey, 1984; Lane, 1994). When family members are deeply involved in the treatment and/or care of an individual with a mood disorder, it may be difficult for the researcher to determine whether the individual consenting to participation in the research is doing so of his or her own volition or is feeling pressure to accede to it.

Other Considerations

Confidentiality of the Data

The level of confidentiality protection of the information that is disclosed to the researcher may be of concern for a number of reasons. First, confidentiality may be difficult to maintain if interviews or other procedures are conducted in the context of an institutional residence (such as a nursing home or mental health care facility) as a result of the physical layout of the institution, a scarcity of private space, and the possibility that the participant may have impaired hearing ability, thereby requiring that the researcher speak at a level that is audible to others (Cassel, 1985, 1988).

Depending upon the nature of the study, attempts to access the study data could be made through the legal system. For instance, assume that an investigator is conducting a behavioral intervention trial designed to increase medication adherence and decrease illicit substance use among individuals diagnosed with bipolar disorder. The investigator knows, through interviews with the participant, that the participant has been abusing illicit substances and is selling them as a means of support. The police learn somehow that he is a participant in a study and the prosecuting attorney wishes to have the research records subpoenaed to establish further the individual's possession and sale of the illegal drugs. Without a certificate of confidentiality, the attorney might well gain access to these records. Such access would impact not only the specific participant and study involved, but could well affect adversely the validity of any research conducted that might provoke the interest of law enforcement officials or plaintiffs in civil litigation, as well as the ability of researcher to recruit and retain participants. It is critical that the investigator apply, prior to the collection of data, for a federal certificate of confidentiality to protect their data from subpoena if they are collecting data that may be of some interest to law enforcement or lawyers (National Institutes of Health, 2005).

Assessing and Balancing Risks and Benefits

A decision relating to participation in a research protocol requires that the decision maker, usually the prospective participant him- or herself, balance the risks and benefits of participation. (A balancing of risks and benefits must also be done by the researcher proposing the study prior to its initiation and must also be conducted by the institutional review board [IRB] of the researcher's institution in its initial and continuing reviews of the research protocol [Code of Federal Regulations, 2007].)

Commentators have identified four categories into which research protocols may be classified:

1. Research in which there is the potential for a direct therapeutic benefit to the participant and minimal risk is involved
2. Research in which the participant may obtain some direct therapeutic benefit, but more than minimal risk is involved
3. Research in which there is no expected benefit for the individual participating, but there is no more than minimal risk
4. Research in which there is no expected therapeutic benefit to the participant and there is more than minimal risk (Kapp, 1998; LeBlang & Kirchner, 1996)

Minimal risk is often interpreted to mean that the risks of participation are no greater than those that would be experienced in the everyday course of living (Levine, 1988).

The study design itself may entail significant risks. *Challenge studies* are designed to expand our understanding of the pathophysiological mechanisms that underlie the symptomatic expression of psychiatric illnesses (Miller & Rosenstein, 1997). Such study protocols demand the intentional inducement of disease symptoms. It is not clear that the relationship between the risks and potential benefits of participation can ever justify enrolling individuals in studies such as these, when under any other circumstances the instigation of symptoms would be considered harmful. Additionally, it is unclear whether informed consent is ever obtainable in studies that, by their very design, are intended to provoke symptoms of illness (National Bioethics Advisory Commission, 1998).

Clinical trials and crossover trials may involve the use of washout periods and/or placebo controls. Washout periods, during which an individual is deprived of his or her medication, may be utilized at baseline or between phases of a crossover trial to return the research participant to a medication-free baseline to facilitate evaluation of a new or different drug's effects on symptoms or behavior. However, the sudden or rapid withdrawal of medication to accomplish this washout may result in harm to the individual, raising substantial ethical concerns (National Bioethics Advisory Commission, 1998). The use of placebo controls may also be ethically problematic as a result of individuals' possibly fluctuating ability to comprehend information and the erroneous belief that the administration of any medication must be treatment designed to benefit the individual (National Bioethics Advisory Commission, 1998).

Often, as noted earlier, risks have been conceived of as potential risks to participants' physical and mental well-being related to the administration of experimental drugs or the utilization of experimental procedures. However, participation in a study may entail additional risks that may differ across subgroups. As an example, a diagnosis of mental illness is highly stigmatizing in many cultures (Finzen, 1996; Goffman, 1962). Accordingly, recruitment efforts within specified communities may need to be sensitive to these issues and refer to symptoms, without necessarily referring to the mental illness diagnosis in public forums. As an example, efforts to recruit Latinas into a study that requires the diagnosis of bipolar disorder or depression, may refer instead in its recruitment studies to *ataques de nervios*, a common idiom of distress among many Latino groups that encompasses many of the same symptoms that would be encompassed by such formal diagnoses (Loue, in press). In such instances, further details and assessment can be conducted with the individuals who indicate interest in participation.

Direct benefits may include short- or long-term improvement in the individual's condition, an improvement in the individual's symptoms, and the slowing of the degenerative process (Keyserlingk et al., 1995). Indirect benefits may include enhanced opportunities for social interaction, increased attention from health and ancillary health professionals, and a feeling of contributing in a way that may help others. Examples of risks include the physiological effects of an experimental drug or procedure and increased levels of anxiety associated with study questions or procedures (Dresser, 2001).

It is a common misperception that observational studies do not entail any potential risks or benefits to study participants because these studies do not involve an intervention. However, this view overlooks the fact that observation itself may constitute an intervention, however unintended and unmeasurable its effects may be. As a consequence of participation, individuals may experience attachments to members of the study team, and emotional trauma at the study's conclusion. Because many individuals with severe mood disorders often experience unstable relationships, the maintenance of a stable connection with study team members during the course of the study may constitute a potential benefit. The loss of this connection at the study's conclusion may, however, constitute a risk that should be anticipated at the outset and for which ameliorative protections must be devised.

In many studies, individuals who are suicidal or who are experiencing suicidal thoughts are automatically excluded, although some studies include them if the individual is not at increased risk (such as someone who might be hospitalized). This is an issue of ongoing difficulty, with competing interests of not including those with potential bad outcome (even in "humanitarian" trials) versus the need to learn more about what types of treatments might help these most sick individuals.

Research suggests that even when risks of study participation are divulged to prospective participants, individuals may have difficulty comprehending the risks. In one clinical trial of a drug, respondents were found to be well informed about the study design and general risks of participation, but 39% were unable to enumerate specific minor side effects of the drug, and 64% were unable to identify the serious risks of the medication that had been divulged to them (Howard, DeMets, & The BHAT Research Group, 1981). In yet another study, few of the respondents recognized the possibility of unknown risk, meaning that there could be risks that had not been anticipated prior to the initiation of the study (Gray, 1975).

There is always the possibility that individuals participating in any study, whether a clinical trial or observation, may experience a deterioration of their mental status during the course of the study, including heightened suicidal ideation and suicide attempts. It is critical that research participants be monitored throughout the course of the study for such changes. It may be necessary in some cases to terminate their participation involuntarily if it appears that the risks of participating exceed the potential benefits resulting from such changes.

There is no formula that will dictate how the benefits and risks of a particular individual's participation are to be weighed against each other. In fact, there is no consensus among researchers or ethicists regarding the level of risk or benefit that must be present for a surrogate decision maker to be able to consent to research participation by a cognitively impaired individual (Dresser, 2001).

MECHANISMS FOR EXPRESSING CHOICE DURING INCAPACITY

Advance Directives for Research

Because of the intermittent nature of mood disorders and their potential impact on decision-making ability, it may be advisable for individuals diagnosed with such disorders to indicate in advance whether they wish to participate in research. For instance, an individual diagnosed with bipolar disorder may strongly believe that he or she would like to participate in research if the opportunity were to arise, but may fear that he or she will be unable to give consent at a future date because of an acute exacerbation of symptoms. Accordingly, the individual might want to express this intent at a time when he or she is still able to do so, when legally that expression will be recognized as valid.

One mechanism that has been suggested is an advance directive for research. Similar to an advance directive for health care, such a document would allow the individual to make his or her wishes known at a time when the individual retains decision-making capacity. Alternatively, the individual might execute a durable power of attorney for health care and specify that his or her designated agent should have the legal authority to decide for him or her whether participation in a particular research study would be advisable, and to provide or withhold consent accordingly.

This type of advance decision making may be an option, depending upon the state in which the individual resides. Not all states provide for such a document or recognize an agent as having the authority to make research-related decisions. Even where this possibility exists, many individuals may be unaware of the mechanism. Even in the context of health care, it appears that only a minority of elderly patients execute durable powers of attorney for health care, often because of a lack of knowledge about the mechanism or the erroneous assumption that a relative will automatically be able to make health care decisions for them if they are unable to do so (Cohen–Mansfield, Droge, & Billing, 1991).

There are other difficulties associated with an advance directive for research even if the individual state permits this mechanism. Because the informed consent process is supposed to be ongoing throughout the course of the study, an individual who consents to participate before knowing what a study is about is not really giving *informed* consent.

Questions also arise about the current validity of the prior expression to participate in research because changes in the individual's situation may have occurred during the intervening period of time. For instance, an individual may have indicated, when he or she had the capacity to do so, an intent and desire to participate in research. Some ethicists, distinguishing between the "then-person," the precursor to the person who now lacks capacity, and the "now-person," have argued that, as the individual's capacity decreases, so should the weight to be given to his or her previously expressed wishes in an advance directive decrease (Brock & Buchanan, 1989; Dresser, 1992). This perspective results in the incongruous result whereby the greatest weight is given to the severely demented now-self's needs, who has the least psychological continuity with his or her former competent self (Klepper & Roty, 1999). Others have emphasized the concept of *precedent autonomy* and have argued that past decisions of the competent then-self must be respected even if they are not consistent with the wishes of the cognitively impaired now-self (Dworkin, 1994). Still others have argued for the compassionate application of the principle of precedent autonomy, which would permit the implementation of previously expressed wishes as long as doing so does not result in discomfort to the now-self (Post, 1995). This discussion has occurred most frequently in the context of Alzheimer's disease, in which the loss of individual capacity is progressive. The relevance of concepts addressing the then-person and now-person to individuals with fluctuating capacity, such as those with bipolar disorder, has not been explored.

Surrogate Consent

Even in the absence of a legally executed document, such as an advance directive for research, some have suggested that adults who lack capacity to consent should be able to participate in research through the consent of a surrogate. Federal regulations permit a "legally authorized representative" to provide consent in some circumstances when the prospective participant is unable to do so

(Code of Federal Regulations, 2007, § 46.102(c)). The term *legally authorized representative* is defined in the regulations as "an individual or judicial or other body authorized under applicable law to consent on behalf of a prospective subject to the subject's participation in the procedure(s) involved in the research" (Code of Federal Regulations, 2006).

A number of states have implemented state regulations or statutes that govern in addition to the federal law and that may place severe restrictions on the ability of cognitively impaired individuals to participate in research, on the ability of a legally authorized representative to consent to an individual's participation in research, and/or may require judicial approval for such participation. Restrictions range in scope from Michigan's prohibition against psychosurgery specifically (*Kaimowitz v. Michigan Department of Mental Health*, 1973), to Connecticut's prohibition against participation in any biomedical or behavioral research that is not specifically intended to preserve the life of the individual, to prevent serious impairment, or to restore lost abilities (Connecticut General Statutes Annotated, 1997).

A question arises regarding which individuals are best suited to be appointed as the surrogate decision makers. The National Alliance for the Mentally Ill has proposed family members as the most appropriate surrogates in a research context (Flynn, 1997). Many IRBs allow family members or friends to give consent (LeBlang & Kirchner, 1996). However, some IRBs interpret the term *legally authorized representative* in the federal regulations narrowly and require that the surrogate be a court-appointed guardian, a designated health care agent under a written durable power of attorney for health care, a health care surrogate as defined by the relevant state law, or a combination of these individuals (LeBlang & Kirchner, 1996). At least one commentator has argued that judicial approval must be obtained any time an individual is to be involved in research if that individual is unable to consent for him- or herself (Bein, 1991).

A number of commentators have pointed out the dangers to an individual of having decisions made by a surrogate, regardless of whether the surrogate is appointed through the execution of a document. First, family members may be inappropriate because of their own lack of capacity, unavailability, or inattention to the needs of the cognitively impaired individual (High et al., 1994). Second, the surrogate may act in his or her own interest, rather than that of the individual (Sachs, 1994). Accordingly, it has been suggested that an appropriate surrogate be an individual who (a) is chosen, known, and trusted by the individual; (b) participates with the cognitively impaired individual in the informed consent process; (c) is familiar with the individual's medical and psychiatric history; (d) is familiar with the prodromal signs and symptoms indicative of a relapse; (e) is informed about and is willing to assume the responsibilities of a surrogate decision maker; (f) is willing to overrule the individual's previously expressed desire to participate in research if the participation could adversely affect the individual; and (g) is willing and able to ensure appropriate medical and/or psychiatric follow-up care if needed (Backlar, 1998).

Assuming that a surrogate, legally appointed or not, is able to decide for the individual who lacks capacity to decide for him- or herself, there remains the question of how the surrogate should make that determination. Two processes have been suggested: the best interest test and the substituted judgment test. The best interest test requires an assessment of what is in the individual's best interest at the time that the decision by the surrogate is to be made. This perspective allows a surrogate to disregard more easily any previously expressed desire or intent of the mentally ill individual, because what was once expressed may no longer be in his or her best interest, as determined by the surrogate. The substituted judgment test requires that the surrogate decide the issue of research participation in a manner consistent with what the individual would have chosen for him- or herself if he or she had remained able to do so. This perspective allows the surrogate to preserve to a greater degree the psychological continuity between the once-capable then-self and the now-self. In situations in which an IRB permits reliance on the substituted judgment test, the IRB may require, in addition to the surrogate's consent, the assent of the mentally ill individual to participate, meaning that, to the best of that individual's ability, he or she must indicate some preference, although that indication does not rise to the level of legal consent (cf. Sachs et al., 1994).

CONCLUSION

Individuals diagnosed with mood disorders should not be categorically excluded from participation in research because of a presumed lack of decision-making capacity. Rather, the ethical principles of respect for persons and justice require that a careful assessment be conducted with each prospective participant to ensure that eligible individuals are permitted to participate and that, when necessary, special protections be implemented to reduce potential risks. Concomitantly, the ethical principle of nonmaleficence requires that those who are found ineligible, as a result of an inability to provide informed consent, be appropriately excluded. The participation of individuals with mood disorders in mood disorder research is necessary if we are ever to understand fully the causal mechanisms that underlie these illnesses and mechanisms for their alleviation and cure.

REFERENCES

Abramsky, S. & Fellner, J. (2003). *Ill-equipped: U.S. prisons and offenders with mental illness*. New York: Human Rights Watch.

Advisory Committee on Human Radiation Experiments. (1996). *Final report*. Washington, DC: Advisory Committee on Human Radiation Experiments.

American Psychiatric Association. (2000). *Diagnostic and statistical manual of mental disorders* (4th ed., text rev.). Washington, DC: American Psychiatric Association.

Annas, G. J., & Glantz, L. H. (1997). Informed consent to research on institutionalized mentally disabled persons: The dual problems of incapacity and voluntariness. In A. E. Shamoo (Ed.), *Ethics in neurobiological research with human subjects: The*

Baltimore Conference on Ethics (pp. 55–79). Amsterdam: Gordon and Breach Publishers.

Backlar, P. (1998). Anticipatory planning for research participants with psychotic disorders like schizophrenia. *Psychology, Public Policy, and Law, 4,* 829–848.

Baker, J. E., & Channon, S. (1995). Reasoning in depression: Impairment on a concept discrimination learning task. *Cognition and Emotion, 9,* 579–597.

Barker, P. R., et al. (1992). Serious mental illness and disability in the adult household population: United States, 1989. In R. W. Manderscheid & M. A. Sonnenschein (Eds.), *Advance data from vital and health statistics of the National Center for Health Statistics* (no. 218, pp. 1–11). Washington, DC: Department of Health and Human Services.

Bein, P. M. (1991). Surrogate consent and the incompetent experimental subject. *Food, Drug and Cosmetic Law Journal, 46*(5), 739–771.

Beit-Hallahami, B. (1997). *The psychology of religious behavior, belief, and experience.* New York: Routledge.

Benson, P. R., Roth, L. H., Appelbaum, P. S., Lidz, C. W., & Winslade, W. J. (1988). Information disclosure, subject understanding, and informed consent in psychiatric research. *Law and Human Behavior, 12*(4), 455–475.

Bergler, J. H., Pennington, A. C., Metcalfe, M., & Freis, E. D. (1980). Informed consent: How much does the patient understand? *Clinical Pharmacology and Therapeutics, 27,* 435–440.

Bisbing, S., McMenamin, J., & Granville, R. (1995). Competency, capacity, and immunity. In ACLM Textbook Committee (Ed.), *Legal medicine* (3rd ed., pp. 27–45). St. Louis, MO: Mosby-Year Book.

Bonnie, R. J. (1997). Research with cognitively impaired subjects: Unfinished business in the regulation of human research. *Archives of General Psychiatry, 54*(2), 105–111.

Brock, D., & Buchanan, A. (1989). *Deciding for others.* Cambridge, U.K.: Cambridge University Press.

Cassel, C. (1985). Research in nursing homes: Ethical issues. *Journal of the American Geriatrics Society, 33,* 795–799.

Cassel, C. (1988). Ethical issues in the conduct of research in long term care. *Gerontologist, 28,* 90–96.

Code of Federal Regulations. (2006). Title 45, §§ 46.101, 46.102(c), 46.111(a)(4), 46.116.

Cohen–Mansfield, J., Droge, J. A., & Billing, N. (1991). The utilization of the durable power of attorney for health care among hospitalized elderly patients. *Journal of the American Geriatrics Society, 39,* 1174–1178.

Connecticut General Statutes Annotated. (1997). § 45a-677(e)(West Supp. 1997).

Council of Organizations for Medical Sciences. (2002). *International ethical guidelines for the conduct of biomedical research involving human beings.* Geneva, Switzerland: Council of Organizations for Medical Sciences.

Ditton, P. M. (1999). *Special report: Mental health and treatment of inmates and probationers.* Washington, DC: United States Department of Justice, Bureau of Justice Statistics.

Dresser, R. S. (1992). Autonomy revisited: The limits of anticipatory choices. In R. H. Binstock, S. G. Post, & P. J. Whitehouse (Eds.), *Ethics, values, and policy choices* (pp. 71–85). Baltimore, MD: Johns Hopkins University Press.

Dresser, R. (2001). Dementia research: Ethics and policy for the twenty-first century. *Georgia Law Review, 35,* 661–690.

Dworkin, R. (1994). *Life's dominion: An argument against abortion, euthanasia, and individual freedom.* New York: Vintage.

Elliott, C. (1997). Caring about risks: Are severely depressed patients competent to consent to research? *Archives of General Psychiatry, 54*, 113–116.

Faden, R., & Beauchamp, T. (1986). *A history and theory of informed consent.* New York: Oxford University Press.

Finzen, A. (1996). *Der Verwaltungsrat ist schizophren. Die Krankheit und das Stigma.* Bonn: Psychiatrie-Verlag.

Flanery, M., Gravdal, J., Hendrix., P., et al. (1978). Just sign here. . . . *South Dakota Journal of Medicine, 31*(5), 33–37.

Fletcher, J.C. (1973). Realities of patient consent to medical research. *Studies-Hastings Center, 1*, 39–40.

Flynn, L. M. (1997). Statement. *Issues concerning informed consent and protections of human subjects in research: Hearings before the Subcommittee on Human Resources of the House Committee on Government Reform and Oversight,* 105th Cong.

Fox, R., & Swazey, J. (1984). Medical morality is not bioethics: Medical ethics in China and the United States. *Perspectives in Biology and Medicine, 27*, 336–360.

Garnett, R. W. (1996). Why informed consent? Human experimentation and the ethics of autonomy. *Catholic Lawyer, 36*, 455–511.

Goffman, E. (1962). *Asylums: Essays on the social situation of mental patients and other inmates.* New York: Doubleday Anchor.

Gray, B. (1975). *Human subjects in medical experimentation: A sociological study of the conduct and regulation of clinical research.* New York: Wiley.

Grisso, T., & Appelbaum, P. (1998). *Assessing competence to consent to treatment: A guide for physicians and other health professionals.* New York: Oxford University Press.

Grisso, T., & Appelbaum, P. S. (1995). The MacArthur Treatment Competence Study III: Abilities of patients to consent to psychiatric and medical treatment. *Law and Human Behavior, 19*, 149–174.

Hartlage, S., Alloy, L. B., Vazquez, C., & Dykman, B. (1993). Automatic and effortful processing in depression. *Psychological Bulletin, 113*, 247–278.

Hassar, M., & Weintraub, M. (1976). "Uninformed" consent and the wealthy volunteer: An analysis of patient volunteers in a clinical trial of a new anti-inflammatory drug. *Clinical Pharmacology & Therapeutics, 20*, 379–386.

High, D. M., Whitehouse, P. J., Post, S. G., & Berg, L. (1994). Guidelines for addressing ethical and legal issues in Alzheimer disease research: A position statement. *Alzheimer's Disease & Associated Disorders, 8*(Suppl. 4), 66–74.

Howard, J. M., DeMets, D., & The BHAT Research Group. (1981). How informed is informed consent? *Controlled Clinical Trials, 2*, 287–303.

Isaac, R. J., & Armat, V. C. (1990). *Madness in the streets: How psychiatry and the law abandoned the mentally ill.* New York: Free Press.

Kaimowitz v. Michigan Department of Mental Health. (1973). *U.S. Law Week, 42*, 2063 (Circuit Court, Wayne County, MI).

Kapp, M. (1998). Decisional capacity, older human research subjects, and IRBs: Beyond forms and guidelines. *Stanford Law and Policy Review, 9*, 359–365.

Kennedy, G. J. (2000). *Geriatric mental health care: A treatment guide for health professionals.* New York: Guilford Press.

Keyserlingk, E. W., Glass, K., Kogan, S., & Gauthier, S. (1995). Proposed guidelines for the participation of persons with dementia as research subjects. *Perspectives in Biology and Medicine, 38*, 319–361.

Kildahl, J. P. (1972). *The psychology of speaking in tongues.* New York: Harper and Row.

Klepper, H., & Roty, M. (1999). Personal identity, advance directives, and genetic testing for Alzheimer disease. *Genetic Testing, 3*, 99–106.

Lane, S. D. (1994). Research bioethics in Egypt. In R. Gillon (Ed.), *Principles of health care ethics* (pp. 885–894). New York: John Wiley.

LeBlang, T. R., & Kirchner, J. L. (1996). Informed consent and Alzheimer disease research: Institutional review board policies and practices. In R. Becker & E. Giacobini (Eds.), *Alzheimer's disease from molecular biology to therapy* (pp. 529–534). Boston: Birkhauser.

Lee, M. A., & Ganzini, L. (1992). Depression in the elderly: Effect on patient attitudes toward life-sustaining therapy. *Journal of the American Geriatric Society, 40,* 983–988.

Levine, R. J. (1988). *Ethics and regulation of clinical research.* New Haven, CT: Yale University Press.

Loue, S. (2001). Elder abuse and neglect in medicine and law: The need for reform. *Journal of Legal Medicine, 22,* 159–209.

Loue, S. (2007). HIV prevention research among severely mentally ill Latinas: An examination of ethical issues in the context of gender and culture. *Acta Bioetica, 13,* 81–97.

Lubasch, A. H. (1982, September 14).Trial ruled in 1953 death case. *New York Times,* p. A-14.

Malony, H. N., & Lovekin, A. A. (1985). *Glossolalia: Behavioral science perspectives on speaking in tongues.* New York: Oxford University Press.

McCollum, A. T., & Schwartz, A. H. (1969). Pediatric research hospitalization: Its meaning to parents. *Pediatric Research, 3,* 199–204.

Meisel, A., Roth, L. H., & Lidz, C. W. (1977). Toward a model of the legal doctrine of informed consent. *American Journal of Psychiatry, 134,* 285–289.

Metzner, J. L., Cohen, F., Grossman, L. S., & Wettstein, R. M. (1998). Treatment in jails and prisons. In R. M. Wittstein (Ed.), *Treatment of offenders with mental disorders* (pp. 211–264). New York: Guilford Press.

Miller, F.G. & Rosenstein, D.L. (1997). Psychiatric symptom-provoking studies: An ethical appraisal. *Biological Psychiatry, 42,* 403–409.

Morrow, G., Gootnick, J., & Schmale, A. (1978). A simple technique for increasing cancer patients' knowledge of informed consent to treatment. *Cancer, 42,* 793–799.

National Bioethics Advisory Commission. (2001). *Ethical and policy issues in research involving human participants, vol. 1.* Rockville, MD: National Bioethics Advisory Commission.

National Bioethics Advisory Commission. (1998). *Research involving persons with mental disorders that may affect decision making capacity.* Rockville, MD: National Bioethics Advisory Commission.

National Institutes of Health. (2005). *Certificates of confidentiality kiosk* [Online]. Available: http://grants1.nih.gov/grants/policy/coc/index.htm

Park, L. C., Slaughter, R. S., Covi, L., & Kniffin, H. G., Jr. (1966). The subjective experience of the research patient: An investigation of psychiatric outpatients' reactions to the research treatment situation. *Journal of Nervous and Mental Disease, 143,* 199–206.

Post, S. G. (1995). Alzheimer disease and the "then" self. *Kennedy Institute of Ethics Journal, 4,* 307–321.

Riecken, H. W., & Ravich, R. (1982). Informed consent to biomedical research in Veterans Administration hospitals. *Journal of the American Medical Association, 248*(3), 344–348.

Roth, L. H., Lidz, C. W., Meisel, A., Soloff, P. H., Kaufman, K., Spiker, D. G., & Foster, F. G. (1982). Competency to decide about treatment or research: An overview of some empirical data. *International Journal of Law and Psychiatry, 5,* 29–50.

Rothman, D. J. (1991). *Strangers at the bedside: A history of how law and bioethics transformed medical decision making*. New York: Basic Books.

Routledge, P. A., O'Mahony, M. S., & Woodhouse, K. W. (2004). Adverse drug reactions in elderly patients. *British Journal of Clinical Pharmacology, 57*(2), 121–126.

Sachs, R.S. (1994). Ethical aspects of dementia research: Informed consent and proxy consent. *Clinical Research, 42,* 403–412.

Sachs, G., & Cassel, C. (1989). Ethical aspects of dementia. *Neurologic Clinics, 7,* 845–858.

Scott v. Casey. (1983). 562 F. Supp. 475 (N.D. Ga.).

Valenti v. Prudden. (1977). 58 A.D.2d 956, 397 N.Y.S.2d 181.

Williams, R. L., Rieckmann, K. H., Trenholme, G. M., Frischer, H., & Carson, P. E. (1977). The use of a test to determine that consent is informed. *Military Medicine, 142,* 542–545.

14

Strategies for Recruitment and Retention of Minorities in Research of Mood Disorders

ESPERANZA DIAZ & CRISTINA I. HUEBNER

Paradoxically, although minority groups have greater morbidity and mortality than the general population, they continue to be underrepresented in research studies. Without research data it becomes difficult to evaluate minority health status and treatments. Research on recruitment and retention methods of minorities in studies is growing (Keller, Gonzales, et al., 2005; Yancey, Ortega, et al., 2006); however, there is still a paucity of literature in mental health research investigating or reporting on these issues (Thompson, Neighbors, et al., 1996). The literature reveals that some researchers find recruitment and retention of minorities in research particularly challenging whereas others find that minorities are willing to participate but they are not invited as needed (Cabral, Napoles–Springer, et al., 2003; Keller et al., 2005; Markens, Fox, et al., 2002; Meinert, Blehar, et al., 2003; Norton & Manson, 1996; O'Brien, Kosoko–Lasaki, et al., 2006; Olin, Dagerman, et al., 2002; Staffileno & Coke, 2006; Thompson et al., 1996; Wendler, Kington, et al., 2006).

This chapter provides a brief review of barriers and strategies to improve recruitment and retention in mood disorder research of minorities. Barriers and strategies for recruitment and retention are summarized, but most of the data had to be taken from general medical health research because specific reports on mood disorder research are scarce. We utilize illustrative examples from our own experience recruiting research subjects in medical and mental health settings.

To the best of our knowledge, this is the first report of minority recruitment and retention for clinical research on mood disorders. The literature reviewed was identified by doing a combined Medline and PsycINFO search of articles published from 1996 to the present. Combining the keywords *mood disorders,*

Table 14.1 Summary of Published Studies Addressing Recruitment of Minorities in Mental Health Research

Author, Year	Mental Disorder Type, Study Type, Gender, Age	African Americans	Hispanics	Native Americans	Whites
Steffens, Artigues, et al., 1997[a]	Depression, intervention, elderly	Yes	—	—	Yes
Meinert, Blehar, et al., 2003	Mental health, outreach intervention pregnant women	Yes	—	—	—
Cardemil, Kim, et al., 2005[a]	Depression, intervention trial, mothers	—	Yes	—	—
Breland–Noble, Bell, et al., 2006	Depression, review adolescents	Yes	—	—	—
Thompson, Neighbors, et al., 1996[a]	Severe mental disorders, inpatient treatment	Yes	—	—	Yes
Aranda, 2001	Alzheimer's, review	—	Yes	—	—
Arean & Gallagher–Thompson, 1996	Mental health, review, elderly	Yes	Yes	—	Yes
Arean, Alvidrez, et al., 2003[a]	Mental health, intervention, elderly	Yes	Yes	—	—
Ballard, Nash, et al., 1993[a]	Dementia, survey, intervention	Yes	—	—	—
Connell, 2001	Alzheimer's, focus groups, caregivers	Yes	—	—	—
Fritsch, 2006[a]	Alzheimer's, intervention, elderly	Yes	—	—	—
Gallagher–Thompson, 2004[a]	Dementia, intervention, elderly/caregivers	—	Yes	—	Yes
Levkoff, 2000[a]	Dementia, intervention, elderly	Yes	Yes	—	Yes
Olin et al., 2002	Dementia, review, elderly	Yes	Yes	—	Yes
Olin, 1997[a]	Dementia, clinical trial, elderly	—	Yes	—	—
Sano, 1997[a]	Dementia, Spanish instruments development, elderly	—	Yes	—	—

— Data not reported.
[a]Empirical study.

minorities, and *recruitment* resulted in zero articles. Combining the keywords *minority, recruitment,* and *clinical research* resulted in 27 articles. Combining the words *mental disorders, recruitment,* and *research enrollment* resulted in 31 articles, 27 of which were the same as the previous search. We also repeated the search specifically for each minority group (African Americans, Hispanics, and Native Americans) and did not find any new articles. The 31 articles were read and reviewed for historical accounts of minorities in clinical research, barriers to recruitment and retention, strategies for recruitment and retention, outcomes of recruitment methods, and aims and suggestions for future research in minority populations. Confirmation of the leading articles and studies, and several additional references, were found by reviewing the cited literature of these 31 articles. We also looked at comprehensive reviews on recruitment for minorities in general health studies (Swanson & Ward, 1995; Wendler et al., 2006; Yancey et al., 2006).

Ultimately 16 articles, listed in Table 14.1, were directly applicable to the themes of recruitment and retention of minorities in mental health research, but very few were empirical studies specifically of recruitment. Of these 16 articles, four directly address depression, one addresses severe mental disorders, and 11 address dementia and related disorders in elderly minorities. There were no articles meeting our criteria for Native Americans.

Table 14.1 is a summary of the published studies, listed by author and year, that address the recruitment of minorities in mental health research. The table identifies each article's particular focus regarding the type of mental disorder studied, the type of study done, and the gender and/or developmental stage of the populations studied. The table identifies whether African Americans, Hispanics, Native Americans, and Whites, are included in the study.

BACKGROUND

On reviewing the literature it becomes evident that there are major gaps related to recruiting minorities in mental health research. Frequently the reports lack crucial information to analyze and make further recommendations:

1. Report of race/ethnicity is uncommon, uneven, and not consistent.
2. Keyword terminology differs from study to study and key words are often not well defined (e.g., enrollment, refusal, attrition).
3. Study designs and aims are widely varied. For example, Yancey and colleagues (2006) identify the type of study (e.g., observational, experimental), the types of disease, the health target or domain, the type of sampling used (e.g. probabilistic, nonprobabilistic), sample demographics, the level of burden to participate, the recruitment setting, and U.S. region/residential characteristics (e.g. urban, rural).
4. Most studies have been observational and lack systematic designs to test and report statistically significant evidence of the most efficacious strategies to recruit and retain minorities in clinical research.

Yancey and colleagues (2006) and Swanson and Ward (1995) have compiled two comprehensive studies each reviewing nearly 100 studies, giving an exhaustive analysis of the literature at different time frames of recruitment and retention of minorities into clinical research studies. Other comprehensive studies (Arean & Gallagher–Thompson, 1996; Levkoff & Sanchez, 2003; Moreno–John, Gachie, et al., 2004; Olin et al., 2002) and still more smaller scale studies examine various aspects of including minorities in clinical research, particularly regarding recruitment and retention barriers and solutions. The majority of these studies, however, are observational, and thus statistical evidence of the most efficacious practices is extremely limited.

Recruitment and retention of minority populations in clinical mental health studies comprise only 2% of the literature from 1998 to the present (Yancey et al., 2006). The underreporting of methods, barriers, and solutions at all levels of engagement, including potential, contacted, eligible, and enrolled participants, and attrition in clinical mental health studies poses the greatest barrier to reducing, successfully, well-documented health disparities among minorities.

REASONS FOR MINORITIES TO AVOID RESEARCH

Historically, clinical research has discriminated against minorities and has engaged in abhorrent inhumane acts against them. There are two main examples of these atrocities: the abusive experiments performed by Nazi physicians and scientists revealed by the Nuremburg trials and the Tuskegee Syphilis Study in Alabama, during which researchers studied untreated syphilis in hundreds of poor African American men who had adverse consequences and died despite available treatment (Seto, 2001). Minority distrust of researchers and medical research has its roots in these horrible abuses. However, the history of abuse is not the only reason for nonparticipation in research (Yancey et al., 2006).

Cultural incompetence causing uncertainty in the interpretation of symptoms in minorities might mislead clinicians. Their clinical judgments in minorities compared with whites lead to differences in care—a dynamic referred to as *statistical discrimination* (Balsa & McGuire, 2001). This dynamic has been shown to affect diagnosis of depression, hypertension, and diabetes (Balsa, McGuire, et al., 2005). Language barriers could be sources of mistrust if appropriate efforts to understand are not in place. In a pediatric population, language barriers between physician and family caused significantly higher charges related to diagnostic tests than those for whom no language barrier existed (Hampers, Cha, et al., 1999).

One study of minority willingness to participate in research studies found 20 health research studies reporting consent rates by ethnicity. Eighteen of those studies were conducted in the United States. The consent rate of non-Hispanic Americans was compared with that of Hispanics and African Americans, resulting in a nonsignificant difference. The authors concluded that minorities are not unwilling to participate, but rather that there is underrepresentation among the invited participants (Wendler et al., 2006). The study included articles that have cited consent rates by ethnicity. Unfortunately, for our chapter only one of those studies was related to mental health and was focused on schizophrenia (Robinson, Woerner, et al., 1996). The study was a multicenter clinical trial of schizophrenia studying the effect of selection biases on the generalizability of the findings. The authors recommend that investigators should consider collecting data on the recruitment process to estimate the selection bias if any.

Women and minority health were marginalized in clinical research, supposedly out of the protective legislation that was meant to protect them from medical disasters like Tuskegee and like the Food and Drug Administration's thalidomide tragedy. Thalidomide was commonly used as an effective sedative in Germany in the late 1950s and early 1960s. It became common as well to treat nausea and sleep issues in pregnant women. However, when thousands of babies were born with similar deformities, thalidomide was finally pulled from the market in 1962 (Seto, 2001). Not surprisingly, however, low to no enrollment of minorities and women in clinical research throughout the years has led to major health disparities. Regarding the Native American and Alaskan native populations, Norton and Manson (1996) warn that the potential for such abuses are still significant, and researchers must stringently adhere to NIH guidelines for inclusion of minorities into clinical research while carefully monitoring and assessing the cost–benefit ratio for the target community's needs (Norton & Manson, 1996, p. 859). These efforts are limited to clinical research funded by NIH and other sources with similar guidelines. A large part of clinical research, however, is privately funded and is not subject to inclusion requirements for minorities (Olin et al., 2002).

BARRIERS TO RECRUITMENT AND RETENTION OF MINORITY POPULATIONS IN CLINICAL RESEARCH

Today, the elimination of health disparities among minorities has become a central investigative theme in clinical research focus nationwide (O'Brien et al., 2006). However, to improve the opportunity for reducing health disparities, researchers must first apply strategies reported to minimize the barriers experienced by minority populations. Therefore, recruitment and retention of minority populations is a process that requires the researchers to learn what barriers exist for community members and how best to eliminate those barriers (Staffileno & Coke, 2006; Taylor, 2003).

An added complexity to this analysis is the major gap of reports on these issues in clinical mental health research. Although it may be possible to apply strategies to reduce barriers across differing chronic medical conditions, clinical mental health research faces an additional level of complexity, particularly among minority communities, of the social stigma associated with seeking mental health care and/or believing in mental health services diagnosis, treatment, and research (Meinert et al., 2003). Therefore, this is an important step toward increasing minority participation, decreasing minority health disparities, and addressing issues of stigma and culturally relative concerns strongly rooted in minority communities regarding research and mental health.

Ten main barriers to recruitment were identified by Yancey and colleagues (2006) (see Table 14.2). All could facilitate recruitment if strategically addressed

Table 14.2 Ten Main Barriers to Recruitment

1. Attitudes toward and perceptions of the scientific and medical community, particularly among African Americans
2. Sampling approach
3. Study design
4. Disease-specific knowledge and perceptions of prospective participants
5. Prospective participant psychosocial issues such as self-efficacy, depressiveness, distress, hostility, social support, and readiness to change
6. Study incentives and logistics
7. Community involvement
8. Sociodemographic characteristics of prospective participants
9. Participant beliefs (e.g., religiosity)
10. Cultural adaptations or targeting

Source: Yancey et al., 2006.

and accounted for in the initial study design (Daunt, 2003). In addition to the 10 major barriers cited were distrust of research and researchers (particularly white researchers); lack of ethnic minority researchers (Levkoff & Sanchez, 2003; Yancey et al., 2006); institutional racism; variations in cultural values and cultural perceptions of health and disease (Olin et al., 2002, p. 675); language; issues related to socioeconomic status such as transportation, time, childcare, and cost of missing work; invasive, lengthy, or burdensome requirements for participation; and stigma (Keller et al., 2005; O'Brien et al., 2006; Olin et al., 2002; Thompson et al., 1996). Table 14.2 provides the complete list of the ten main barriers to recruitment as identified by Yancey et al. 2006.

Distrust of research, researchers, medical and academic institutions, as well as the resulting fear of being mistreated or used as "guinea pigs" for experimentation are the most commonly reported barriers across all the studies representing African Americans, Latinos, and Native Americans and Alaskan natives (Arean & Gallagher–Thompson, 1996; Cabral et al., 2003; Daunt, 2003; Gillis, Lee, et al., 2001; Harris, Ahluwalia, et al., 2003; Hughes, Peterson, et al., 2004; Keller et al., 2005; Levkoff & Sanchez, 2003; Markens et al., 2002; Meinert et al., 2003; Moreno–John et al., 2004; Norton & Manson, 1996; O'Brien et al., 2006; Seto, 2001; Staffileno & Coke, 2006; Steinke, 2004; Taylor, 2003; Thompson et al., 1996; Welsh, Adam, et al., 2002; Yancey et al., 2006). The following is an excerpt of an interviewer's experience recruiting patients from a regular community mental health center and from the satellite Hispanic clinic of the center that is culturally appropriate for monolingual Latinos for the Medication Adherence in Latinos Study (Diaz, Woods, et al., 2005):

> The monolingual Latino patients were the hardest patients to get to participate in the study. Many cannot read and so putting up fliers alone was not enough. Further, those that could read didn't like the idea of being in a study because they perceived it as an experiment. Some expressed to me their concern of being used as a guinea pig. So the way I approached the Hispanic clients was in a more

personal matter, going to their meetings with their therapist after they have agreed to have me. By approaching the patients in this way it will be more time-consuming but well worth it. (Diaz, 2003)

Institutional racism and its effects impact many lower income ethnic minority populations who typically have less access to health care insurance and other health-promoting resources (e.g., balanced diet, regular checkups). As noted by Thompson and colleagues (1996) and Olin and associates (2002), institutional racism plays a major role in low numbers of African Americans and other minorities recruited to participate in clinical research. In his study of increasing ethnic minorities in clinical research on Alzheimer's disease, Olin and colleagues (2002) cite the effects of institutional racism in cases in which industry-sponsored clinical trials recruit by entering study criteria into Alzheimer's disease patient registries that are designed to select white, wealthier, and more highly educated subjects.

A combination of the NIH requirement to include minorities and women with the fact that many times research studies are conducted out of the same locale (e.g., hospital clinics) has also resulted in researchers conducting multiple studies on the same population. This process has also contributed to minority population's distrust of clinical research, because it is experienced as the researchers are only taking from the community to fulfill their needs, without giving anything that could benefit the minority community (Levkoff & Sanchez, 2003).

As introduced earlier, mental health clinical research faces the additional barrier of social stigma toward mental health care, psychotherapy, and mental illness, particularly in the African American, Latino, and Native American and Alaskan native communities, making recruitment a slightly different challenge than in other clinical research fields (Arean & Gallagher–Thompson, 1996; Norton & Manson, 1996; Thompson et al., 1996). Each of these minority groups culturally have a collective identity and tend to be less likely and less willing to seek help or services from someone not affiliated directly with their community, are less likely to share information about their families and communities, are more likely to have negative attitudes toward mental health, and are more likely to seek alternative sources of social support (Arean & Gallagher–Thompson, 1996; Markens et al., 2002; Norton & Manson, 1996; Thompson et al., 1996).

Similarly, African American communities tend to rely more on community-based support networks through their local churches, family, and primary health care providers (Thompson et al., 1996) rather than seeking mental health support. Stigma toward mental health services in Latinos, who tend to be more private, results in a preference for the treatment to be individualized, making group therapy and participation in clinical research less desirable. Arean and Gallagher–Thompson (1996) have found, when trying to recruit older minority adults into clinical research, that building trust by developing relationships with the target community, their families, and their community leaders as potential sources for referral is a critical first step. She and her colleagues found that excluding family members from the recruitment process will lead to greater distrust in research, research institutions, and research individuals (Arean

& Gallagher–Thompson, 1996). Therefore, particularly in Latino populations, it is critical to allow the potential participant to include family members in the decision-making process, because it has been found that decision making is rarely an individual process and more likely includes family and providers' input (Steinke, 2004). The following example is an excerpt from a research associate's unpublished research design notes that illustrates useful changes made to increase recruitment of minority women for a clinical obstetric/gynecological study on preterm delivery conducted at a hospital clinic serving women with minimal or no health insurance:

> Participation was quite burdensome on the woman and required several, fairly invasive clinical visits. After analyzing the daily recruitment log and the reasons entered for refusal, it became apparent to the recruiters that many women were refusing participation because they did not want to have to endure these additional procedures or the additional time it would add to their already long appointments for which they were missing work or without appropriate childcare. The clinical research team modified the study requirements and procedures, and after the modifications were approved by the IRB, implemented the changes. The new design added a maximum 10 minutes to the women's routine prenatal clinical visits and enabled the women to self-administer the specimen collections, making the entire procedure significantly easier on the participants. These modifications greatly reduced skepticism and increased recruitment and retention of participants into the study. Throughout the study, participants mentioned other solutions to barriers that have made participation viable: 1) Unsigned consent forms could be taken home to read, review, and discuss with family before being asked to decide whether to enter the study at their next prenatal visit. This flexible and family-inclusive approach to recruitment lessened mistrust or fear of the research and made potential subjects more comfortable to make a fully informed decision to consent or not. 2) Participants were reminded at each follow-up clinical visit that they had the right to refuse participation in that particular visit, giving them complete control over their participation. 3) Research staff scheduled study visits around clinical visits so that patient care was always the primary focus of any visit, reducing travel costs and time, and making participation convenient based on location. (Huebner, 2005)

Practical barriers when conducting clinical mental health research involve challenges in patient mental/emotional capacity to give informed consent. It is suggested that the level of cognition impairment and whether it is appropriate to proceed with the consenting process be assessed if the potential study participant is experiencing severe depression (Steinke, 2004). The following case example is from a research associate's unpublished notes about recruitment and retention into a medication adherence study among monolingual Latinos and illustrates that study methods can, at times, interfere with trust whereas other methods can enhance trust:

> The adherence study utilized an electronic monitor in the bottle cap (a "MEMS" cap: Medical Event Monitoring System) to track adherence. One consented patient believed that the MEMS cap was actually a surveillance device and she was suspicious of the motivation and purpose of the study. This participant chose to

withdraw from the study. Other characteristics of the study, however, facilitated recruitment and retention: The instruments used were modified to be culturally and linguistically sensitive and appropriate. The research team was bilingual and bicultural and all steps of the study were able to be carried out in Spanish. The study was located at a widely known and trusted community mental health center whose care was specifically available for the local monolingual Latino population. The research team made themselves available to conduct interviews and have clinical visits on weekends, in the evenings, and at two clinical locations, depending on which was more convenient for the participant. All participants were fairly compensated for any costs related to the study and for their time. (Huebner, 2003)

STRATEGIES FOR RECRUITMENT AND RETENTION OF MINORITIES INTO CLINICAL RESEARCH

It was not until the National Institute of Health Revitalization Act of 1993 that researchers were required to include women and minorities (underrepresented minorities defined as African Americans, Latinos, and Native Americans) in NIH-funded clinical research (Seto, 2001; Yancey et al., 2006). In 1997, minority research ethics was further promoted as part of a formal apology to the Tuskegee study survivors, acknowledging that the ethics of a study are central in the scientific design of the study (Seto, 2001). Unfortunately, the suggestion of a review on minorities' willingness to participate in research studies suggests that minorities are not appropriately outreached despite the NIH mandates (Wendler et al., 2006).

Barriers to participation must be met with culturally appropriate and effective solutions (Taylor, 2003). The research team is 100% responsible for initiating and carrying out this problem-solving approach. Barriers cannot be justified as problems of the target community, but rather must be understood within the institutional and systemic structures that cause them.

To achieve adequate and representative samples of current U.S. demographics, clinical research studies need to be done in areas where multiple ethnic groups are located, and it may require oversampling to produce proportions of minorities beyond their levels of representation in a population to achieve adequate numbers (Wendler et al., 2006; Yancey et al., 2006).

In general, engagement strategies for recruitment have been documented to be most successful when they include both passive/reactive and active/proactive strategies. Passive/reactive strategies include any type of mass publication, handing out of fliers, or media/public service announcement to reach a wide audience. Active/proactive methods include face-to-face encounters of research staff members with potential participants and include community-based or community-action research methods such as attending health fairs, acquiring referrals from health providers, approaching community leaders or "gatekeepers" to endorse study initiatives, and creating and seeking the help of a community advisory board or group, or community consultants (Spilker & Cramer, 1992; Yancey et al., 2006).

When implementing passive/reactive recruitment methods, studies report the most success with regard to publishing ads and articles in local papers read by the target community. Population-based methods that rely on phone calls have varied outcomes. Telephoning may reduce barriers produced by racial differences between researcher and participant. However, if telephoning is required by the study's IRB, it can be a barrier because many disadvantaged minorities do not have a telephone or have intermittent telephone service (Daunt, 2003). Telephoning is also often experienced as invasive, impersonal, and a method that increases the potential participant's distrust of research and researcher's motivations for calling. Limited or lack of success through passive/reactive recruitment methods has led to the implementation of face-to-face proactive, community-based methods (Gillis et al., 2001).

Clinical researchers can transfer and modify methods of social scientists' recruitment and retention methods because they, too, have faced similar challenges. Health promotion programs that serve minority populations should take a cultural relativist orientation toward the design and delivery of treatment interventions to ensure that they meet the needs of minority groups, thereby improving chances of retention. (Keller et al., 2005).

Cultural competence is cited as the most important issue to consider when researching an ethnic minority population. Identified requirements for achieving a culturally competent research design are the following: the setting must be embedded in the cultural community, the staff administering the research protocols and interview packages must be bilingual/bicultural, and the staff must be sensitive to the cultural nuances within the ethnic group (Arean, Alvidrez, et al., 2003; Arean & Gallagher–Thompson, 1996, p. 878; Hughes et al., 2004).

One of the most commonly cited strategies to increase cultural competency and thereby improve recruitment and retention within minority communities is community-based recruitment efforts, also reported as being the most effective way to minimize distrust and increase awareness of the purpose and practice of clinical research among minority populations. By relying on proven methods and data from community-based research models, researchers can have success in recruiting minority populations (Cabral et al., 2003; Keller et al., 2005; Markens et al., 2002; Meinert et al., 2003; Norton & Manson, 1996; Olin et al., 2002; Staffileno & Coke, 2006; Thompson et al., 1996). Although the majority of the studies are observational and few empirical data have been reported to prove the efficacy of community-based recruitment strategy outcomes (Olin et al., 2002), these findings can hardly be discounted.

To improve efforts, evidence-based research generated from systematic designs to measure and report outcomes of recruitment and retention strategies are needed to test the efficacy of some of the most frequently reported community-based research methods, including becoming familiar with and a participant in local businesses, organizations, churches, and events (Keller et al., 2005; Thompson et al., 1996); establishing a community advisory board and/or community consultants network comprised of community members, key community leaders or gatekeepers, and trusted community service providers (Levkoff & Sanchez, 2003; Markens et al., 2002; Staffileno & Coke, 2006); coordinating focus groups with each target population to understand better their views toward research and how they would most like to be approached and included; identifying the community's direct needs as identified by members of the community; hiring outreach staff and interviewers who speak the same language of the target population (in the Latino population these outreach workers are called *promotoras*) (Harris et al., 2003; Keller et al., 2005, p. 293); and having principal investigators of the same ethnic minority as the population being studied (Arean & Gallagher–Thompson, 1996; Levkoff & Sanchez, 2003; Yancey et al., 2006). Both sufficient time and financial resources must be budgeted to establish culturally appropriate research models and methods for recruitment and retention (Thompson et al., 1996).

A comparative study of population-based and community-based recruitment strategies and their respective success rates with Latino and African American populations was conducted. The authors found that community-based methods of mobilizing their ethnically diverse research staff to give face-to-face presentations of the study aims and to disseminate fliers at local churches, community centers, and health fairs, and to local health care providers proved more successful than either of the two population-based methods, in which contact with potential participants was initiated by phone (Cabral et al., 2003). The greater success of the community-based methods can, at least in part, be attributed to their ability to concentrate their recruitment efforts on areas of high concentration of the target population (Cabral et al., 2003).

Various descriptive studies report community-based strategies of identifying trusted local organizations and leaders as a means for increasing recruitment of minorities. Particularly among the African American populations, churches and pastors have been central to the community's ability to organize and effect positive political, social, and economic movements within their community (Markens et al., 2002). Therefore, accessing the African American population through establishing a relationship with local churches, pastors, and churchgoers has been one community-based method to increase recruitment and retention of minorities in clinical research (Markens et al., 2002).

Although some of the descriptive data report involvement with churches a facilitator to recruitment (Markens et al., 2002; Meinert et al., 2003), others report it as an additional barrier to recruitment (Yancey et al., 2006). Pastors are the respected gatekeepers to many African American communities; however, they are also incredibly overextended trying to reach the needs of their community, often with insufficient resources. Therefore, it is essential that recruitment strategies and studies that intend to involve the church as a means for increasing community comfort, trust, and cultural relativity consider the limitations of the pastors and be creative in designing methods that do not impede religious and community work that is already being done (Markens et al., 2002). Markens and colleagues (2002) utilized this knowledge to create a successful research design for their community-based mammography health promotion program that relied on pastor delegates to serve as coordinators between the study and their church to minimize any burdens felt by the pastors.

To address African American women's health, researchers utilized several community-based strategies. As a starting point they established a relationship with a well-respected and trusted African American women's center. Through that connection they began to attend meetings regularly and, per the suggestion of the leader of that community group, they developed a community-based conference for African American women. Because of the cultural strength and value placed on religiosity and spirituality, the conference incorporated themes of mental health and spirituality as two intertwined and interacting forces that provide healing. By incorporating the language, cultural beliefs and values of the community, they were able to increase awareness of mental health resources and increase knowledge of the role of research in addressing health disparities that are impacting their community (Meinert et al., 2003).

In another study, recruiting minority elders through printed ads in local newspapers (1% of respondents) was not successful, and investigators chose to contact the leaders of local senior centers to establish a relationship and to schedule meetings that occurred throughout the rest of the study periodically to discuss the barriers they could anticipate and any suggestions for improved recruitment. They also met with members of the target population. This community-based method greatly enhanced recruitment outcome (Arean & Gallagher–Thompson, 1996).

Socioeconomic status of many of the underrepresented populations often impacts access to health care and services. Studies that provide free educational materials and opportunities to learn more about health conditions prevalent in certain communities facilitate individuals' access to resources otherwise unavailable. Potential study participants may become more interested and comfortable with a research study that makes such efforts (Arean & Gallagher–Thompson, 1996).

It is clear from the literature that interviewers are integral to a study's recruitment and retention success (Thompson et al., 1996). Therefore, interviewers should be trained on how to approach potential study subjects and how to conduct the informed consent procedure. Matching of interviewer with interviewee based on visible ethnic and racial traits, including skin color and language dialect, have been studied; however, the outcomes are varied regarding the significance of matching.

In a similar vein, using culturally appropriate survey instruments and the potential need to adapt or modify survey instruments so that they are applicable to different minority populations has been found to impact retention (Steinke, 2004; Yancey et al., 2006). For example, survey questions using Likert scale descriptors can confuse Latino participants because they cannot be directly translated. Instead of answers like "strongly agree," a more meaningful answer in Spanish would be "I feel very sure" (Steinke, 2004). Similarly, scales that measure a numeric rating of positive and negative will elicit more accurate responses if positive is associated with higher numbers and negative with lower numbers (Steinke, 2004).

Staffileno and Coke (2006) summarize the strategies most commonly reported in the literature to reduce barriers into four overarching themes. Most of the methods reported in each theme have been discussed; however, several additional methods are also included:

1. *Importance of community:* (a) situate research site location near public transportation and target population work/community spaces; (b) publish health articles and ads with culturally appropriate pictures, themes, in local newspapers; (c) utilize local cable channels, radio stations, and community centers to relay research to community while making an initial bond; (d) create a community advisory board representative of leaders, residents, and activists; (e) hire staff from the community or of the same ethnic background as the target community; (f) train staff in cultural sensitivity and local day-to-day living in the community.
2. *Establish trust:* (a) disseminate mass mailings through well-respected, trusted centers/organizations/and schools; (b) ensure all staff are visibly participating in community functions, as community patrons, and attending local churches and events; (c) conduct house to house community canvassing and do telephone recruitment with a local community member.
3. *Cultural sensitivity:* (a) design recruitment materials and methods that are reflective of the target community's beliefs, values, and customs; (b) rely on "community consultants" to review and edit fliers and other study materials; (c) utilize "new knowledge" that is gained from interviews, focus groups, and other community engagements to acknowledge the target community's expertise of being the most knowledgeable of their own needs and experiences.
4. *Caring:* implement face-to-face personalized acts of recruiting, listening to individuals stories, and following up frequently with phone calls (after trust has been established) or mailings (including reminder postcards, birthday cards, and appreciation for participation cards).

The following case example comes from an ethnographer's unpublished field notes while conducting qualitative research on the transitions in drug use among urban drug-using and drug-selling youth and youth networks:

In order to access drug using and selling youth, field ethnography and recruitment were conducted on the streets and in the nightclubs of the city. Being on foot in the streets every day during early afternoon to early evening hours assured [sic] coming in contact with youth. Both on the street and in the clubs, I would clearly identify myself as a community researcher so as to dispel any suspicious that I was associated with the police or any other crime reduction or law enforcement agencies. By walking through the streets of several neighborhoods on a daily basis and in the nightclubs four nights a week, I have become a familiar face, with no needs or expectations other than my interest in learning from the youth and youth networks. This process not only led to successful recruitment of youth to participate in the study survey, but it also resulted in youths' desire to participate in "key informant" in-depth interviews and focus groups in which the youths' voice became the expert knowledge of their individual and collective experience of drug trends and culture in the city. Instead of being criminalized or stigmatized, the youth became actively engaged in "knowing," thereby increasing the knowledge gained in the research but also increasing the youths' experience of being knowledgeable and interested in participating in research. Many of the youth's contact information changes frequently. Being a constant presence in their community, I am able to keep up to date with new cellphone and beeper numbers, telephone numbers of family members or friends who can always find the individual if they have no phone, and new residential addresses. This recruitment method and presence in the community has led to an opportunity to teach at a local adult education program in which all of the information learned about street drugs, their composition, their physiological and psychological effects, and their role in youth culture is shared with students over a six-month period. (Huebner, 2000)

Levkoff and Sanchez (2003) identify community involvement in the research initiative as central to its success. They identify potential barriers and solutions to recruitment and retention for both the community members and the researchers at the macro level (community clinics/organization and academic/research institution, respectively), the mediator level (respected community gatekeepers and research team, respectively) and at the micro/individual level (potential study subject and researcher, respectively). Ultimately the success of a research study will result when the goals and motivation of the researchers match the goals of the community. Any disagreement of goals at any one of these three levels can dismantle the success of the study (Levkoff & Sanchez, 2003; Yancey et al., 2006).

When successfully recruited, researchers must also ensure retention of minority participants. Successful recruitment and retention methods must be established in the initial research design and, by sufficiently investing in the time and resources needed to implement barrier-reducing strategies for recruitment, retention rates are more likely to increase. Organizing focus groups with each of the targeted minority populations during the research design stage is a way of identifying potential participants' perceived barriers, concerns, and general beliefs about mental health and research. General engagement strategies for retention are similar to those for recruitment. A combination of proactive and reactive recruitment strategies will likely produce the best results for successfully recruiting and retaining the most minority participants from the widest socioeconomic status demographic range (Harris et al., 2003). Yancey and colleagues (2006) identify 12 main themes of retention criteria in the literature:

1. Communication of respect and benefits (personal and common good) without coercion
2. Minimal risk
3. Convenience (evening/weekend hours, childcare, transportation, schedule flexibility, accessibility)
4. Compensation for expenses related to participation (parking, mass-transit passes, cab vouchers)
5. Private space for data collection
6. Communication of appreciation for investment of time and effort (verbal recognition, certificates of participation, letters of gratitude)
7. Disclosure of electronic recording
8. Ensuring anonymity and confidentiality
9. Full informed consent
10. Ethical conduct

11. Provision of incentives (monetary honoraria, food, raffle tickets)
12. Maintenance of follow-up contact (birthday cards, reminder postcards)

Inclusion of minority ("cultural insider") investigators was also advanced as a community engagement strategy integral to a study's successful recruitment and retention of minorities. Having ethnic minority research staff, particularly a principal investigator who matches the studied population, can increase trust and instill ease in potential participants (Arean & Gallagher–Thompson, 1996; Hughes et al., 2004; Levkoff & Sanchez, 2003). However, there is a significant absence of ethnic minority researchers compared with white American, particularly principal, investigators. This indicates a significant power imbalance in the system of who is generating information about whom, and also indicates systemic barriers based on socioeconomic status and racial marginalization of ethnic minorities that, until it shifts, will continue to feed feelings of mistrust that resonate from more macro elements of institutional racism. All aspects of clinical research would be enhanced and outcomes strengthened if there were more ethnic minorities in lead research positions (Yancey et al., 2006).

LACK OF MINORITY-SPECIFIC RECRUITMENT AND RETENTION REPORTING

In trying to compile a representative breakdown of recruitment and retention outcome data by ethnicity and race, it became apparent that what is more significant is the paucity of such data. There has been far greater focus in the literature on African Americans than any other minority population and an increase in studies specifically on elderly minority populations as an age-specific category, as indicated in the data in this chapter. However, according to findings by Yancey and colleagues (2006), analysis of Latino populations makes up only 20% and Native Americans only 5% of all reported data. The relatively recent spike in research on recruitment and retention of minorities is mostly in medical clinical research and is spread out across various major medical issues, such as breast cancer, hypertension, adverse pregnancy outcomes, and Alzheimer's disease, therefore making generalizability of findings challenging (Yancey et al., 2006). Equally important, however, is the need not to stereotype recruitment methods based on race and ethnicity, but it is very possible that methods used to increase recruitment and retention of minorities may be applicable to broader populations as well (Olin et al., 2002).

The lack of participation in clinical research is suggested as one of the causes for the scarcity of efficacy studies on depression in Hispanics (Evelyn, Toigo, et al., 2001). Most of the studies have been conducted on white populations, and those results have been applied to Hispanics (Delgado, Alegria, et al., 2006). A recent review on mental illness in Hispanics reports only one randomized, placebo-controlled study and four open-label studies on the efficacy of pharmacological treatment of depression that included Hispanics. The randomized trial included 17 Hispanics from a total of 118 (Marin, Escobar, et al., 2006). The authors were unable to reach any conclusions.

Clinical research reports of Native American and Alaskan native participation are even fewer. In our review only one article was identified that specifically addressed research in Native American and Alaskan native communities, and it highlighted the mistrust associated with research because of past abuses with no recognizable benefits (Norton & Manson, 1996). As a result, the Indian Health Service (IHS) IRB requires that all research, regardless of whether it is IHS funded, obtain informed consent from local tribes and individuals (Norton & Manson, 1996). Issues such as community confidentiality, obtaining tribal consent, tribal compensation rather than individual compensation, and reporting of findings to tribal councils are unique cultural specifications that must be respected and honored when conducting research, and reflect the collectivist nature of the Native American and Alaskan native communities.

FUTURE RECOMMENDATIONS

The publication and dissemination of outcome reports on strategies for the recruitment and retention of minorities, successful or not, is a critical first step to addressing mental health disparities in minorities successfully and is the most instrumental way to ensure more effective research designs that benefit research goals and the mental health needs of minority communities. Many of the successful strategies may be able to be applied to other areas of clinical research with minorities, further reducing health disparities. Candid reporting of recruitment methods and outcomes must include all potential, eligible, and refusing subjects, and, for refusing subjects, must include the reasons why qualified potential participants choose not to participate to adjust future research designs better to resolve barriers.

The U.S. population will soon be a minority majority, and it is estimated that by the year 2060 there will no longer be a majority ethnic/racial group (Yancey et al., 2006). The successful elimination or reduction of health disparities among minorities depends on increased enrollment of minorities in mental health research. Successful recruitment and retention of minorities in research depends on researchers and research designs that establish solutions to the barriers. Comprehensive efforts identifying areas requiring research are important, but more important still is identifying the strategies that will facilitate how to accomplish these projects in a culturally sensitive and appropriate manner. Beyond strategies, it will also be critical to involve potential participants in identifying community health concerns to increase the potential for having study goals match community goals. Without these efforts, there often results a split between researchers and clinicians, and potential participants—a gap that needs addressing.

The literature has indicated that although there has been a significant increase in research on recruitment and retention of minorities into clinical medical research during the past decade, there are still major gaps. One major gap is the lack of reports on mental health research methods and outcomes for research with minorities. Another major gap is the representation of ethnic minorities in leading research positions, particularly as principal investigators. The impacts of socioeconomic status, racial oppression, and institutional racism are glaringly apparent factors to this imbalance of leadership and scientific innovation. And finally, in addition to descriptive reporting, systematic and quantitative analysis of recruitment methods, in particular community-based methods, is needed to generate evidence-based data that identify the most efficacious methods of recruitment and retention.

A culturally relative and sensitive combination of active and passive recruitment methods that is flexible to create adaptive solutions to community-identified barriers is best suited to recruit successfully a wide-ranging demographic spectrum of minority populations into clinical research. Particular to mental health clinical research, it is critical that research designs incorporate culturally relevant health and healing belief systems and language in combination with traditional mental health paradigms, as well as provide educational forums that are cofacilitated between community members and the research team to increase trust, increase disease and treatment awareness, and increase individual and community-based perception of research "giving back" to the community from which it is learning.

ACKNOWLEDGMENT

This research was supported in part by grants NIMH P20 MH074634-02 (Escobar and Gara Co-Principal Investigators), NIMH MH01912 (Esperanza Diaz, Principal Investigator), #20-FY98-698 (Charles J. Lockwood, Principal Investigator), and #DA 1142 from the National Institute on Drug Abuse (Jean Schensul, Principal Investigator; Merrill Singer and Margaret Weeks, Co-Investigators).

REFERENCES

Aranda, M. P. (2001). Racial and ethnic factors in dementia care-giving research in the US. *Aging & Mental Health, 5*(Suppl. 2), 116–123.

Arean, P. A., Alvidrez, J., et al. (2003). Recruitment and retention of older minorities in mental health services research. *Gerontologist, 43*(1), 36–44.

Arean, P. A., & Gallagher–Thompson, D. (1996). Issues and recommendations for the recruitment and retention of older ethnic minority adults into clinical research. *Journal of Consulting & Clinical Psychology, 64*(5), 875–880.

Ballard, E. L., Nash, F., et al. (1993). Recruitment of black elderly for clinical research studies of dementia: The CERAD experience. *Gerontologist, 33*(4), 561–565.

Balsa, A., & McGuire, T. G. (2001). Statistical discrimination in health care. *Journal of Health Economics, 20*, 881–907.

Balsa, A., McGuire, T. G., et al. (2005). Testing for statistical discrimination in health care. *Health Services Research, 40*(1), 227–252.

Breland–Noble, A. M., Bell, C., et al. (2006). Family first: The development of an evidence-based family intervention for increasing participation in psychiatric clinical care and research in depressed African American adolescents. *Family Process, 45*(2), 153–169.

Cabral, D. N., Napoles–Springer, A. M., et al. (2003). Population- and community-based recruitment of African Americans and Latinos: The San Francisco Bay Area Lung Cancer Study. *American Journal of Epidemiology, 158*(3), 272–279.

Cardemil, E. V., Kim, S., et al. (2005). Developing a culturally appropriate depression prevention program: The Family Coping Skills Program. *Cultural Diversity & Ethnic Minority Psychology, 11*(2), 99–112.

Connell, C.M., Shaw, B.A. et al. (2001). Caregivers' attitudes toward their family members' participantion in Alzheimer disease research: Implications for recruitment and retention. *Alzhimer Disease & Associated Disorders, 15*(3), 137–145.

Daunt, D. J. (2003). Ethnicity and recruitment rates in clinical research studies. *Applied Nursing Research, 16*(3), 189–195.

Delgado, P., Alegria, M., et al. (2006). Depression and access to treatment among US Hispanics: Review of the literature and recommendations for policy and research. *Focus, IV*, 38–47.

Diaz, E. (2003). *[Field notes from adherence study]*.Unpublished raw data.

Diaz, E., Woods, S. W., et al. (2005). Effects of ethnicity on psychotropic medication adherence. *Community Mental Health Journal, 41*(5), 521–537.

Evelyn, B., Toigo, T., et al. (2001). Participation of racial/ethnic groups in clinical trials and race-related labeling: A review of new molecular entities approved 1995–1999. *Journal of the National Medical Association, 93*(12 Suppl.), 18S–24S.

Fritsch, T., Adams, K.B., et al. (2006). Use of live theater to increase minority participation in Alzheimer Disease Research. *Alzheimer Disease & Associated Disorders, 20*(2), 105–111.

Gillis, C. L., Lee, K. A., et al. (2001). Recruitment and retention of healthy minority women into community-based longitudinal research. *Journal of Women's Health & Gender-Based Medicine, 10*(1), 77–85.

Hampers, L. C., Cha, S., et al. (1999). Language barriers and resource utilization in a pediatric emergency department. *Pediatrics, 103*(6), 1253–1256.

Harris, K. J., Ahluwalia, J. S., et al. (2003). Successful recruitment of minorities into clinical trials: The Kick It at Swope Project. *Nicotine & Tobacco Research, 5*(4), 575–584.

Huebner, C. I. (2000). *[Field notes from a drug use study]*.Unpublished raw data.

Huebner, C. I. (2003). *[Field notes from adherence study]*.Unpublished raw data.

Huebner, C. I. (2005). *[Field notes from a preterm delivery study]*.Unpublished raw data.

Hughes, C., Peterson, S. K., et al. (2004). Minority recruitment in hereditary breast cancer research. *Cancer Epidemiology, Biomarkers and Prevention, 13*(7), 1146–1155.

Keller, C. S., Gonzales, A., et al. (2005). Retention of minority participants in clinical research studies. *Western Journal of Nursing Research, 27*(3), 292–306.

Levkoff, S., Levy B.R., et al. (2000). The matching model of recruitment. *Journal of Mental Health and Aging, 6*(1), 29–38.

Levkoff, S., & Sanchez, H. (2003). Lessons learned about minority recruitment and retention from the Centers on Minority Aging and Health Promotion. *Gerontologist, 43*(1), 18–26.

Marin, H., Escobar, J. I., et al. (2006). Mental illness in Hispanics: A review of the literature. *Focus*, *IV*(1), 23–37.

Markens, S., Fox, S. A., et al. (2002). Role of black churches in health promotion programs: Lessons from the Los Angeles Mammography Promotion in Churches Program. *American Journal of Public Health*, 92(5), 805–810.

Meinert, J. A., Blehar M. C., et al. (2003). Bridging the gap: Recruitment of African-American women into mental health research studies.*Academic Psychiatry*, 27(1), 21–28.

Moreno–John, G., Gachie, A., et al. (2004). Ethnic minority older adults participating in clinical research: Developing trust. *Journal of Aging & Health*, 16(5 Suppl.), 93S–123S.

Norton, I. M., & Manson, S. M. (1996). Research in American Indian and Alaska native communities: Navigating the cultural universe of values and process. *Journal of Consulting and Clinical Psychology*, 64(5), 856–860.

O'Brien, R. L., Kosoko–Lasaki, O., et al. (2006). Self-assessment of cultural attitudes and competence of clinical investigators to enhance recruitment and participation of minority populations in research. *Journal of the National Medical Association*, 98(5), 674–682.

Olin, J. T., Dagerman, K. S., et al. (2002). Increasing ethnic minority participation in Alzheimer disease research. *Alzheimer Disease & Associated Disorders*, 16(Suppl. 2), S82–S85.

Olin, J. T., Pawluczyk, S., et al. (1997). A comparative analysis of Spanish- and English-speaking Alzheimer's disease patients: Eligibility and interest in clinical drug trials. *Journal of Clinical Geropsychology*, 3(3), 183–190.

Robinson, D., Woerner M. G., et al. (1996). Subject selection biases in clinical trials: Data from a multicenter schizophrenia treatment study. *Journal of Clinical Psychopharmacology*, 16(2), 170–176.

Sano, M., Mackell, J., et al. (1997). The Spanish Instrument Protocol: Design and implementation of a study to evaluate treatment efficacy instruments for Spanish-speaking patients with Alzheimer's disease. *Alzheimer Disease & Associated Disorders*, 11(Suppl. 12), S57–S64.

Seto, B. (2001). History of medical ethics and perspectives on disparities in minority recruitment and involvement in health research [republished]. *American Journal of Medical Science*, 322(5), 248–252.

Spilker, B., & Cramer, J. A. (1992). *Patient recruitment in clinical trials*. New York: Raven Press.

Staffileno, B. A., & Coke, L. A. (2006). Recruiting and retaining young, sedentary, hypertension-prone African American women in a physical activity intervention study. *Journal of Cardiovascular Nursing*, 21(3), 208–216.

Steffens, D. C., Artigues, D. L., et al. (1997). A review of racial differences in geriatric depression: Implications for care and clinical research. *Journal of the National Medical Association*, 89(11), 731–736.

Steinke, E. E. (2004). Research ethics, informed consent, and participant recruitment. *Clinical Nurse Specialist*, 18(2), 88–95; quiz, 96–97.

Swanson, G. M., & Ward, A. J. (1995). Recruiting minorities into clinical trials: Toward a participant-friendly system. *Journal of the National Cancer Institute*, 87(23), 1747–1759.

Taylor, R. E. (2003). Pharmacological and cultural considerations in alcohol treatment clinical trials: Issues in clinical research related to race and ethnicity. *Alcoholism: Clinical and Experimental Research*, 27(8), 1345–1348.

Thompson, E. E., Neighbors, H. W., et al. (1996). Recruitment and retention of African American patients for clinical research: An exploration of response rates in an urban psychiatric hospital. *Journal of Consulting & Clinical Psychology, 64*(5), 861–867.

Welsh, J. L., Adam, P., et al. (2002). Recruiting for a randomized controlled trial from an ethnically diverse population: Lessons from the Maternal Infection and Preterm Labor Study. *Journal of Family Practice, 51*(9), 760.

Wendler, D., Kington, R., et al. (2006, February 1). Are racial and ethnic minorities less willing to participate in health research? *Public Library of Science, 3*(2), Article e19. Retrieved December 15, 2007, from http://medicine.plosjournals.org/perlserv/?request =get-document&doi=10.1371/journal.pmed.0030019

Yancey, A. K., Ortega, A. N., et al. (2006). Effective recruitment and retention of minority research participants. *Annual Review of Public Health, 27,* 1–28.

15

Training the Next Generation of Health Care Professionals

Awareness and Appreciation of Cultural Issues in Mental Health

ELIZABETH J. KRAMER, CYNTHIA I. RESENDEZ,
& IQBAL AHMED

Differential population growth throughout the world, and widespread migration, both voluntary and involuntary, make it essential that health care providers be keenly aware of cultural and ethnic issues relating to the patients they serve, regardless of where they practice. For example, according to the U.S. Census Bureau in 2006, ethnic minority individuals comprise about 33% of the U.S. population, and 12.5% of those people are immigrants (U.S. Census Bureau, 2006b). These individuals experience mental health problems at rates similar to those of whites and they need to be appropriately addressed in a culturally competent manner. By 2020, depression, which frequently is not recognized and not treated (Simon & Von Korff, 1995) is expected to be the second leading cause of death and disability, and is anticipated to impose the greatest burden of ill health worldwide (Murray & Lopez, 1997). Prior to the NESARC there was a paucity of data on the prevalence of mood and other mental health disorders in ethnic minority patients. The NESARC, which was large enough to include all the major ethnic groups, found an overall 12 month *DSM-IV* prevalence of major depressive disorder of 5.3% and a lifetime prevalence of 13.2% Those rates are summarized by race/ethnicity in Table 15.1.

Although these rates are lower for Asian and Pacific Islanders, Hispanics, and blacks than those for whites, Native Americans have the highest rates of any ethnic group. Furthermore, these figures do not include dysthymic disorder, which tends to be higher in minorities, at least in Hispanics, more than in whites (Marin, Escobar, & Vega, 2006).

The widespread use of psychotropic medication, the community mental health movement, and managed care have all contributed significantly to making the diagnosis and treatment of mental illness a team effort rather than the sole

Table 15.1 Prevalence of 12-Month and Lifetime *DSM-IV* Major Depressive Disorder (MDD) by Race/Ethnicity

Race/Ethnicity	12-Month MDD	Lifetime MDD	MDD Odds Ratio
White	5.5	14.6	1.0
Black	4.5	8.9	0.7
Native American	8.9	19.2	1.5
Asian or Pacific Islander	4.1	8.8	0.6
Hispanic	4.3	9.6	0.6

Source: Hasin et al. (2005).

purview of psychiatrists and clinical psychologists. Because there are critical shortages of professional mental health care providers, particularly psychiatrists, in all major ethnic groups, services to members of those groups usually are delivered primarily by personnel other than psychiatrists. Furthermore, because members of a number of ethnic minority groups tend to somatize their psychological distress, most of their initial contacts regarding mental health problems are with primary care providers. This results in primary care providers treating more than 50% of patients with depression and makes them essential members of the mental health care team. This is especially the case with ethnic minority patients because primary care providers also often have the greatest linguistic and cultural competency. When bilingual/bicultural personnel do not exist, primary care providers are most likely to be the point of entry into the health care system. This chapter is about cultural competency and what all providers have to know to provide appropriate, high-quality care to members of ethnic minority groups, especially those who do not speak English.

Cultural competency training is becoming increasingly more important for several reasons: (a) changing demographics, which by 2050 will result in whites being a minority in the United States; (b) a dearth of linguistically and culturally competent mental health personnel to treat minority populations, resulting from both a shortage of ethnic minority providers and from inadequate training in culturally competent care; and (c) the recognition of health care disparities, which leads to examination of public policy and recommendations (Smedley, 2003), and resultant professional education requirements in most disciplines for all providers. In fact, New York, New Jersey, and California, three states with the most ethnically diverse populations, now require that all practicing physicians complete mandated amounts of cultural competency training. Training should transcend all disciplines. Integrated training prepares learners to work as members of multidisciplinary teams.

In the subsequent sections we focus on critical concepts and core requirements for training, mental health needs of ethnic minority groups, mandates required by accreditation agencies, education and training methods, utilization of an educational sample of an Asian family, and evaluation of cultural competency, including a sample evaluation tool.

CULTURE, ETHNICITY, AND RACE

Culture has been defined in a number of different ways, an indication that even the most comprehensive definitions cannot encompass all of its attributed meanings. Culture is a set of meanings, norms, beliefs, and values that are shared by a group of people. It is dynamic and it evolves over time, with each generation (Matsumoto, 1996). Culture is learned. Therefore it can be taught and reproduced. Culture shapes how individuals make sense of the social and natural world. It also includes both subjective and objective components of human behavior. (Lim, 2006).

Culture shapes the expression and recognition of psychiatric problems. It influences the meanings that are attributed to symptoms and what a society defines as appropriate or inappropriate behavior. It also provides the matrix for clinician–patient dialog, and it can be the source of both risk and protective factors of mental illness.

Culture influences illness and health-seeking behavior in four ways:

1. It defines what is "normal" compared with what is "abnormal" in symptoms and functioning.
2. It provides people with ideas about causality.
3. It determines who the patient is as well as the health care decision-making hierarchy.
4. It defines the steps that are taken in seeking health care (Ferran, Tracy, Gany, & Kramer, 1999).

The terms *culture, ethnicity,* and *race* often are used interchangeably. Ethnicity refers to an individual's sense of belonging to a group of people who share a common history, origin, and culture. It may imply nationality, geographic location, and/or religion. Race, on the other hand, usually refers to a group of people who share biological similarities (Lu, Lim, & Mezzich, 1995).

CULTURAL COMPETENCE AND HEALTH
CARE PROFESSIONALS

Many definitions of cultural competence have been put forward, but the one that follows probably is the most widely accepted. Cultural and linguistic competence is a set of congruent behaviors, knowledge, attitudes, and policies that come together in a system, organization, or among professionals that enables effective work in cross-cultural situations. *Culture* refers to integrated patterns of human behavior that include the language, thoughts, actions, customs, beliefs, and institutions of racial, ethnic, social, or religious groups. *Competence* implies having the capacity to function effectively as an individual or an organization within the context of the cultural beliefs, practices, and needs presented by patients and their communities (Cross et al., 1989).

Lavizzo–Mourey and MacKenzie (1995) define cultural competence as "the demonstrated integration of population-specific related cultural values, disease incidence, prevalence, or mortality rates, and population-specific treatment outcomes." (p.226) They argue that the integration of the three components is as necessary to meet the health care needs of defined populations and subpopulations as are the patients' values and needs.

Culturally competent care includes awareness of one's own value system, understanding of culture and its role in health care, cultural sensitivity to patients, and skill in using methods to address cultural issues in multiple interactions. Recognition of one's own ethnocentrism, including Western ideas about health and medicine, and sensitivity to stereotyping, which is important to avoid poor patient communication, poor alliance, and ultimately poor diagnosis/treatment or treatment adherence are equally important traits of a culturally competent provider.

Provision of culturally competent services requires that clinicians and institutions know the cultural norms for appropriate delivery of services to the various ethnic groups they serve. This includes being responsive to sociopolitical issues, such as the impact of racism, discrimination, immigration, and poverty that can impact patients' health, and adapting services to differences in family structure, expectations, preferences, help-seeking behavior, and worldviews. These points help to elucidate (a) why the patient chooses to seek help at a particular point in time, (b) what coping skills and stresses of daily living the patient brings to the encounter. and (c) what the family strengths and stressors are and how they contribute to the patient's help seeking behaviors (Kramer, Ivey, & Ying, 1999).

Becoming culturally competent is a developmental process in which one learns to recognize diversity, value diversity, adapt to diversity, assess one's own knowledge attitudes and beliefs about others' cultures, and incorporate the patient's beliefs and practices into the health care encounter. Patients perceive services as being culturally competent when they are appropriate for their problems and helpful in achieving desired outcomes according to their explanatory belief models (Dana, 1993).

Culturally competent health care practitioners must be able to differentiate between behavioral and ideological ethnicity. Behavioral ethnicity is characterized by traits such as recent immigration to the United States at an older age, frequent trips back to the "old country," emigration from a rural area, lack of or limited formal education, lower socioeconomic status, segregation in an ethnic subculture in this country, inexperience with Western health care systems, and major differences in language, dress, and diet. Ideological ethnicity is characterized by nominal identification with the group of origin (Johnson, Hardt, & Kleinman, 1995).

Basic clinical approaches should include understanding the patient's explanatory model, agenda, and illness behavior; understanding environmental constraints, environmental changes, social stressors, support network, language and literacy issues; and negotiating explanatory models and management options.

ETHNIC MINORITY POPULATIONS
AND THEIR MENTAL HEALTH NEEDS

Asian Americans

Asian Americans are one of the fastest growing racial groups in the United States. They include at least 43 different ethnic groups who speak more than 100 languages and dialects, many of which are not spoken outside their own communities (Kramer, Kwong, Lee & Chung, 2002). Between 1980 and 1990, the Asian American population in the United States increased 107.8% compared with 6% for whites, 13% for blacks, and 53% for Hispanics (Bureau of the Census, 1991). Between July 2004 and July 2005, the Asian American population grew by 3% or 420,000 to 14.4 million (U.S. Census Bureau, 2006b). Fifty-seven percent of the increase was the result of immigration. Collectively, Asian Americans comprise more than 4% of the current U.S. population, a figure that is expected to double by 2025. About 71% of Asian Americans are foreign born (Kramer, Kwong, Lee & Chung, 2002). Proportionately, according to the 2000 census, the major groups of Asian Americans in the United States are Chinese, Filipino, Asian Indian, Vietnamese, Korean, and Japanese (U.S. Census Bureau, 2001). Each group has a different immigration history, is at a different stage of acculturation, and has varying levels of education and income. Nationally, 40% or more of Chinese, Vietnamese, and Korean Americans are linguistically isolated, meaning that no one in the household age 14 years or older speaks English very well (President's Advisory Commission on Asian Americans and Pacific Islanders, 2001). In the New York metropolitan area in 2000, more than 60% of Chinese, 66% of Koreans, and about 44% of Japanese had limited English proficiency (Asian American Federation of New York Census Information Center, 2004). In that same year, approximately 25% of Asian senior citizens and children in New York City lived in poverty (Asian American Federation of New York Census Information Center, 2004). Limited English proficiency and linguistic diversity are major barriers to health promotion and access to services in this rapidly growing population.

Of the few epidemiological studies on the prevalence of mental disorders in Asian Americans, a study by Takeuchi and colleagues (1998) in Los Angeles County found that the lifetime prevalence rate of depressive disorders in Chinese Americans is about 12% (6.9% major depression, 5.2% dysthymia), and the 12-month prevalence rate is about 5.3% (4.9% major depression, 0.9% dysthymia), both of which appear to be lower than that of the general U.S. population. However, other studies that used depression-specific screening measures, such as the CES-D, demonstrate that depressive symptomatology in Asian Americans may be higher than in whites, but lower than in Latinos and African Americans (Kuo, 1984; Kuo & Tsai, 1986; Ying, 1988). A more recent study performed in one primary care setting found that 40% of Asians had significant depressive symptoms (Chung, Teresi, Guarnaccia, Olfson, Meyers, Holmes, et al., 2003). The findings of that study must be interpreted with caution because the study population consisted entirely of people who had sought medical care, many of whom may have been somatizing their emotional distress. Underdetection may occur because of the lack of psychological complaints, which usually must be specifically elicited by the provider.

Asian Americans have mental health needs that are similar to or greater than those of whites (USDHHS, 2001). To wit, Asian American and Pacific Islander women age 65 years and older have the highest suicide rates of any racial group, and Asian American women age 15 to 24 have the highest suicide rates of all races for that age group (Centers for Disease Control and Prevention, 2004). Suicide rates among men age 65 years and older have declined for all groups except Asian American and Pacific Islanders. Death and suicidal ideation rates for elderly Asian Americans seeking primary care are higher than for any other racial group (Bartels et al., 2002). A school-based study of Korean adolescents in New York City found that 16.2% suffered from depression and 17% had social phobia (Shin & Lukens, 2002). Depression rates among Asian Americans are between 15% and 20%, figures similar to those of white European Americans, but Asian Americans are more likely to seek help through venues other than mental health providers (Lin & Cheung, 1999). The reasons for this include stigma; the belief that psyche and soma are one, with a resulting tendency to somatize behavioral symptoms; insurance discrimination; language discrimination; and a severe dearth of culturally competent bilingual services. The result of these beliefs and practices is that there is greater delay in seeking care, and Asian patients tend to be much more severely ill when they reach the mental health care delivery system.

Hispanics

Hispanics are the largest minority group in the United States (U.S. Census Bureau, 2006b), and this group continues to grow. Between July 2004 and July 2005, Hispanics as a group grew by 3.3% (or 1.3 million) to 42.7 million. Fifty-seven percent of the population includes immigrants. The United States has the fifth largest Spanish-speaking population in the world, exceeded only by Mexico, Colombia, Spain, and Argentina. Currently, Hispanics account for 50% of the national population growth, and by 2050 they are expected to number 102.6 million, or 24.4% of the U.S. population (U.S. Census Bureau, 2004). The dominant Hispanic groups in the United States are from Mexico (66%); Central and South America, most notably El Salvador and the Dominican Republic (14%); Puerto Rico (9%); and Cuba (4%). These subgroups have differing life experiences, natural histories, and risks of psychiatric disorders. Of special significance are their experiences with war and trauma.

The terms *Hispanic* and *Latino* often are used interchangeably to refer to people who have cultural identities based on language and geography. Neither term is perfect, because Hispanic gives priority to Spanish origins or language, and Latino implies Latin descent. Nonetheless, according to the 2002 National Survey of Latinos, the proportion of Hispanics who defined themselves as Latino or Hispanic was 85% for the first generation, 77% for the second generation, and 72% for the third and later generations.

Despite a common ethnic identification, Hispanics are heterogeneous in aspects such as birthplace, acculturation, genetics and race, health care access and utilization, and language. The Hispanic Americans include groups that are predominantly Native American, black, or white, plus mixtures of any of these three. They are younger, poorer, less educated, and more likely to be foreign born than whites. They also are more likely to live with family and are less likely to speak English and have health insurance. Forty percent of Hispanic Americans are foreign born. Most Hispanics share the Spanish language. However, there are dramatic variations in the Spanish spoken by different subgroups, for example Cubans and Mexicans. Some elders do not speak Spanish at all; for example, some indigenous elders who have emigrated from Mexico speak only Nahuatl or other native languages. Approximately 45% of Hispanic Americans have limited English proficiency (Kochlar, Suro, & Tafoya, 2005).

Some studies suggest that Hispanics are more likely than whites to receive diagnoses of psychotic disorders and are less likely to be diagnosed as having mood disorders (Marin et al., 2006). They are more likely to somatize distress than whites. Somatization and preoccupation with somatic concerns among Hispanics have been widely described in the literature (Escobar, 1987, 1995; Escobar, Randolph, & Hill, 1986). Somatic symptoms are culturally sanctioned expressions for seeking and receiving care and treatment, and are reported by patients with and without axis I diagnoses (Barrio, Yamada, Atuel, Hough, Lee, Berthot, & Russo, 2003; Escobar et al., 1986; Weisman, Lopez, Ventura, Nuechterlein, Goldstein, & Hwang, 2000). It would be stigmatizing to express psychological distress explicitly, because this would indicate mental illness. Thus for Hispanics, especially elderly Hispanic women, somatic symptoms may be manifestations of psychological distress (Angel & Guarnaccia, 1989). Hispanics have tended to present to primary care providers for assistance with mental health issues such as depression, rather than seek out mental health specialty care (Vega, Kolody, Aguilar–Gaxiola, & Catalano, 1999).

Acculturation seems to work against the immigrant advantage. The Mexican American Prevalence and Services Survey showed that the estimated lifetime mental disorder rate for immigrants who had lived in the United States for more than 13 years was nearly double that for newer immigrants (Vega et al, 1998). Several studies have consistently shown lower rates of diagnosable disorders among immigrant Hispanics than among those who were born in the United States (Canino, Bird, Shrout, Rubio–Stipec, Bravo, Martinez, et al., 1987; Karno, Hough, Burnham, Escobar, Timbers, Santana, et al., 1987; Moscicki, Rae, Regier & Locke, 1987). A study of beliefs about the cause of mental illness among the elderly found that Hispanics were less likely than whites or African Americans to endorse biopsychosocial causes of depression (Ayalon, Alvidrez, & Arien, 2005).

U.S. Puerto Ricans appear to face greater mental health risks and lifetime depression rates that are more than double those for Mexican Americans and Cuban Americans, and they are almost twice as likely as whites to have depression in a given year (Oquendo, Ellis, Greenwald, Malone, Weissman, & Mann, 2001).

African Americans

Between July 2004 and July 2005, the U.S. African American population grew by 1.3% (or 420,000) to 39.7 million (U.S. Census Bureau, 2006b). Eighteen percent of the increase was the result of immigration. Most African Americans are a heterogeneous group of people whose ancestry can be traced to Africa. U.S. residents with African ancestry include both the descendants of slaves, primarily of West African origin who were born here, and relatively recent immigrants from other nations. Immigrants from Caribbean nations, Central and South America (who may or may not consider themselves Hispanic), and South and East Africa add diversity to these groups. In addition to multiple variations in national origin, these groups have diverse cultural and religious beliefs and customs.

Although African Americans are a very diverse group ethnically, many face the same unique socioeconomic challenges. In 2000, 79% of African Americans age 25 years or older were high school graduates, and 17% had bachelor or graduate degrees (U.S. Census Bureau, 2002). Nearly 25% of all African Americans had incomes more than $50,000 in 1997, and the median income of African Americans living in married couple households was 87% of that of comparable white households. Nearly one third of African Americans lived in the suburbs. Yet, in 1999, approximately 22% of African American families had incomes below the poverty level. African Americans are more likely to move in and out of poverty because they have few assets to protect them when they are unemployed; as a result, many become homeless.

Studies have shown that African Americans prefer to seek help from health professionals of the same race (Johnson, Saha, Arbelaez, Beach, & Cooper, 2004; Malat & Hamilton, 2006). Given that only 2% of psychiatrists, 2% of psychologists, and 4% of social workers in the United States are African Americans, this is a very difficult feat. This limited access largely underscores the concept in the black community: fear of double discrimination (i.e., being black and mentally ill). Despite making strides in stamping out more obvious forms of discrimination since the Civil Rights Movement of the 1950s and 1960s, African Americans still report the experience of racism on an ongoing basis. Furthermore, African Americans have historically endured misdiagnoses, inadequate treatment, and a lack of awareness of the ethnocultural differences in the presentation of psychiatric symptoms. To wit, they are more likely to receive a diagnosis of schizophrenia when they really are suffering from depressive disorder and they are less likely to receive accurate diagnoses when they are suffering from depression and are seen by primary care providers (Primm, 2006).

African Americans are also more likely to see emotional disturbances and their treatment through a spiritual framework, and to seek help from family and their surrounding community (Taylor, Ellison, Chatters, Levin, & Lincoln, 2000). With African Americans comprising 40% of the homeless population, 45% of the public foster care population, and nearly half of the prison system, this social network is both at risk and largely fragmented. As such, the church plays a large role in the provision of support and education (Blank, Mahmood,

Fox, & Guterboc, 2002). Because many of its leaders often lack a full understanding of mental disorders, there is often an unbalanced focus on prayer *alone* and a shunning of secular models of treatment.

Resilience in African Americans has been well documented, and in general the community identifies with this strength. African Americans highlight their ability to overcome slavery and some even believe that suffering is a part of the black experience. Because there is limited education about mental disorders in this community, the lack of understanding only fuels the many other negative ideas about causes and solutions for emotional symptoms. This misunderstanding goes two ways. The manifestation of physical symptoms related to mental health problems is 15% in African Americans, compared with 9% in whites—a fact that is often unknown by the treating provider or the community (Das, Olfson, McCurtis, & Weissman, 2006).

Native Americans and Alaskan Natives

There are many terms of reference for the indigenous populations of North America, including American Indians, Alaskan Natives, Native Americans, Native Indians, Native American Indians, Indians, Natives, and First Nations. The Native American and Alaskan native population rose by 1% (or 43,000) from 2004 to 2005 to 4.5 million (about 1.5% of the total U.S. population) (U.S. Census Bureau, 2006a). Most of these people live in Western states, primarily California, Arizona, New Mexico, South Dakota, Alaska, and Montana, and 42% live in rural areas (Rural Policy Research Institute, 1997). Despite widespread availability of reservations and trust lands for Native Americans, 62% reside in urban, suburban, or rural nonreservation areas (US Census Bureau, 2006b). However, most maintain close family and political ties with reservations and trust land communities.

Native American and Alaskan native populations are younger than their white counterparts because of higher overall mortality, less education, and lower incomes. Thirty-eight percent of Native Americans and Alaskan natives are children, 20% live in families in which no adult graduated from high school, and 55% have incomes below the federal poverty level. Like all other minority groups, Native Americans and Alaskan natives experience severe barriers to access to mental health services. Despite their small numbers, Native Americans are a heterogeneous group, with subgroups that are defined by the different geographic regions in which they live. These regions have defined the following North American Native American cultural areas that are unique and complex: Arctic, Subarctic, Plateau, Northwest Coast, California, Great Basin, Southwest Plains, Northeast, and Southeast. Indigenous groups that shared environments tended to develop similar skills, knowledge, beliefs, and customs. There are more than 560 federally recognized tribes and more than 100 state recognized tribes, each of which has its own unique culture. Thus, there is great diversity within the Native American and Alaskan native people's political, social, cultural, and spiritual communities (U.S. Census Bureau, 2002). Native American language families (Algonquian, Athapascan, Siouian, Iroquoian, and Eskimo–

Aleut) are an additional hallmark of diversity. Scholars have estimated that at the beginning of European colonization of North America there were between 200 and 300 distinct native languages. Today, more than half of these are extinct, and another large group is nearly extinct. The transmission of the nuances of cultural beliefs and ways is severely compromised when a native language is not widely spoken within a Native American community. As a result, literacy in native languages has become a high priority for contemporary tribal nations.

Mental and emotional distress among Native American and Alaskan native individuals is best understood in the context of the multigenerational trauma that native people have experienced (Duran & Duran, 1995). These psychological patterns of colonization may be transmitted through family dynamics even while rapid social change is occurring (Yellow Horse Brave Heart & DeBruyn, 1998). The trauma dates back to colonial and military subrogation that contributed to the loss of connection to tribal lands, separation of family members, and the disappearance of tribal languages. This trauma is closely associated with high rates of alcohol and drug use, interpersonal violence, and suicide among Native American and Alaskan native peoples. Native Americans and Alaskan natives are considerably more likely to be hospitalized for psychiatric illness than Asian Americans/Pacific Islanders and whites (Snowden & Cheung, 1990). Major problems include depression, and alcohol and substance use (Hasin, Goodwin, Stinson, & Grant, 2005).

Often Native Americans and Alaskan natives have great mistrust of formal health care systems. Many contemporary native communities have longstanding traditional healing and support for personal and family development. Usually family leaders arrange access to this healing. Native Americans commonly use native healers. The medicinal use of plants and roots is common in some Native American communities. Several targeted studies suggest that Native Americans and Alaskan natives use alternative therapies at rates that are equal to or greater than the rates for whites (Fleming, 2006).

EDUCATIONAL MANDATES FOR CULTURAL TRAINING AND COMPETENCY

In 1995, and again in 2001, the Accreditation Council for Graduate Medical Education (2006) added a requirement that residency programs address cultural training and diversity issues. The Residency Review Committee of the Accreditation Council for Graduate Medical Education special requirement reads as follows:

> Each resident must have supervised experience in the evaluation and treatment of patients of different ages throughout the life cycle and from a variety of ethnic, racial, sociocultural and economic backgrounds. . . . The residency program should provide its residents with instruction about American culture and subcultures, particularly those found in the patient community associated with the training program. . . . This instruction should include such issues as gender, race, ethnicity, socioeconomic status, religion/spirituality, and sexual orientation. (pp. 18–20)

Accreditation Council for Graduate Medical Education requirements emphasize six core competencies: patient care, knowledge, practice-based learning, interpersonal communication, professionalism, and systems-based practice. Cultural competency should be an inherent part of at least four of those competencies, specifically patient care, knowledge, interpersonal communication, and systems-based practice. Learning objectives and evaluation tools can be developed around these competencies, as demonstrated in a recent cultural competency curriculum (American Psychiatric Association Ethnic Minority Elderly Curriculum 2006).

In a similar vein the Association of American Medical Colleges has introduced cultural competence in medical student education and developed the Tool for Assessing Cultural Competence Training and other resources, all of which are available at the Association of American Medical Colleges website (Association of American Medical Colleges, 2006). In addition, some states such as New York, New Jersey, and California have begun to require cultural competency continuing medical education for all practicing providers in their states.

There are several barriers to implementing cultural competence training. They include limited time for new coursework, lack of expertise in multiculturalism in most programs, and lack of interest in teaching in this area by faculty in most programs. In addition, some programs may serve very few minority patients, and the skewed clinical case experience with minority patients may not be generalizable because only the most severely psychotic or behaviorally disturbed are seen. Finally, training about a single ethnic group (e.g., African Americans) will not be transferable to other groups, and general guidelines may be too superficial to be useful.

Faculty members in all institutions need to develop multicultural competency. In general, the few minority faculty members at many institutions tend to be researchers who are not the most competent to teach in this area. There should be Continuing Medical Education-approved cross-cultural clinical programs that include faculty participation, and evaluations of programs should be analyzed to ensure adequate depth of presentations. Faculty development workshops also should be offered.

Materials that can aid in the development of curriculum include publications such as the *National Standards for Culturally and Linguistically Appropriate Services in Health Care* and *Curriculum Guides and Resources* (Office of Minority Health, Department of Health and Human Services, 2006), and *Resources in Cultural Competence Education for Health Care Professionals* (Gilbert, 2003). The format of the California endowment guide is similar to the initial American Psychiatric Association curriculum guide, but it is more detailed.

Some progressive institutions such as UC-Davis School of Medicine are developing longitudinal, integrative curricula for undergraduate medical education. The goal of the program at UC-Davis is to have all graduating medical students be culturally proficient. Cultural competence education will be integrated into experiential community-based activities, didactics, standardized patient cases, and teaching opportunities during four years of medical training (Ton H, personal communication, August 2006).

TEACHING METHODS AND APPROACHES

We advocate and use a multidisciplinary approach to cultural competency training, which includes physicians (including residents and medical students), nurses, social workers, psychologists and, when appropriate, case managers. Cultural competency training requires the acquisition of knowledge, attitudes, and skills. Attitudes are modified by exposure; skills are acquired by practice. The most effective way to increase cultural sensitivity and, ultimately, develop cultural competency is to emphasize experiential learning, supplemented by reading, videos, and other passive learning activities that are useful for the acquisition of cognitive knowledge.

Experiential Techniques

Experience is the best teacher. This includes the use of techniques that encourage learners to examine their own cultural attitudes and values, which might affect their interactions with others from diverse backgrounds. This can be done through self-reflective papers, journaling, and discussions in which each learner describes him- or herself to a group, and the group then discusses commonalities and differences among the members. We encourage the use of discussion sessions in which learners are asked to share the health beliefs of their own families based on cultural and religious backgrounds, and then explore the similarities and differences, and respect differing values and beliefs. Inviting people from diverse ethnic populations to discuss the important historical events in their lives and the health beliefs that they and others of their ethnic group hold generally stimulates lively discussion. Whenever possible, visits to traditional medicine practitioners (e.g., TCM practitioners or *curanderos*), herbal pharmacies, and even just a walk through an indigenous community can be an eye-opener. A home visit to a family of another culture can be a humbling and enlightening educational experience. Although it is not usually possible to create total-immersion learning experiences in our academic and clinical learning environments, the more "real world" the learning experiences can be, the better it will be for the learner.

The first skill that must be taught is patient assessment. The initial interview should follow the *DSM-IV* "Outline for Cultural Formulation," a five-part tool for familiarizing the clinician with the patient's cultural background. An excellent discussion of how to use this tool can be found in the first chapter of Russell Lim's *Clinical Manual of Cultural Psychiatry* (Lim, 2006), which contains an appendix written by residents *for* residents on how to use the cultural formulation. The tool by Lim (2006) is easy to use and is useful not only for psychiatric residents but also for trainees in social work, psychology, and nursing. Whenever possible, learners should have the opportunity to use the cultural formulation with people from several cultures. That way they can compare the patients they see in their own cohorts as well as those seen by their peers.

For beginning learners, Arthur Kleinman's health explanatory belief model (Kleinman, Eisenberg, & Good, 1978) provides a simple way of eliciting

Table 15.2 Kleinman's Health Explanatory
Belief Model

1. What do you call your problem?
2. What do you think causes your problem?
3. Why do you think it started when it did?
4. How does it work? What is going on inside of you?
5. What kind of treatment do you think would be best
   for this problem?
6. How has this problem affected your life?
7. What frightens or concerns you most about this
   problem and its treatment?

cultural information. Although there are a number of variations on the questions proposed by Kleinman (1978), one of us (EJK) prefers to use seven questions, which are summarized in Table 15.2.

Videos and Biographical Resources

Viewing films of various ethnic groups, asking learners to place their patient in a specific cohort, and discussing the possible influences on their clinical care is a great teaching tool. The films may be those playing in theaters or educational videos. It also is helpful to encourage students and residents to read biographies of people from different ethnic backgrounds and discuss them. The concept of acculturation can be taught by comparing two or three generations of immigrants from the same family in terms of their responses to their illness, diagnosis, and the health care system.

Small-Group Learning Techniques

A number of small-group learning techniques can be used to provide meaningful educational experiences. These include problem-based discussions of, for example, cultural, ethnic, socioeconomic, and diversity issues. One example is to discuss barriers to access to care and then have learners develop and test an educational program designed to reduce those barriers. Developing demographic and community profiles of different ethnic populations can be a fun experience, especially for medical, nursing, social work, and psychology students. Residents/fellows can analyze the system-level indicators of cultural competence within a health care system in their own community, perhaps even the system in which they work, and the entire team can discuss public policy and public advocacy related to disadvantaged groups as it impacts psychiatric care issues. Additional learning experiences can include focusing on ways to reduce disparities in access to psychiatric care, and creating and using a cultural competence training manual that focuses on use of culturally appropriate assessment tools for patients from one or more cultural backgrounds.

Clinical Supervision and Teaching

Clinical teaching pulls together all the community experiences and reading that learners have acquired and gives them exposure to the "real thing" while being supervised by experienced cultural practitioners. Clinical supervision to teach cultural sensitivity and observe student and resident interactions in dealing with patients, families, and other caregivers is a necessary prerequisite to a successful teaching program. Role-modeling by faculty in their professional interactions with patients, families, colleagues, staff, "consultees," students, trainees, employees, and so on, should be an overarching activity.

Learning to work with interpreters is very important, especially in those settings in which there is a large number of patients with limited English proficiency. Having learners conduct assessments using interpreters, followed by discussion of the benefits, difficulties, and strategies to promote communication, is an important educational experience. If possible, learners should compare notes as well as obtain mentors' feedback.

Cultural psychiatry case conferences that include demonstration of the cultural formulation in case discussions, and cultural competency rounds are excellent venues for multidisciplinary teaching and often, particularly on inpatient services, for problem solving. These rounds may begin with a case presentation by a resident, but they can be equally useful to an entire inpatient or outpatient unit when a problem is presented. For example, when patients refuse to do what they are requested to do by nurses and the nurses become frustrated and communications break down, cultural competency rounds can serve as a forum for the entire patient care team to discuss problems.

Clinical teaching can be multidisciplinary and serves the function of helping learners from various disciplines hone their skills and share their unique knowledge with other members of the team. For example, physicians can talk about psychopharmacology and titration of doses, while nurses talk about adherence and what to teach patients. Social workers' contributions usually focus on community resources and issues relating to the patient's return to the community as well as follow-up care, and psychologists can address issues related to testing and, perhaps, psychotherapy.

Research and Literature-Based Teaching

A journal club that features papers with a particular focus on cultural and ethnic issues in psychiatry, and grand rounds presented by researchers who are studying culture or ethnic minorities are excellent ways to expose learners to the current state of research in this area. Those institutions that are fortunate enough to have faculty who pursue research in this area can offer electives to medical and nursing students, residents, social workers, and psychology students. Topics that might be included are health beliefs, customs, family systems of different ethnicities, developing culturally relevant research instruments and consent forms, improving skills in obtaining informed consent, and so on.

Learning Exercises with a Specific Ethnic Group Focus

There should be certain core learning requirements for all major ethnic groups, regardless of whether members of those groups are among the patient populations seen at individual institutions. Some of the methods include (a) visiting a local community health center that specializes in the care of different ethnic minority groups for a prearranged question-and-answer session about the history of the target group's health and health care; (b) participating in and observing grand rounds and/or conferences to develop and reinforce insights into conceptions of illness and treatment approaches; (c) visiting a traditional medicine practitioner and an herbal medicine shop to discuss the practitioner's conceptions of illness, treatment, and health; and (d) observing a case conference of an interdisciplinary team meeting with a focus on an ethnic minority patient.

Additionally, assigned readings, lectures, and discussions can be augmented with the following assignments: (a) downloading the latest health care data for different ethnic populations from Web sites such as http://www.cdc.gov/nchs/ and making comparisons; (b) interviewing ethnic minorities on the help they give and receive, or other specific topics; (c) presenting the results of the interviews in class to compare and discuss similarities and differences; (d) conducting group projects that address differences in ethnic groups of diseases such as depression, dementia, suicide, and differences in treatment approaches such as use of psychotropic drugs and their risks of complications such as tardive dyskinesia, diabetes, hypercholesterolemia, and stroke; (e) participating in a field trip to a historical museum dealing with the ethnic group to see film, pictorial displays, and other objects pertinent to the health history of the ethnic group; and (f) viewing film and video depiction of issues relevant to the ethnic group such as *Celebrating African-American Culture* (1994) or *The Culture of Emotions* (Koskoff, 2002).

A number of general concepts must be mastered to make learners competent in cross-cultural psychiatry, and they are listed in Table 15.3. Most of these concepts, which can be taught through reading, small-group discussion, films and video, and case studies, are described in textbooks on cross-cultural psychiatry (Gaw, 1993, 2001; Lim, 2006; Tseng & Streltzer, 2000, 2004).

Table 15.3 Core Conceptual Content of Cultural Competency Training

• Culture	• Health care and health care givers	• Diagnostic issues
• Race	• Health beliefs and health practices, and health care-seeking behaviors	• Unique risk and protective factors
• Ethnicity		• Diagnostic bias
• Cultural sensitivity	• Stigma	• Use of interpreters
• Acculturation	• Health care utilization	
• Diversity	• Importance of the family	
• Cultural competency	• Religion and religiosity	
• Disadvantaged populations	• Treatment issues including ethnopsychopharmacology and the use of indigenous or traditional healing practices	
• Genetic issues		
• Immigration issues	• Access to care	

CULTURE-SPECIFIC CONCEPTS

Some ethnic groups have additional important concepts. For example, the family is extremely important and is the focus of most activities and major decision making in many non-American cultures. An important part of becoming culturally competent is learning about the roles and responsibilities of the family in the patient's culture and the importance that they play in his or her life. Understanding culture-specific concepts about mental states or conditions also is important.

Hispanics

The concepts noted in the following paragraphs must be understood when working with individuals from Hispanic cultures.

Familismo is the emphasis on close relationships with extended family and friends. The family is viewed as the center of one's experience, and the family's needs are more important than those of the individual. Family loyalty, reciprocity, and solidarity are highly valued. (Anez, Paris, Bedregal, Davidson, & Grilo, 2005; Gloria & Peregoy, 1996; Hoppe & Martin, 1986; Marin & Marin, 1991)

Personalismo is the valuing of interpersonal harmony and relating to others on a personal level.

Simpatía is the general tendency toward avoiding interpersonal conflict, emphasizing positive behaviors in agreeable situations, and deemphasizing negative behaviors in conflict-ridden circumstances. It emphasizes the need for behaviors that promote smooth and pleasant social relationships.

Respeto is the adherence to a hierarchical structure, in which individuals defer to authority and to elders (Anez et al., 2005; Santiago–Rivera, Arrendondo, & Gallardo–Cooper, 2002).

Traditional gender roles suggest that, in *machismo*, men are expected to be strong and provide for the family whereas, in *marianismo*, women are expected to be nurturing, take care of children at home, devote themselves to caring for their children and husband, be self-sacrificing, and be submissive to men. They are viewed as the "emotional heart of the family" (Dreby, 2006).

Presentismo is a tendency to be focused on the present, and current problems.

Fatalismo is the expectation of adversity, the notion that life's outcomes may not be fully under one's control, suggesting a belief that outcomes may be decided by fate, luck, or a higher power such as God.

Vergüenza (shame) may limit Latinos' willingness to seek outside help for problems within the family. It is vital to be aware of this, because Latinos will attempt to avoid bringing shame upon their families (Gloria & Peregoy, 1996).

Curanderismo is a diverse folk-healing system practiced by many Mexican Americans that includes beliefs originating from Greek humoral medicine, early Judeo-Christian healing traditions, the Moors, and Native American traditions. A main tenet of this belief system is that natural forces, supernatural forces, or a combination of these cause illness. Examples of beliefs include *suerte* (luck), *susto* (soul or spirit loss resulting from a traumatic event), *mal de ojo* (the evil eye), and *caida de la mollera* (fallen fontanel). Healing practices may include physical and supernatural healings via *limpias* (spiritual cleansings), prayer, massage, and herbal preparations (Gafner & Duckett, 1992; Keegan, 2000; Luna, 2003; Padilla, Gomez, Biggerstaff, & Mehler, 2001). Healing is administered by *curanderos*, who have a divine gift (*don*) for healing (Applewhite, 1995).

Santeria is a religious system that blends African (Yoruba tribe) and Catholic beliefs, and is practiced by many Cuban Americans. It may also include elements of spiritualism and magic. Beliefs include that *oricha* saints (identities based on a combination of African deities and Catholic saints) may influence people on earth, *embrujamiento* (casting spells), and *mal ojo* (evil eye). Healing practices include *despojamientos* (expelling bad spirits), amulets, magic medicines, animal sacrifice, and care of blessed animals. *Santero* group beliefs and practices may vary, based on the needs of the group or the *santero* priest (Alonso & Jeffrey, 1988; Baez & Hernandez, 2001; Suarez, Raffaelli, & O'Leary, 1996).

Espiritismo is a spiritual belief system practiced by many Puerto Ricans in Puerto Rico and in the United States. It includes beliefs in reincarnation and the power of mediums. Individuals are affected by fluids, which are spiritual emanations that surround the body. These fluids are derived from a combination of the individual's spirit, spirits of the deceased, and the spirits of others close to the individual. Mental and physical illnesses are the result of fluids being either sick or disturbed. Fluids may be negatively affected by karma (past actions influencing the present), religious negligence, *brujeria* (witchcraft), spirits, *mal ojo* (evil eye), and inexperienced mediums. Healing practices include prayer, group healings, house cleansings, personal cleansings with herbal baths, and possession trance (Baez & Hernandez, 2001; Harwood, 1977; Hohmann, Richeport, Marriott, Canino, Rubio–Stipec, & Bird, 1990).

Religiosity serves as a resource for support and coping among Latino elders (Beyene, Becker, & Mayen, 2002;). Latino elders who participate in church activities have been shown to manage better than those who are socially isolated (Angel & Angel, 1992). Latinos may see God as the source of stressful events, including mental illness (Lefley, 1990); thus, Latinos may feel obligated to be compassionate and tolerant for those with mental illnesses (Guarnaccia et al., 1992). It is also hypothesized that if there is belief in an afterlife, that suffering during the current life may be easier to endure (Hovey, 1999).

Asians

Culturally competent assessment and treatment of mental health problems in Asian Americans requires that physicians and mental health professionals ask patients and their family members to share their cultural views on the cause of the problem, past coping patterns, health care-seeking behaviors, and treatment expectations (Lee & Lu, 1990). Asians are much more aware of the context of "the moment" than Westerners. For example, in the context of health care, rather than viewing the physician–patient relationship as a partnership, the doctor is the authority. The patient will answer questions, but is not likely to raise issues. He or she will tell you what they think you want to hear. It is the provider's responsibility to define the context for the patient so that he or she perceives that it is all right to talk about his or her problems and that no judgments about the patient and/or his or her family will be made.

Asian American culture often has many strengths in the Confucian teaching of the "middle way," the Buddhist teaching of compassion, the strong focus on the importance of family harmony and interpersonal relationships, and the high value of education and hard work. Asian cultures emphasize family, friends, and ethnic community. During a crisis, Asian American families can usually count on support from extended family members, friends/villagers, and community network and organizations. With appropriate consent, it therefore is helpful explore, recognize, and make use of these support systems in the treatment process.

In summary, successful assessment of mental health problems in the Asian American patient is based on provider awareness of individual patient demography, the patient's beliefs about health and mental health, elicitation of an explanatory model from the patient, negotiation around acceptable diagnosis and treatment, and use of the family support system to increase adherence to treatment and to reduce barriers.

MENTAL HEALTH AND THE ASIAN AMERICAN FAMILY: SAMPLE EDUCATIONAL MATERIAL

The following summary about Asian American families is an example of the type of information that should be provided for each culture as part of a syllabus.

In Asian Americans, the influence of the teachings and philosophies of a Confucian, collectivist tradition discourages open displays of emotions to maintain social and familial harmony or to avoid exposure of personal weakness. Saving face, the ability to preserve the public appearance of the patient and family for the sake of community propriety, is extremely important to most Asian groups. Patients may not be willing to discuss their moods or psychological states for fear of social stigma and shame. Mental illness is highly stigmatizing in many Asian cultures. It reflects poorly on one's family lineage and can influence others' beliefs about the suitability of an individual for marriage. These factors make it more acceptable for psychological distress to be expressed through the body rather than through the mind (Chun, Enomoto, & Sue, 1996, Gaw, 1993; Kleinman, 1977; Nguyen, 1982; USDHHS, 2001; Tseng, 1975).

In contrast to the rugged individualism valued by Western society, traditional Asians place a high value on the family as a unit. Each individual has a clearly defined role and position in the family hierarchy (which is determined by age, gender, and social class), and he or she is expected to function within that role. The individual is expected to submit to the larger needs of the family and is seen as the product of all the generations of his or her family. Rituals and customs such as ancestor worship, family celebrations, funeral rites, and genealogy records reinforce this concept. The result is that an individual's personal action reflects on his extended family and ancestors as well as himself. To achieve peaceful coexistence with the family and others, emphasis is placed on harmonious interpersonal relationships and interdependence. Mutual obligations and shame are the mechanisms that help to reinforce societal expectations and proper behavior.

Extended families are common among Asian Americans, and two or three generations often live in the same household. Nuclear families become more prevalent as acculturation progresses and economic circumstances permit. Traditional Asian American families are patrilineal. Major decision making is the purview of the father, followed by the oldest son, who receives preferential treatment on the assumption that he will accept greater responsibility in the care of the family. The mother's job is to nurture and care for her husband and children. Female children have a lower status within the family than male. In some cultures, such as the Chinese, the wife is expected to become part of her husband's family.

Gender Roles

Chinese males usually are more highly respected and valued than females, who usually are responsible for the caring role. Japanese women usually are involved in the decision-making process, but men tend to be the family spokespersons. Korean men and women both provide financial support for the family. However, some traditional roles continue to prevail. Women serve as caretakers of the home and children, and primary decision-making responsibilities are the domain of the husband/father. Traditional roles for males and females prevail among the Vietnamese. Women usually maintain the attitude that their husbands have a legitimate right to make final decisions, and they usually will withdraw from spousal conflict to maintain harmony within the family.

Women are at particularly high risk for the development of psychiatric disorders during their lifetimes. In fact, practically all major mood and anxiety disorders, with the exception of obsessive–compulsive disorder, occur more frequently in women. It is beyond the scope of this chapter to discuss the various biological, social, and cultural hypotheses that have been advanced to explain this phenomenon.

Among Asian women, culture affects the presentation, course, and treatment of mental health and substance use disorders. Male gender is more highly valued in traditional Asian families. Not only is the authority structure within families patrilineal, but continuity of the family line and its honor resides in males. The number of Asian girls placed in orphanages in Asian countries, and the skewed gender ratio of 1.5 males to 1 female in China with its strict population control policies exemplifies a drastic example of the value placed on males compared with females. It has been estimated that this ratio will continue to increase. The continued influence of Confucian principles in traditional East Asian thinking keeps females in a highly subservient role. For example, according to Confucian principles, one of the primary virtues that all women should possess is obedience, first to one's parents, then to the husband (and by extension, to the in-laws), and lastly to the first-born son. In the Japanese culture, the expression *sh-kataganai* ("it cannot be helped") encourages women to tolerate life's suffering without complaint or help from others.

In the United States, these traditional expectations can severely conflict with Western ideals, which place emphasis on independent thinking, achievement, and self-sufficiency, even at the expense of others feelings and needs. These conflicting values can play out in several ways: untreated depression and anxiety in teenagers, which can lead to isolation and withdrawal or acting-out behaviors; spousal conflict as women work and interact within a Western paradigm that elevates their status compared with their husbands'; and resistance or refusal of treatment because chronic low self-esteem leads to a sense of fatalism.

Children and Adolescents

Children are highly valued in Asian American families because they represent the future of the family. They are taught to be polite, quiet, shy, and humble, and to defer to their elders. Conformity to expectations is emphasized, and emotional outbursts are discouraged. Failure to meet the family's expectations brings shame and loss of face both to the children and their parents. Parents are seldom forthcoming with affection and praise, for fear that such demonstrations will encourage laziness. Education is highly valued and children who do not do well in school bring shame to their families. Positive reinforcement and discussion of one's achievements are uncommon. Usually children acculturate more readily than their parents and other elders. Often, the older generations benefit from this rapid acculturation because the children become culture brokers, serving as interpreters and negotiators for them in the new culture. Although parents expect their children to acquire the language and skills that will enable them to be successful in their new country, they often are reluctant to have them become American. This results in confusing messages to the child and leads to transgenerational conflict. For example, parents may encourage their children to learn English to succeed in American society, but may refuse to allow them to speak English at home.

In Asian cultures, one derives a sense of identity from the family group identity rather than one's individual position within it. The Asian American adolescent's school and peer group may expose him or her to the generational conflicts characteristic of parents and adolescents in mainstream American society. As he or she becomes increasingly aware of identity and the range of behaviors that accompany adolescence, the contrast between the culture of origin and the mainstream culture becomes sharper. This results in a combination of acculturation and intergenerational conflicts, which may cause the adolescent to act out or to withdraw.

Young Adults

For many Asians, young adulthood means achieving for the family. However with increased exposure to or immersion in Western cultures and values, and conflict between peer pressure and family expectations, many young adult Asian Americans begin to question their family values. Interpersonal relationships become more of a challenge, and interracial relationships may cause serious conflicts because parents usually fear that biracial children will diffuse the family lineage and culture. Asian males may feel pressured to date only females from their specific ethnic group.

Many adult Asians may misunderstand the meaning, experience self-doubt, or feel personally devalued and exploited when personal relationships are brief and transient—a common occurrence in urban Western settings. Decisions concerning the group with which one wants to be identified can cause serious dilemmas, as can having one identity at home and another when out in public—a phenomenon known as *dual identity*.

Often the obligation to parents takes precedence over the individual's choice of career. If one chooses a career that is different from the one chosen by his or her parents, there can be loss of emotional and financial support.

Another stressful situation for the young Asian adult occurs when he or she must serve as negotiator between parents and the host culture, a situation that occurs among those whose parents are monolingual or experience great discomfort in dealing with Western ways. This is also stressful and uncomfortable for the parents, who may not wish to share personal matters with their children or rely on them with regard to their non-Asian environment.

The Elderly

Although American elders emphasize independence as a means to maintain their self-esteem and avoid becoming burdens on their children, Asian elders look forward to having their grown children care for them. Traditional elders tend to have full control over family and financial decisions, regardless of whether they live with their children. Most Chinese elderly immigrants prefer to have their children move in with them, rather than move in with their children. They are not inclined to value independence and, when they live separately from their children, it is to avoid conflict over family roles.

Elders are highly respected and honored by all Asian cultures. In Chinese extended families, grandparents often are responsible for the care of grandchildren. Families are expected to care for their children and elders. Japanese Americans frequently maintain separate households from their children and grandchildren. Korean and Vietnamese elders are welcomed to live with their children for the rest of their lives. Those who reside with children and grandchildren are viewed as having been rewarded for everything they have provided to younger generations.

Clinical Caveats in the Diagnosis and Treatment of Asian Patients With Depression

The evaluation of depressed Asian patients should include the following: *First, ask about both physical and psychological symptoms.* Asian patients tend to present with somatic complaints. Unexplained symptoms that have been worked up and treated in other settings and remain unresolved may be considered "red flags" for further probing. At least one study has found that Asian patients with high levels of depressive symptoms in primary care may be at greater risk for not having their symptoms detected than Latino patients, even when there is language and ethnic congruence (Chung et al., 2003). A list of phrases commonly used by Asian Americans that potentially indicate their underlying depression is presented in Table 15.4.

Yeung and colleagues (2004) investigated the illness beliefs of depressed Chinese American patients, using the Exploratory Model Interview Catalogue and found that 76% complained of somatic symptoms, and 14% reported psychological symptoms including irritability, rumination, and poor memory. No patients spontaneously reported depressed moods. Seventy-two percent of the patients did not know the name of their illness or did not consider it a diagnosable medical problem. Only 10% labeled their problems psychiatric. Help was sought from general hospitals (69%), laypeople (62%), alternative treatments (55%), spiritual treatment (14%), self-administered alternative treatments (10.5%), and mental health practitioners (3.5%). Yeung and colleagues (2004) concluded that many Chinese Americans do not consider depressed mood a symptom to report to their physicians, and many are unfamiliar with depression as a treatable psychiatric disorder.

Second, determine onset, duration, and course of symptoms. It appears that asking the first two questions of the *DSM-IV* criteria related to depressed mood and anhedonia (For the past two weeks have you had depressed mood or lack of interest or pleasure in usual activities? Have you felt down, depressed or hopeless?) are sensitive for depression screenings, at least in Chinese patients (Chen, Chen, & Chung, 2002). The criteria have been translated into Chinese as part of a large-scale study of the elderly. We recommend that clinicians learn to ask these questions in the patient's vernacular, using a skilled culture broker to develop the questions and frame them as important for determining an accurate diagnosis.

Third, determine past psychiatric and medical history, especially any prior history of depression, anxiety, and/or substance use. In general, about 50% to 85% of individuals who have had one episode of major depression will suffer another episode. Alcohol use may cause or worsen existing depression. Anxiety disorders may coexist with depression. In addition, untreated anxiety disorders can often lead to recurring depression. Unfortunately, no culture-specific data are available on this point.

Fourth, identify risk factors. Bereavement, divorce, and loss of job are life events that can predispose individuals to depression. Low socioeconomic status,

Table 15.4 East Asian Idioms of Distress That May Indicate Depression

• Stress	• Poor sleep	• Worried, crazy	• Lonely
• Nervous	• Poor appetite	• Restless	• Sad
• Tired	• Bothered, annoyed	• Feel low	• Irritable

lack of social support, or social isolation also increase the vulnerability of an individual to depression.

Fifth, assess functional impairment. The patient should be asked in what ways symptoms have caused physical, social, or role impairment. For Asian Americans, who typically underreport their mood symptoms, a visible and persistent decrease in the level of function can be an important motivating factor for depression treatment. Although Asian patients may not volunteer loss of functioning readily because of shame or loss of face, obtaining collateral history from family members can often be helpful.

Sixth, assess suicide risk. Research during the past four decades consistently indicates that Asian women have the highest suicide rate compared with all other women in the United States (Kalish, 1968; Lester, 1994). Asian American women between the ages of 15 and 24, and older than age 65 are particularly vulnerable compared with other racial and ethnic groups in the same age range (Chen, Chen & Chung, 2002. Committing suicide in many Asian cultures is considered an immoral and disrespectful act to one's parents and antecedents. Many Asian patients with depression will express passive suicidal thoughts when questioned sensitively. It is important to frame the question by asking the following: "Other patients with these symptoms sometimes lose hope. Do you have thoughts of giving up?" This type of probe avoids the confrontational and shameful statements that patients feel about having suicidal thoughts. It is imperative to probe further for suicidal ideas with intent and plan. Suicidal thoughts are part of the depressive illness, and inquiry about suicide will not provoke it in depressed patients. We have observed that Asian patients and families often will deny past history of suicide attempts for fear of shame and stigma. We ask frequently about history of unusual injuries or accidents occurring to family members to cull suicidal or parasuicidal behavior.

Seventh, assess medical history and medications. The use of medications, including some herbal remedies, alcohol, and illicit drugs, also can trigger symptoms of depression. Because some East Asian (Chinese, Japanese, and Taiwanese) physicians commonly prescribe benzodiazepines to treat anxiety symptoms associated with depression, many recently immigrated Asian patients have been taking large doses of benzodiazepines for long periods. Long-term benzodiazepine use can trigger or worsen depressive symptoms and also increase the risks of physical dependence (Chen, Chen, & Chung, 2002).

Eighth, complete a mental status examination. Hearing reassuring voices from deceased ancestors, especially around the anniversary of their deaths, may reflect a cultural phenomenon and not psychotic ideation. Nonetheless, all patients who hear voices should generally be referred to a culturally competent psychotherapist for further evaluation.

Ninth, establish a differential diagnosis. We have noted that most Asian patients who present in the primary care setting have prominent anxiety symptoms that can coexist with depression or may be representative of having more than one psychiatric disorder (e.g., depression and PTSD).

Lastly, make appropriate referrals. Because of cultural bias and stigma Asians tend to view depression as a personal weakness or moral failing. Communication with Asian patients with depression is critical for successful diagnosis and treatment of their depression. Because of their holistic orientation, primary care providers have an important opportunity to undercut the stigma and intervene positively. They can use their valued position in the community to help build a trusting relationship with patients and, with the patient's permission, participate in conjoint management. Depression should generally be framed as a medical illness with specific signs and symptoms caused by a neurochemical imbalance in the brain. It is essential to emphasize that having depression is not indicative of a personal weakness or failure. Maintaining culturally competent continuity helps to build the rapport and trust necessary to help with referral if needed. Even if the patient refuses to engage in formal psychotherapy or psychiatric treatment, he or she may be emboldened to use more indigenous forms of treatment such as pastoral counseling, acupuncture, peer counseling, fortune telling, and so on, that are generally low cost and not harmful. Patients should be cautioned gently about using large quantities of herbal pharmaceuticals, particularly herbs in concentrated pill forms, which may contain toxic ingredients such as lead, arsenic, and so forth, that may worsen symptoms. This sensitive approach maintains the alliance without the patient feeling rejected and then in turn rejecting further help.

Case Example

The following case of a young Chinese man, who presented to his primary care provider with what proved to be depression, illustrates some of the material that needs to be taught.

Mr. X is a 25-year-old Chinese man who immigrated to the United States from China nine months earlier with the hope of attaining financial security and bringing his family to this country. He presented to a primary care clinician with complaints of severe fatigue and sharp, fleeting chest discomfort, which had been occurring for the past six months, most often when he tried to fall asleep at night. He had become increasingly concerned and apprehensive about the meaning of this pain. His sleep was disturbed, his appetite was poor, and he had difficulty concentrating at work. He had been working as a waiter in a restaurant 12 hours a day, 6 days a week since he arrived here. Mr. X attributed his physical symptoms (especially fatigue) to long working hours. This physical exhaustion made him stay in bed more than he wanted to. When asked if the symptoms caused him to feel sad or lose interest in his usual activities, he stated that he no longer watched videotapes or spent time with his coworkers on days off because he just couldn't concentrate and did not want to be a burden to his friends. He stated that these problems have affected his hopes for the future, and he admitted that he felt hopeless and desperate. A complete medical workup, including physical examination, basic blood chemistries with liver function tests to rule out hepatitis, and electrocardiogram were within normal limits.

The findings of the medical workup were reviewed with Mr. X, and the possibility that his physical symptoms were the result of an underlying depression was suggested to him. He was surprised and refused to accept depression as a possible diagnosis. He declined the recommendation that he see a psychotherapist, but agreed to take some medication to get help with his fatigue and improve his sleep. The physician started him on an SSRI antidepressant, expressing confidence that if he took his medication daily he would improve. He also was told that side effects such as nausea and headache could occur, but that they usually are mild and go away within a week or so. He was informed that his sleep would improve, but that he would not notice this until the second or third week of taking the antidepressant daily. The patient was asked to return in two weeks to reassess his condition, and was told that he could call in the interim if he had any questions or concerns.

Although he had doubts, Mr. X took the antidepressant and returned for his two-week visit, where he admitted that he was beginning to feel a little bit better. By his third visit, he was starting to feel like his old self again. His chest pain had disappeared, and he was sleeping through the night. His ability to concentrate also had increased. At the end of six months, he was completely asymptomatic, and the side effects of his medication had disappeared.

EVALUATION OF CULTURAL COMPETENCY

Although evaluation of trainees should be an ongoing process with timely feedback, formal tools for evaluation can be used. This can be done using objective structured clinical examinations, a standardized patient interview, or the evaluation tool Geriatric Psychiatry Cultural Competency Evaluation Form (Form 1). This form is based on core competencies outlined by the Accreditation Council for Graduate Medical Education (American Psychiatric Association Cultural Competency Curriculum for the Elderly, 2006). Use of the form should be considered only a part of an ongoing process of evaluation and feedback in the context of teaching and training activities. Trainees should also be encouraged to evaluate themselves and their peers. A number of additional possible evaluation tools that can be adapted for the evaluation of cultural competency are described by accrediting bodies such as the Accreditation Council for Graduate Medical Education (2006).

REFERENCES

Accreditation Council for Graduate Medical Education. (2006a). *ACGME Outcome Project: Assessment* [Online]. Available: http://www.acgme.org/outcome/assess/assHome.asp

Accreditation Council for Graduate Medical Education. (2006b). *Psychiatry program requirements* [Online]. Available: http://www.acgme.org/acWebsite/downloads/RRC_progReq/400pr1104.pdf

Ahmed, I., & Kramer, E. (Eds.). (2006). *American Psychiatric Association ethnic minority elderly curriculum: A product of the APA EME Committee, 2004–2006.*Washington, DC.

Alonso, L., & Jeffrey, W. D. (1988). Mental illness complicated by the santeria belief in spirit possession. *Hospital and Community Psychiatry, 39*(11), 1188–1191.

American Psychiatric Association. (1994). *Diagnostic and statistical manual of mental disorders* (4th ed.) Primary care version. Washington, DC: American Psychiatric Association.

Anez, L. M., Paris, M., Jr., Bedregal, L. E., Davidson, L., & Grilo, C. M. (2005). Application of cultural constructs in the care of first generation Latino clients in a community mental health setting. *Journal of Psychiatric Practice, 11*(4), 221–230.

Angel, J. L., & R. J. Angel. (1992). Age at migration, social connections, and well-being among elderly Hispanics. *Journal of Aging Health* 4: 480–499.

Angel, R., & Guarnaccia, P. J. (1989). Mind, body, and culture: Somatization among Hispanics. *Social Science and Medicine, 28*(12), 1229–1238.

Applewhite, S. L. (1995). *Curanderismo*: Demystifying the health beliefs and practices of elderly Mexican Americans. *Health and Social Work, 20*(4), 247–253.

Asian American Federation of New York Census Information Center. (2004). *Census profiles: New York City's Chinese population, Japanese population.* Asian American Federation, New York, NY.

Association of American Medical Colleges. (2006). *Tool for Assessing Cultural Competence Training (TACCT)* [Online]. Available: http://www.aamc.org/meded/tacct/start.htm

Ayalon, L., Alvidrez, J., & Arien, P. (2005, November). *Beliefs about the causes of mental illness explains the low levels of mental health service use in ethnic minority older adults.* Presented at the Critical Research Issues in Latino Mental Health Conference, Princeton NJ.

Baez, A., & Hernandez, D. (2001). Complementary spiritual beliefs in the Latino community: The interface with psychotherapy. *American Journal of Orthopsychiatry, 71*(4), 408–415.

Barrio, C., Yamada, A. M., Atuel, H., Hough, R. L., Yee, S., Berthot, B., & Russo, P. A. (2003). A tri-ethnic examination of symptom expression on the Positive and Negative Syndrome Scale in schizophrenia spectrum disorders. *Schizophrenia Research, 60*(2–3), 259–269.

Bartels, S. J., Coakley, E., Oxman, T. E., Constantino, G., Oslin, D., Chen, H., Zubritsky, C., Cheal, K., Durai, U. N., Gallo, J. J., Llorente, M., & Sanchez, H. (2002). Suicidal and death ideation in older primary care patients with depression, anxiety, and at-risk alcohol use. *American Journal of Geriatric Psychiatry, 10*(4), 417–427.

Beyene, Y., Becker, G., & Mayen, N. (2002). Perception of aging and sense of well-being among Latino elderly. *Journal of Cross-Cultural Gerontology, 17*(2), 155–172.

Blank, M. B, Mahmood, M., Fox, J. C., & Guterboc, T. (2002). Alternative mental health services: The role of the black church in the South. *American Journal of Public Health,* 92, 1668–1672.

Bureau of the Census. (1991, August). *Census of population and housing, 1990.* No. XIV-38. U.S. Bureau of the Census, Data User Services Division, Data Developments. Suitland, MD.

Canino, G. J., Bird, H. R., Shrout, P. E., Rubio–Stipec, M., Bravo, M., Martinez, R., et al. (1987). The prevalence of specific psychiatric disorders in Puerto Rico. *Archives of General Psychiatry,* 44, 727–735.

Celebrating African-American culture [videocassette]. (1994). Salt Lake City, UT: Innovative Caregiving Resources.

Centers for Disease Control and Prevention. (2004). *National Center for Injury Prevention and Control (NCIPC) Suicide: Fact sheet* [Online]. Available: http://www.cdc.gov/ncipc/factsheets/suifacts.htm

Chen, J. P., Chen, H., & Chung, H. (2002). Depressive disorders in Asian American adults. *Western Journal of Medicine, 176*(4), 239–244.

Chun, C., Enomoto, K., & Sue, S. (1996). Health care issues among Asian Americans: Implications of somatization. In P.M. Kato & T. Mann (Eds.), *Handbook of diversity issues in health psychology* (pp. 327–366). New York: Plenum.

Chung, H., Teresi, J., Guarnaccia, P., Olfson, M., Meyers, B., Holmes, D., et al. (2003). Depressive symptoms and psychiatric distress in low income Asian and Latino primary care patients: Prevalence and recognition. *Community Mental Health Journal*, 39(1), 33–46.

Cross, T. L., et al. (1989). *Towards a culturally competent system of care: A monograph on effective services for minority children* [Online]. National Center for Cultural Competence, Georgetown University. Available: http://www.stanford.edu/group/ethnoger/

Dana, R. (1993). *Multicultural Assessment Perspectives for Professional Psychology*. Needham Heights, MA. Allan & Bacon.

Das, A. K., Olfson, M., McCurtis, H. L., & Weissman, M. M. (2006). Depression in African Americans: Breaking barriers to detection and treatment. *Journal of Family Practice*, 55(1), 30–39.

Dreby, J. (2006). Honor and virtue: Mexican parenting in the transnational context. *Gender & Society*, 20(1), 32–59.

Duran, E., & Duran, B. (1995). *Native American postcolonial psychology*. Albany: State University of New York Press.

Escobar, J.I., Burnam, M.A., Karno, M., Forsythe, A. & Golding, J.M. (1987). Somatization in the community. *Archives of General Psychiatry*. 44(8): 713–718.

Escobar, J. I. (1995). Transcultural aspects of dissociative and somatoform disorders. *Psychiatric Clinics of North America*, 18(3), 555–569.

Escobar, J. I., Randolph, E. T., & Hill, M. (1986). Symptoms of schizophrenia in Hispanic and Anglo veterans. *Culture, Medicine and Psychiatry*, 10(3), 259–276.

Ferran, E., Tracy, L. C., Gany, F. M., & Kramer, E. J. (1999). Culture and multicultural competence. In E. J. Ivey (Ed.), *Immigrant women's health: Problems and solutions*. San Francisco, CA: Josey-Bass, 19–34.

Fleming, C. M. (2006). American Indian and Alaska Native patients. In R. Lim (Ed.), *Clinical manual of cultural psychiatry* (pp. 175–203). Washington, DC: APPI Press.

Gafner, G., & Duckett, S. (1992). Treating the sequelae of a curse in elderly Mexican-Americans. *Clinical Gerontologist*, 11(3–4), 145–153.

Gaw, A. C. (Ed.). (1993). *Culture, ethnicity, and mental illness*. Washington, DC: American Psychiatric Press.

Gaw, A. C. (Ed.). (2001). *Concise guide to cross-cultural psychiatry*. Washington, DC: American Psychiatric Press.

Gilbert, M. J. (Ed.). (2003). *Principles and recommended standards for cultural competence education of health care professionals* [Online]. Available http://www.calendow.org/reference/publications/pdf/cultural/TCE0218-2003_Resources_in_C.pdf

Gloria, A. M., & Peregoy, J. J. (1996). Counseling Latino alcohol and other substance users/abusers: Cultural considerations for counselors. *Journal of Substance Abuse and Treatment*, 13(2), 119–126.

Grant, B. F., Stinson, F. S., Hasin, D. S., Dawson, D. A., Chou, S. P., & Anderson, K. (2004). Immigration and lifetime prevalence of DSM-IV psychiatric disorders among Mexican Americans and non-Hispanic whites in the United States: Results from the National Epidemiologic Survey on Alcohol and Related Conditions. *Archives of General Psychiatry*, 61, 1226–1233.

Guarnaccia, P. J., Canino, G., Rubio–Stipec, M., & Bravo, M. (1993). The prevalence of *ataques de nervios* in the Puerto Rico disaster study. The role of culture in psychiatric epidemiology. *Journal of Nervous and Mental Diseases*, 181(3), 157–165.

Guarnaccia, P., Guevara, L., González, G., Canino, G., & Bird, H. (1992). Cross cultural aspects of psychotic symptoms in Puerto Rico. Research in Community Mental Health, 7, 99–110.

Harwood, A. (1977). Rx: Spiritist as needed: A study of a Puerto Rican community mental health resource. New York: Wiley.

Hasin, D. S., Goodwin, R. D., Stinson, F. S., & Grant, B. F. (2005). The epidemiology of major depressive disorder: Results from the National Epidemiologic Survey on Alcohol and Related Conditions. Archives of General Psychiatry, 62, 1097–1106.

Hohmann, A. A., Richeport, M., Marriott, B. M., Canino, G. J., Rubio–Stipec, M., & Bird, H. (1990). Spiritism in Puerto Rico. Results of an island-wide community study. British Journal of Psychiatry, 156, 328–335.

Hoppe, S. K., & Martin, H. W. (1986). Patterns of suicide among Mexican Americans and Anglos, 1960–1980. Social Psychiatry, 21(2), 83–88.

Hovey, J. D. (1999). Religion and suicidal ideation in a sample of Latin American immigrants. Psychology Reports, 85(1), 171–177.

Johnson, T., Hardt, E., & Kleinman, A. (1995). Cultural factors in the medical interview. In M. Lipkin, S. Putnam, & A. Lazare (Eds.), The medical interview. New York: Springer-Verlag., 153–162.

Johnson, R. L., Saha, S., Arbelaez, J. J., Beach, M. C., & Cooper, L. A. (2004). Racial and ethnic differences in patient perceptions of bias and cultural competence in health care. Journal of General Internal Medicine, 19(2), 101–110.

Kalish, R. A. (1968). Suicide: An ethnic comparison in Hawaii. Bulletin of Suicidology, 4, 37–43.

Karno, M., Hough, R. L., Burnham, M. A., Escobar, J. I., Timbers, D. M., Santana, F., et al. (1987). Lifetime prevalence of specific psychiatric disorders among Mexican Americans and non-Hispanic whites in Los Angeles. Archives of General Psychiatry, 44, 695–701.

Kramer, E., Ivey, S. & Ying, Y.,(1999). Immigrant Women's Health. San Francisco, CA. Jossey-Bass.

Keegan, L. (2000). A comparison of the use of alternative therapies among Mexican Americans and Anglo-Americans in the Texas Rio Grande Valley. Journal of Holistic Nursing, 18(3), 280–295.

Kleinman, A. (1977). Depression, somatization and the "new cross cultural psychiatry." Social Science and Medicine, 11, 3–10.

Kleinman, A., Eisenberg, L., & Good, B. (1978). Culture, illness and care: Clinical lessons from cross-cultural research. Annals of Internal Medicine, 88(2), 351–358.

Kochlar, R., Suro, R., & Tafoya, S. (2005, July 26). The New Latino South: The context and consequences of rapid population growth. Pew Hispanic Center, 12.

Koskoff, H. (Producer). (2002). The Culture of Emotions. DSM-IV Outline for cultural formulation. Fanlight Productions Media Library [Online]. Available: http://www.fanlight.com/catalog/films/361_coe.php

Kramer, E. J., Kwong, K., Lee, E., & Chung, H. (2002). Cultural factors influencing the mental health of Asian Americans. Western Journal of Medicine, 176(4), 227–231.

Kuo, W. H. (1984). Prevalence of depression among Asian Americans. Journal of Nervous and Mental Disease, 172, 449–457.

Kuo, W. H., & Tsai, Y. M. (1986). Social networking, hardiness and immigrants' mental health. Journal of Health and Social Behavior, 27, 133–149.

Lavizzo–Mourey, R., & MacKenzie, E. (1995). Cultural competence: An essential hybrid for delivering high quality care in the 1990's and beyond. Transactions of the American Clinical and Climatological Association, 107, 226–237.

Lee, E. & Lu, F. (1990). Family therapy with Southeast Asian families. In M.P. Mirkin (ed.), *The social and political context of family therapy* (pp 331-354). Boston: Allyn & Bacon, Inc.

Lefley, H. P. (1990). Culture and chronic mental illness. *Hospital Community Psychiatry, 41*(3), 277–286.

Lester, D. (1994). Differences in the epidemiology of suicide in Asian Americans by nation of origin. *OMEGA, 29,* 89–93.

Lim, R. (Ed.). (2006). *Clinical manual of cultural psychiatry.* Washington, DC: American Psychiatric Press.

Lin, K. M., & Cheung, F. (1999). Mental health issues for Asian Americans. *Psychiatric Services, 50,* 774–780.

Lu, F. G., Lim, R. F., & Mezzich, J. E. (1995). Issues in the assessment and diagnosis of culturally diverse individuals. In J. M. Oldham & M. B. Riba (Eds.), *American Psychiatric Press review of psychiatry* (Vol. 14, pp. 477–510). Washington, DC: American Psychiatric Press.

Luna, E. (2003). *Las que curan* at the heart of Hispanic culture. *Journal of Holistic Nursing, 21*(4), 326–342.

Malat, J., & Hamilton, M. A. (2006). Preference for same-race health care providers and perceptions of interpersonal discrimination in health care. *Journal of Health and Social Behavior, 47*(2), 173–187.

Marin, G., & Marin, B. (1991). *Research with Hispanic populations.* Newbury Park, CA: Sage Publications.

Marin, H., Escobar, J. I., & Vega, W. A. (2006). Mental illness in Hispanics: A review of the literature. *Focus, IV*(1), 23–37.

Matsumoto, D. (1996). *Culture and psychology.* San Francisco, CA: Brooks/Cole.

Moscicki, E. K., Rae, D. S., Regier, D. A., & Locke, B. Z. (1987). The Hispanic health and nutrition survey: Depression among Mexican Americans, Cuban Americans and Puerto Ricans. In M. Garcia & J. Arana (Eds.), *Research agenda for Hispanics* (pp. 145–149). Chicago: University of Illinois Press.

Mueller, T. I., Leon., A. C., Keller, M. B., Solomon, D. A., Endicott, J., Coryell, W., et al. (1999). Recurrence after recovery from major depressive disorder during 15 years of observational follow-up. *American Journal of J Psychiatry, 156,* 1000–1006.

Murray, C. J., & Lopez, A. D. (1997). Global mortality, disability, and the contribution of risk factors: Global burden of disease study. *Lancet, 349,* 1436–1442.

Nguyen, S. D. (1982). Psychiatric and psychosomatic problems among Southeast Asian refugees. *Psychiatric Journal of the University of Ottawa, 7,* 163–172.

Office of Minority Health, Department of Health and Human Services. (2006). *Cultural competency* [Online]. Available: http://www.omhrc.gov/

Oquendo, M. A., Ellis, S. P., Greenwald, S., Malone, K. M., Weissman, M. M., & Mann, J. J. (2001). Ethnic and sex differences in suicide rates relative to major depression in the United States. *American Journal of Psychiatry, 158,* 1652–1658.

Oquendo, M. A., Lizardi, D., Greenwald, S., Weissman, M. M., & Mann, J. J. (2004). Rates of lifetime suicide attempt and rates of lifetime major depression in different ethnic groups in the United States. *Acta Psychiatrica Scandinavica, 110,* 446–451.

Padilla, R., Gomez, V., Biggerstaff, S. L., & Mehler, P. S. (2001). Use of *curanderismo* in a public health care system. *Archives of Internal Medicine, 161*(10), 1336–1340.

President's Advisory Commission on Asian Americans and Pacific Islanders. (2001). *A people looking forward: Action for access and partnerships in the 21st century. An interim report to the President.* Washington, DC: Government Printing Office.

Primm, A. B. (2006). African American patients. In R. F. Lim (Ed.), *Clinical manual of cultural psychiatry*. Washington, DC: APPI Press, 35–66.

Rural Policy Research Institute. (1997). *Rural by the numbers: Information about rural America* [Online]. Available: www.rupri.org/resources/rnumbers/demopop/demo.html

Santiago–Rivera, A., Arredondo, P., & Gallardo–Cooper, M. (2002). *Counseling Latinos and la familia: A practitioner's guide*. Thousand Oaks, CA: Sage.

Shin, S. K., & Lukens, E. P. (2002). Effects of psychoeducation for Korean Americans with chronic mental illness. *Psychiatric Services, 53*, 1125–1131.

Simon, G. E., & VonKorff, M. (1995). Recognition, management and outcomes of depression in primary care. *Archives of Family Medicine, 4*, 99–105.

Smedley, B. (Ed.). (2003). *Unequal treatment: Confronting racial and ethnic disparities in health care*. Washington, DC: The National Academies Press.

Snowden, L. R., & Cheung, F. K. (1990). Use of inpatient mental health services by members of ethnic minority groups. *American Psychologist, 45*(3), 347–355.

Suarez, M., Raffaelli, M., & O'Leary, A. (1996). Use of folk healing practices by HIV-infected Hispanics living in the United States. *AIDS Care, 8*(6), 683–690.

Takeuchi, D., Chung, R. C. Y., Lin, K. M., Shen, H., Kurasaki, K., Chun, C. A., et al. (1998). Lifetime and twelve-month prevalence rates of major depressive episodes and dysthymia among Chinese Americans in Los Angeles. *American Journal of Psychiatry, 155*, 1407–1414.

Taylor, R. J., Ellison, C. G., Chatters, L. M., Levin, J. S., & Lincoln, K. D. (2000). Mental health services in faith communities: The role of clergy in black churches. *Social Work, 45*(1), 73–87.

Tseng, W. S. (1975). The nature of somatic complaints among psychiatric patients: the Chinese case. *Comprehensive. Psychiatry 16*(3) 237–245.

Tseng, W. S., & Streltzer, J. (Eds.). (2000). *Culture and psychotherapy: A guide to clinical practice*. Washington, DC: American Psychiatric Press.

Tseng, W. S., & Streltzer, J. (Eds.). (2004). *Cultural competency in clinical psychiatry*. Washington, DC: American Psychiatric Press.

U.S. Census Bureau. (2002). *2001 Statistical abstract of the United States* [Online]. Available: http://www.census.gov/prod/2002pubs/01statab/pop.pdf

U.S. Census Bureau. (2004). *US interim projections by age, sex, race and Hispanic origin* [Online]. Available: http://www.census.gov/ipc/www/useinterimproj

U.S. Census Bureau. (2006a). *American Indian and Alaska Natives (AIAN) data and links* [Online]. Available: http://factfinder.census.gov/home/aian/index.html

U.S. Census Bureau. (2006b). *Nation's population one-third minority* [Online]. Available: http://www.census.gov/Press-Release/www/releases/archives/population/006808.html

U.S. Department of Health and Human Services. (2001). *Mental health: Culture, race and ethnicity—A supplement to mental health: A report of the Surgeon General*. Rockville, MD: U.S. Department of Health and Human Services.

Vega, W. A., Kolody, B., Aguilar-Gaxiola, S., Alderete, W., Catalano, R., Caraveo-Anduaga, J. (1998). Lifetime prevalence of DSM-III-R psychiatric disorders among urban and rural Mexican Americans in California. *Archives of General Psychiatry, 55*, 771–778.

Vega, W. A., Kolody, B., Aguilar–Gaxiola, S., & Catalano, R. (1999). Gaps in service utilization by Mexican Americans with mental health problems. *American Journal of Psychiatry, 156*(6), 928–934.

Whooley, M. A., Avins, A. L., Miranda, J., & Browner, W. S. (1997). Case finding instruments for depression: Two questions are as good as many. *Journal of General Internal Medicine, 12*, 439–445.

Yellow Horse Brave Heart, M., & DeBruyn, L. M. (1998). The American Indian holocaust: Healing historical unresolved grief. *American Indian and Alaskan Native Mental Health Research, 5,* 56–78.

Yeung, A., Chang, D., Gresham, R., Nirenberg, A., & Fava, M. (2004). Illness beliefs of depressed Chinese American patients in primary care. *Journal of Nervous and Mental Diseases, 192*(4), 324–327.

Ying, Y.-W. (1988). Depressive symptomatology among Chinese-Americans as measured by the CES-D. *Journal of Clinical Psychology, 44,* 739–746.

Index

Acceptance and commitment therapy, 119

Accreditation Council for Graduate Medical Education, 279–280, 294

Acculturation, 19, 21, 23, 27, 63, 87, 102, 168, 174, 274, 276, 282, 284, 288–289

Acupuncture, 112, 114, 122–124, 127–129, 131–134, 147, 293

Adherence, 5, 24, 69, 70, 80, 88, 105, 126, 161, 172, 173, 183, 205, 223, 225, 239, 255, 257, 273, 283, 285, 287

Adolescents, 58, 95, 98, 99, 100, 106, 208, 251, 275, 289

Adoption studies, 59

Advance directives for research, 242

African Americans, 7, 18, 20, 22, 23, 24, 25, 26, 54, 55, 56–57, 63, 81, 83, 87, 88, 96, 98, 99, 100, 102, 103, 104, 105, 113, 144, 165, 166, 167, 169, 178, 179, 181, 182, 217, 218, 222, 223, 224, 225, 226, 251, 252, 253, 255, 256, 258, 260, 261, 264, 274, 276, 277–278, 280, 284
    and bipolar disorder, 24, 57, 178–179, 223–226

elders, 57, 264–265
and prevalence of dysthymia, 56–57
and prevalence of major depression, 23, 55–57

Age, 20, 42, 56, 59, 60–61, 96, 234, 251, 275

Alaskan Natives, 59, 65, 220, 255, 278–279

Alcoholism, 23, 29, 71, 93, 218, 227–229, 268

Allopathic medicine, 111, 113, 115, 126–127

American Indian Depression Schedule, 42

Anorexia, 142, 146

Antidepressants, 76, 88, 105, 123, 127, 158, 180, 184, 187, 215, 217, 218, 222

Antipsychotic medication, 105, 224

Arab Americans, 18

Asians. *See also* specific subgroups, e.g. Chinese, 7, 18, 19, 20, 21–24, 25, 26, 30, 50, 55, 59, 73, 74, 76–77, 84–85, 96, 100, 101, 102, 104–106, 113, 143, 148, 165, 166, 169, 170, 173, 174, 222, 224, 225, 274, 286–294